Study Guide
to
DSM-IV

Study Guide
to
DSM-IV

Michael A. Fauman, Ph.D., M.D.
Associate Professor of Psychiatry
University of Maryland School of Medicine
Baltimore, Maryland

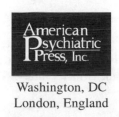

American Psychiatric Press, Inc.

Washington, DC
London, England

Copyright © 1994 American Psychiatric Press, Inc.
ALL RIGHTS RESERVED
Manufactured in the United States of America on acid-free paper
97 96 95 94   4 3
First Edition

American Psychiatric Press, Inc.
1400 K Street, N.W., Washington, DC   20005

Diagnostic criteria included in this book are reprinted, with permission, from the *Diagnostic and Statistical Manual of Mental Disorders,* 4th Edition. Copyright 1994, American Psychiatric Association.

Library of Congress Cataloging-in-Publication Data
Fauman, Michael A., 1942–
    Study guide to DSM-IV   /   Michael A. Fauman.
        p.   cm.
    Includes bibliographical references and index.
    ISBN 0-88048-696-1
    1. Diagnostic and statistical manual of mental disorders.
    2. Diagnosis, Differential.   3. Mental illness—Diagnosis.
    I. Title.   II. Title: DSM-IV.
        [DNLM: 1. Psychiatric Status Rating Scales.   2. Diagnosis,
    Differential.   3. Mental Disorders—diagnosis.   4. Mental
    Disorders—classifcation.   WM 141 F263s 1994]
RC473.D54F38   1994
616.89'075—dc20
DNLM/DLC   94-7366
for Library of Congress   CIP

British Library Cataloguing in Publication Data
A CIP record is available from the British Library.

To My Parents
and
Bonnie, Eric, Susan,
Karen, and Lisa

Contents

C H A P T E R 1

Introduction to DSM-IV

The diagnoses in DSM-IV (American Psychiatric Association 1994) are like ready-made suits that come in a variety of standard styles and sizes. They fit many patients well, others adequately, and some barely at all. The clinician's task, like the clothier's, is to fit individuals with specific characteristics into standard, predefined categories. For the clinician, the specific characteristics are the patient's psychiatric signs and symptoms, and the standard predefined categories are psychiatric diagnoses. When the characteristics and diagnoses match closely, the process is straightforward and rapid. When there is a notable discrepancy between the two, the process becomes complicated and prolonged.

The art of diagnosis depends on the clinician's ability to find and fit the patient into the appropriate diagnostic category even if he or she has atypical signs and symptoms. The resolution of this problem of "diagnostic fit" is one of the most challenging tasks in diagnosis. Briefly, it arises because of the variability of expression of all human disease, and the inadequacy of any diagnostic category to encompass that variability and still retain its specificity. One major goal of this book is to provide a structured approach to the resolution of diagnostic uncertainty that will allow the clinician to make an appropriate diagnostic fit for the patient.

This book was written to address the needs of clinicians at several levels of expertise, from the beginning student to the experienced clinician. On the most superficial level the book serves as an organized introduction to and synopsis of the criteria for the individual diagnoses in DSM-IV. It also provides brief clinical vignettes for most of these diagnoses to help the reader visualize the disorder in the context of a multidimensional patient who is characterized by more than just fulfillment of the individual criteria. On the next level the book offers a guide to making a differential diagnosis for each group of disorders. It also provides *Key Diagnostic Points* to clarify important areas for diagnosis and includes self-test questions to allow the clinician to test his or her understanding of DSM-IV. On the most sophisticated level the book discusses common problems in diagnosis and is designed to help experienced clinicians resolve diagnostic uncertainty and increase diagnostic fit through the use of clinical judgment and the explicit rules of diagnostic precedence contained in DSM-IV.

Because the book is written to cover a wide spectrum of clinical expertise, experienced clinicians may find some portions too elementary, such as the sections titled *Making a Diagnosis* that leads the reader through a step-by-step differential diagnosis. On the other hand, these sections may be very useful to a resident or medical student who doesn't know where to start in the process of diagnosis. Similarly, the sections titled *Common Problems in Making a Diagnosis* should be more useful to the experienced clinician who is trying to determine the diagnosis for a patient who doesn't quite fulfill the necessary criteria for a specific diagnosis or fulfills the criteria for too many diagnoses. The same section may be too complicated for the beginning student. Each reader must decide which sections are most useful for his or her level of expertise.

This chapter provides an introduction to the theory and practice of psychiatric diagnosis using DSM-IV. It will begin with a short discussion of the reasons for making a psychiatric diagnosis followed by a review of the concept of a clinical syndrome and its relationship to DSM-IV diagnostic criteria. Psychiatric syndromes and criteria are clinical categories. As such, they can be understood as a specific product of the general cognitive function of categorization. Therefore, categorization theory will be discussed to determine what it can contribute to a further understanding of the process of psychiatric diagnosis. This process has already been described as a potentially uncertain practice. The source of this uncertainty will be examined along with the role of clinical judgment in its resolution. The use of multiple "Not Otherwise Specified" diagnoses and the establishment of rules of diagnostic precedence will be examined as two examples of methods used to resolve uncertainty. DSM-IV also contains some criteria that apply to most of the diagnostic categories. These general criteria will be briefly presented. Each chapter following the introduction has a similar structure and discusses one DSM-IV diagnostic category in detail. The final segment of this chapter will outline the common organization of the subsequent clinical chapters and discuss the function of each section.

Why Make a Psychiatric Diagnosis?

The main function for a psychiatric diagnosis is to provide a succinct means of communicating a large amount of information about a patient's illness. A diagnosis fulfills this role because it is a shorthand notation for a syndrome or cluster of clinical signs and symptoms that commonly occur together. A psychiatric diagnosis also has a second important function. More than one psychiatric resident has asked, "What difference does it make whether or not you give the patient a diagnosis? If the patient has psychotic symptoms, treat him with an antipsychotic drug. If he's depressed give him an antidepressant." On the surface this argument makes a certain pragmatic sense. However, it ignores the dangers of treating patients solely on the basis of isolated symptoms. For example, a patient who has psychotic symptoms may have Dementia, Major Depressive Disorder, Schizophrenia, Psychotic Disorder Due to a General Medical Condition, or Substance-Induced Psychotic Disorder. These illnesses may look alike on a superficial level but each has a different etiology and prognosis and each may require a different treatment approach. This correlation with treatment and prognosis is the second function of a psychiatric diagnosis.

Syndromes and Criteria

A *syndrome* is a cluster of signs and symptoms that occur together and are characteristic for a specific disorder. Many psychiatric disorders are syndromes. They usually include a core cluster of symptoms that serve as the model or prototype for the syndrome. For example, one common prototype for Major Depressive Episode includes the following symptoms: depressed mood, anorexia and weight loss, insomnia, psychomotor retardation, and feelings of worthlessness or excessive or inappropriate guilt. This is the syndrome that most clinicians think of when they talk about Major Depressive Episode. It probably fits the majority of patients who have the disorder. However, experienced clinicians know that a substantial number of patients vary from this prototypic clinical presentation. A patient who experiences anhedonia, psychomotor agitation, hypersomnia, weight gain, and indecisiveness can also receive a diagnosis of Major Depressive Episode even if he does not have a depressed mood! The same variability is found in many other psychiatric disorders. Unfortunately, there are few pathognomonic signs and symptoms in psychiatry. However, the concept of prototypes is important in the process of psychiatric diagnosis and will be discussed in more detail below.

DSM-IV is a criteria-based diagnostic system. Criteria are rules that describe or define a clinical disorder. They specify the type, intensity, duration, and effect of the various behaviors and symptoms required for the diagnosis. Many criteria also list the alternate disorders that must be excluded before the diagnosis in question can be made. The criteria set for *Alcohol Withdrawal* provides a typical example.

Criteria for the Diagnosis of Alcohol Withdrawal

A. Cessation of (or reduction in) alcohol use that has been heavy and prolonged.

B. Two (or more) of the following, developing within several hours to a few days after Criterion A:

    (1)   autonomic hyperactivity (e.g., sweating or pulse rate greater than 100)
    (2)   increased hand tremor

(3)   insomnia
(4)   nausea or vomiting
(5)   transient visual, tactile, or auditory hallucinations or illusions
(6)   psychomotor agitation
(7)   anxiety
(8)   grand mal seizures

C. The symptoms in Criterion B cause clinically significant distress or impairment in social, occupational, or other important areas of functioning.

D. The symptoms are not due to a general medical condition and are not better accounted for by another mental disorder.

As discussed above, there may be a number of alternative combinations of symptoms that can fulfill the criteria for a specific diagnosis. The diagnosis of Alcohol Withdrawal may be made if the patient has two out of the eight possible physiological and psychological symptoms in part B. This choice of signs and symptoms is necessary to account for the variability inherent in most psychiatric disorders. The criteria must be designed to accommodate both prototypic cases that represent the modal clinical presentation, as well as clinical variants. One disadvantage of this approach is that two patients can look quite different clinically yet have the same diagnosis. In essence, the disorder of Alcohol Withdrawal includes a group of clinical subsyndromes. What they have in common is a subset of symptoms drawn from the larger pool of symptoms associated with the cessation or reduction of heavy alcohol consumption.

Psychiatric Diagnosis and Categorization

Dividing objects in the world into natural categories is a basic human cognitive task. A *natural category* is a concept that defines and groups real world objects such as mammals, birds, or chairs by a set of rules. Natural categories have two characteristics. They are organized around "best examples" or "prototypes" and they often have relatively vague or fuzzy boundaries. Think of two similar categories, cups and bowls. The prototypic description of a cup might include that it is a deep concave object with a handle that is used to hold liquid for drinking. A prototypic bowl, on the other hand, is a large, shallow, concave object without a handle that is used to hold food for eating with a utensil. Now think of a small, deep, concave object with no handle that is used to hold thick pudding. Is it a cup or bowl? There are no rules to guide this decision. The prototypes of each object are easy to envision but the boundary between the two concepts is fuzzy. One could imagine a similar problem distinguishing between a bowl and a plate as the object becomes more shallow and less concave.

The problem of fuzzy boundaries is not true of all categories. For example, the concept of a bird could be defined as an animal that has feathers. The boundaries of this category are distinct and would exclude all other animals because only birds have feathers. However, within this category are some birds that seemed more prototypic or "birdlike" than others. For example, many people would consider a robin or sparrow a more typical bird than an ostrich or penguin.

Why discuss categorization theory in a book on psychiatric diagnosis? Because psychiatric diagnoses are examples of natural categories and suffer from the advantages and disadvantages inherent in the process of categorization. Many diagnostic categories have prototypic members and fuzzy boundaries. For example, one prototype of Schizophrenia is a patient who has auditory hallucinations and psychotic thought processes without significant symptoms of depression or mania. The prototypic patient with Mood Disorder has symptoms of depression or mania without significant concurrent psychotic symptoms. The distinction appears clear cut. However, some patients have symptoms of depression and concurrent psychotic symptoms that meet the basic requirements for the diagnosis of Schizophrenia. Initially, the diagnosis of these patients was uncertain until a new diagnosis of Schizoaffective Disorder was created that included concurrent mood and psychotic symptoms. Nevertheless, the fuzzy boundary still remains between Schizophrenia and Schizoaffective Disorder and between the latter and Major Depressive Episode with psychotic features.

The problem of fuzzy boundaries becomes even more evident in the distinction between normal behavior and thought and its pathological variant observed in many psychiatric disorders. For example, in the diagnosis of Delusional Disorder the patient has a nonbizarre delusion such as being infected or having a disease. Suppose an individual insists that he has been infected with a low-grade virus but displays no obvious detectable symptoms other than feeling ill. Is this a delusion and should the patient be given a diagnosis of Delusional Disorder? In another example, suppose an individual has been mildly dysphoric all her life and is also irritable, indecisive, and chronically tired. Should the patient be given a diagnosis of Dysthymic Disorder? Both examples raise questions about the boundaries between normal and pathological psychological states. This problem is even more apparent in the diagnosis of personality disorders.

Research on categorization theory also provides some insight into the process of diagnosis. Individuals learn categories best if they learn the prototypic example first. This observation makes sense. Based on these findings the education of a diagnostician can be divided into three steps. First, the clinician must learn the various psychiatric diagnoses and their criteria. Second, he or she must learn to recognize the typical patient who fits these criteria. Finally, the clinician must learn how to make a diagnosis for those patients who have an atypical presentation that doesn't quite fit the criteria. This book is structured around this sequence. In each diagnostic category the criteria are synopsized, a prototypic clinical vignette is presented, and the chapter concludes with a discussion of the diagnosis of patients with atypical clinical presentations.

Diagnostic Uncertainty and the Role of Clinical Judgment

If all individuals with the same psychiatric disorder presented with identical symptoms and all clinicians were able to elicit, remember, and interpret the same information in the same way, there would be little diagnostic uncertainty. Unfortunately, as we have seen, that is an unrealistic fantasy. Although some patients have classic clinical presentations, most vary from the prototype to some degree. Furthermore, clinicians differ in the amount of information they collect and the conclusions they draw from that information. All of these factors intensify the problems associated with diagnostic fit. They can be separated into four types of clinical variance.

• *Natural variance* occurs normally in the biological world because every individual differs, to some degree, from every other individual. Therefore, the type, duration, and intensity of psychiatric symptoms varies even for individuals with the same disorder.

• *Information variance* occurs when the amount and type of clinical information collected about a patient varies because different clinicians have different sources for their information or the patient reports different information to each interviewer.

• *Observation and interpretation variance* occurs when clinicians, who are presented with the same information, notice and remember different parts of the information or attach different significance to what they hear. One of the most important distinctions is between normal behavior and pathological behavior, mood, and thought.

• *Criterion variance* occurs when different clinicians use different criteria for their diagnostic decisions.

One or more of these four types of variance are responsible for most of the difficulties that clinicians face in making a psychiatric diagnosis. Three of the more common problems of diagnostic fit are discussed below.

Patients Who Do Not Quite Fit the Criteria

Some patients come close but don't actually fulfill the diagnostic criteria for a specific disorder. The problem arises because the diagnosis requires information that the clinician has not obtained or the patient presents information that is inconsistent with the diagnosis. Further questioning or probing may or may not elicit information that will allow a definitive diagnosis to be made. For example, a patient may fulfill all of the necessary criteria for a diagnosis of Schizophrenia with the exception of the duration requirement of 6 months. The patient may have actually had symptoms for less than 6 months or may be unable to accurately remember how long the symptoms have been present. The clinician is forced to decide whether to adhere strictly to the criteria or make the diagnosis of Schizophrenia despite the uncertain duration.

Another case raises the question of whether some symptoms should be weighed more heavily than others when the criteria are not completely fulfilled. For example, should a patient with severe depression and suicidal ideation receive a diagnosis of Major Depressive Disorder, Single Episode, even if all the criteria for the diagnosis of Major Depressive Episode have not been met. The DSM-IV leaves room for the clinician's judgment. Because many of the criteria for this disorder are soft and quite subjective (e.g., fatigue or loss of energy, indecisiveness, psychomotor retardation), the clinician has room for interpretation and can usually make a diagnosis. However, if the patient was not suicidal the clinician might not be inclined to try as hard for the diagnosis.

Patients Who Fulfill the Criteria for More Than One Disorder in the Same Category

Some patients fulfill the diagnostic criteria for more than one psychiatric disorder in the same diagnostic group during the course of their illness. Often these disorders are mutually exclusive. For example, panic attacks can occur in many Anxiety Disorders. When they occur, the distinction between the various Anxiety Disorders depends, among other things, on whether the panic attacks were cued or uncued. However, patients who initially experience uncued panic attacks may find that the attacks eventually become cued. Therefore, they initially fulfill the criteria for Panic Disorder (uncued) and subsequently fulfill the criteria for another cued Anxiety Disorder such as Specific Phobia or Social Phobia. These problems can often be solved using the rules of diagnostic precedence that are included in most criteria sets. In this case, cued anxiety disorders such as a phobia take precedence over the diagnosis of Panic Disorder.

Patients Who Have Symptoms of More Than One Psychiatric Disorder

Some patients have a mixed clinical presentation with symptoms of more than one psychiatric illness but do not meet the criteria for any specific disorder. A corollary to this problem occurs when a symptom from one diagnostic group occurs in the context of a disorder from another diagnostic group. For example, the various forms of anxiety may appear as symptoms associated with several different psychiatric disorders. When phobias, obsessive thoughts, compulsive behavior, anxiety, fear, or apprehension occur in conjunction with psychotic, mood, or cognitive disorders it is often difficult to determine whether one disorder predominates or whether they represent comorbid disorders. Frequently the rules of diagnostic precedence will also help resolve these problems.

There are few absolute rules for diagnosis in DSM-IV. The criteria are provided as guidelines that represent the clinical judgment of experts in the field. Many patients fulfill the necessary criteria for a specific psychiatric illness. Other patients vary from the criteria as described above. Problems in diagnosis usually occur when the variation is small and the patient has a clinical presentation that is on the boundary between psychiatric disorders or between normal and abnormal. Some clinicians will tolerate a greater deviance from the criteria than others and still make a diagnosis. Other clinicians will adhere strictly to the criteria. DSM-IV allows both approaches. In these circumstances the final decision about a diagnosis requires the judgment of an experienced clinician.

General Criteria in DSM-IV

There are three general criteria that are explicit or implicit in the diagnosis of almost all disorders in DSM-IV. For that reason they will be discussed here and not repeated in the synopses of the individual disorders unless necessary for clarification. They should be considered in every diagnosis.

1. The disorder is not due to the direct effects of a substance.
2. The disorder is not due to the direct effects of a general medical condition.
3. The disorder causes clinically significant distress or impairment in social, occupational, or other important areas of functioning.

The first two criteria guard against the misdiagnosis of identifiable physical causes for psychiatric syndromes. Substance intoxication or withdrawal and a general medical condition always take diagnostic precedence if they can be shown to be the cause of the disorder. Many diagnostic groups include specific diagnoses for substance-induced disorders and disorders due to a general medical condition. The other disorders in the group usually contain criteria that exclude the diagnosis in the presence of a substance or general medical condition that could be etiologically related to the disorder.

All psychiatric disorders are considered to cause clinically significant impairment or distress. Therefore the third general criterion above is redundant. It is an implicit member of the criteria set for all disorders in DSM-IV. It is stated explicitly in the criteria set for certain disorders to emphasize the importance of considering this issue in the diagnosis. It also helps differentiate patients with the disorder from those who exhibit mild symptoms that are not necessarily pathological or who meet the other criteria for the diagnosis and are still able to function normally. For example, a patient who has a phobia about snakes can live normally in an urban environment without ever having to confront this phobia. Similarly, not all individuals with compulsive behavior have significant distress or have Obsessive-Compulsive Disorder or Obsessive-Compulsive

Personality Disorder. The criterion is often omitted in those illnesses, such as Panic Disorder With Agoraphobia, in which the patient's distress and impairment is obvious from the other parts of the criteria set. It is difficult to think of the average patient having Panic Disorder With Agoraphobia who does not have a significant impairment of functioning or have marked distress.

Not Otherwise Specified Diagnoses

Each diagnostic group contains at least one *Not Otherwise Specified* diagnosis (e.g., Psychotic Disorder Not Otherwise Specified, Anxiety Disorder Not Otherwise Specified, Depressive Disorder Not Otherwise Specified). These categories serve as catch-all diagnoses that can be used when a patient does not fit a more specific diagnosis. They represent one way to resolve the problem of diagnostic uncertainty. They essentially plug gaps in the diagnostic system and ensure that there will be a diagnosis, albeit at the least common denominator, for any patient who exhibits the predominant symptoms of a diagnostic group (e.g., psychosis, depression, anxiety) even if their clinical presentation is atypical.

Although it is important to ensure that the diagnostic system is comprehensive, the *Not Otherwise Specified* diagnosis presents a major problem. The patients who receive this diagnosis are a far more heterogeneous group, with respect to symptoms, than patients who are given a more specific diagnosis. Because they are such a heterogeneous group, the diagnosis of *Not Otherwise Specified* has little predictive value for response to treatment or illness prognosis. Therefore, these diagnoses should be used as little as possible. Every effort should be made to gather the necessary clinical information to make a more specific diagnosis. This likelihood is strengthened if the clinician has a good grasp of the acceptable variations in clinical symptomatology for the more specific diagnoses. The goal of diagnosis using DSM-IV is to identify common core syndromes and their variations with the hope that there is some correlation between these syndromes and the appropriate treatment of the patient.

Precedence of Diagnosis

Many of the cases discussed in this book represent diagnostic dilemmas that arise when patients have symptoms consistent with more than one diagnosis. The diagnoses may belong to the same or different diagnostic groups. When these conflicts occur they are often resolved using exclusion criteria that establish rules of diagnostic precedence. The rules establish boundaries between disorders and clarify the differential diagnosis. Exclusion criteria are included in the criteria set for many diagnoses. The general rule in DSM-IV is to give multiple diagnoses to patients who meet the criteria for more than one disorder. There are three exceptions to the use of multiple diagnoses, which are noted below. In each case DSM-IV uses specific wording in the criteria set to describe the exclusions.

1. When a Mental Disorder Due to a General Medical Condition or a Substance-Induced Disorder is responsible for the patient's symptoms, it precludes the diagnosis of any other mental disorder with similar symptoms (e.g., the diagnosis of Phencyclidine Psychotic Disorder precludes the diagnosis of Brief Psychotic Disorder). The following phrase is used in the criteria set to specify this relationship.

   "not due to the direct effects of a substance (e.g., drugs of abuse or medication) or a general medical condition."

2. When a pervasive disorder has among its defining or associated symptoms the defining symptoms of a less pervasive disorder, only the former is diagnosed. The term *pervasive* refers to how extensively the symptoms permeate the patient's life in terms of their type, duration, and intensity. Three phrases are used in the criteria set of the less pervasive disorder to describe the relationship and specify the exclusion.

   "has never met the criteria for . . . "

   The diagnosis of the less pervasive disorder is excluded if the patient *has ever* met the criteria for the more pervasive disorder. The previous diagnosis of Schizophrenia excludes any subsequent diagnosis of Delusional Disorder.

   "does not meet the criteria for . . . "

   The diagnosis of the less pervasive disorder is excluded if the patient has *currently* met the criteria for the more pervasive disorder. The current diagnosis of Schizoaffective Disorder excludes a simultaneous diagnosis of Schizophrenia.

   "does not occur exclusively during the course of . . . "

   The diagnosis of the less pervasive disorder is excluded if it *occurs solely* during the course of the more pervasive disorder. Bulimia Nervosa is not diagnosed if it occurs only during the course of Anorexia Nervosa. Hypochondriasis is not diagnosed if it occurs only during the course of Obsessive-Compulsive Disorder. However, it may be diagnosed if it occurs at other times.

3. When the boundary between certain disorders is particularly difficult to determine, DSM-IV includes as a criterion the indication that clinical judgment

is necessary to determine which diagnosis is the most appropriate. For example, Specific Phobia includes a criterion stating that the symptoms are not better accounted for by Panic Disorder With Agoraphobia and the latter includes a criterion stating the reverse. The following phrase is used to indicate this difficult differential diagnosis.

"not better accounted for by . . . "

Rules of diagnostic precedence are not infallible and should be used as guidelines. They suggest other diagnoses that should be considered before a specific diagnosis is made and they indicate the circumstances under which the diagnosis in question may be excluded if the patient fulfills the criteria for other diagnoses.

Although the distinctions between these exclusionary criteria seem comprehensive and unambiguous in theory, they prove far less so in clinical practice. For example, the criteria for the diagnosis of Dysthymic Disorder indicates that the diagnosis cannot be made if it occurs exclusively during the course of a chronic, pervasive psychotic disorder such as Schizophrenia, presumably when the patient has active symptoms. However, it is often difficult for the patient to remember when the active psychotic symptoms began and whether or not she was depressed at that time. This problem reemphasizes the importance of clinical judgment in the application of DSM-IV.

Key Diagnostic Points

Key Diagnostic Points are statements that highlight important items necessary for a differential diagnosis. They often capture a diagnostic concept in a form that is easy to remember and that facilitates recall of the more detailed aspects of the diagnosis. In this sense they provide a brief summary, a set of handy rules or clinical pearls that help structure and anchor the clinician's approach to the diagnostic process. A Key Diagnostic Point may refer to a specific diagnosis (e.g., the diagnosis of Bulimia Nervosa cannot be made if an individual fulfills the criteria for Anorexia Nervosa) or an entire diagnostic category (e.g., psychopathology occurring within 1 month after substance use may be etiologically related to the substance use). It may describe an aspect of diagnosis that is counterintuitive (e.g., the delusions or auditory hallucinations associated with the diagnosis of Schizophrenia, Paranoid Type, are not required to have a paranoid content).

Key Diagnostic Points can also be used to identify clinical information that is necessary for a differential diagnosis but is often ambiguous or hard to elicit from the patient (e.g., three psychotic disorders form a continuum based on the duration of the episode: Brief Psychotic Disorder [duration 1 day–1 month], Schizophreniform Disorder [duration 1–6 months], and Schizophrenia [duration more than 6 months].

DSM-IV Axes

DSM-IV is a multiaxial system that allows clinical assessment in the following five areas:

- **Axis I:** Clinical Disorders

- **Axis II:** Personality Disorders and Mental Retardation

- **Axis III:** General Medical Conditions

- **Axis IV:** Psychosocial and Environmental Problems

- **Axis V:** Global Assessment of Functioning

This book discusses only Axes I, II, and III. The decision to limit the discussion to these three axes is based on two considerations. First, most clinicians find the differential diagnosis of Axes I and II to be the most difficult component of the diagnostic process. Second, the discussion of Axes IV and V would make the book too long.

Organization of the Book

Chapters 2 through 17 in this book follow the organization of the American Psychiatric Association's DSM-IV, with a separate chapter for each diagnostic group. Although most chapters contain all the sections shown below, some of the sections may be omitted if they are not relevant (e.g., Chapter 4 *Mental Disorders Due to a General Medical Condition* does not contain the section *Criteria Applicable to Multiple Disorders*).

Clinical Vignettes

Each chapter begins with one or two extended clinical vignettes of patients to introduce the clinician to some of the ambiguities of making a diagnosis within the diagnostic group. The vignettes are actual or constructed clinical cases and are discussed in more detail in a later section titled *Discussion of Clinical Vignettes*.

Core Concept of the Diagnostic Group

The core concept of the diagnostic group is summarized in this section. The disorders in most diagnostic groups represent specific clinical syndromes that cluster around a common core concept.

Definitions

This section includes definitions of important terms used in the diagnostic group.

Criteria Applicable to Multiple Disorders

Several diagnostic groups include overarching criteria that are applicable to multiple disorders within that group. They include syndromes or symptom clusters that are a part of several different specific diagnoses. Examples include the core symptoms of Schizophrenia, Mania, Major Depression, and Panic Attacks. This section is omitted if there are no criteria applicable to multiple disorders in the group.

Synopses and Prototypes of the Individual Disorders

This section contains synopses of the specific diagnoses in the diagnostic category. The synopses are meant to provide a brief description of the individual diagnoses, highlighting the important points that distinguish one from another. When the criteria set requires a choice of a subset of symptoms from a larger list (e.g., Panic Disorder) the entire list is included. Many of the synopses are followed by prototypic vignettes that illustrate the diagnosis. The vignettes come from actual clinical cases or are constructed to illustrate the diagnosis.

Necessary Clinical Information

This section includes a list of the clinical information that is normally necessary to make a differential diagnosis within the diagnostic category.

Making a Diagnosis

This section includes a series of questions that guide the clinician through a step-by-step differential diagnosis of disorders in the diagnostic category, using information listed in the previous section.

Common Problems in Making a Diagnosis

This section discusses the common problems that arise during the diagnostic process. Many of these problems were discussed earlier in this chapter in sections on diagnostic uncertainty, the precedence of diagnosis, and the role of the "not otherwise specified" diagnoses. Each of the problems is presented in the form of a brief clinical vignette and question for the reader followed by a discussion of the problem.

Precedence of Diagnosis

This section presents a brief discussion of the precedence of diagnosis for the diagnostic category followed by a table that lists the diagnoses that must be considered or excluded for each diagnosis in the group.

Discussion of Clinical Vignettes

This section includes a discussion of the differential diagnosis of the clinical vignettes in the first section of the chapter.

Key Diagnostic Points

This section lists the Key Diagnostic Points for the diagnostic category.

Common Questions in Making a Diagnosis

This section includes a list of self-test questions in the form of brief vignettes. A detailed discussion of the differential diagnosis follows each question.

Bibliography

American Psychiatric Association: Diagnostic and Statistical Manual of Mental Disorders, 4th Edition. Washington, DC, American Psychiatric Association, 1994

Lakoff G: Women, Fire, and Dangerous Things: What Categories Reveal About the Mind. Chicago, IL, University of Chicago Press, 1987

Matlin MW: Cognition. Holt, Rinehart & Winston, New York, 1989

Smith EE, Medin DL: Categories and Concept. Cambridge, MA, Harvard University Press, 1981

CHAPTER 2

Disorders Usually First Diagnosed in Infancy, Childhood, or Adolescence

Clinical Vignettes

Vignette 1: Sit in Your Seat

Andy is a 6-year-old boy who was referred for a developmental evaluation by his teacher and school counselor. He was brought to the session by his mother. In the waiting room Andy was unable to sit in a chair for more than 2–3 minutes. He fidgeted and squirmed constantly and eventually bounced out of the chair and ran around the room picking up magazines and small objects lying on the table and the receptionist's desk. Several objects were knocked over in the process. His mother was unable to get him seated for more than a few minutes before he hopped up again. When they finally saw the doctor, his mother related the following story.

Andy is the second of three children and was born after a normal pregnancy, labor, and delivery. His siblings were generally quiet, and well behaved and did well in school. As an infant Andy was colicky and irritable. He learned to walk by the end of his first year and then proceeded to disrupt the entire household by opening all of the drawers in the house and emptying their contents on the floor. As he grew older his disruptive behavior continued and the house had to be childproofed to ensure that he did not inadvertently destroy objects that belonged to other members of the family. Andy began talking in his second year and never stopped. He demanded constant attention from his mother and became all the more insistent if he was ignored. If she tried to ignore his demands or refused to give him what he wanted, he began screaming and threw a temper tantrum.

15

Andy had few friends as a child. One particular episode at a friend's house served to illustrate his problems. One day Andy met another small boy in the neighborhood and was invited to his house for lunch. The boy's mother called Andy's mother after an hour to ask her to take Andy home. She explained that Andy and her son had barely entered the house when Andy began running around out of control. He ran from room to room slamming the doors, banging on the piano, and pulling books off the bookshelf. When the friend's mother served lunch she could not get Andy to sit down. He ran by the table, grabbed a sandwich, took two bites, and threw the rest of the sandwich on the ground. By that time her son was overwhelmed by Andy's behavior and close to tears. Andy never played with the child again.

Andy started first grade when he was 6 years old. Within 3 months his mother was asked to meet with the teacher about her son's behavior. The teacher complained that Andy was impossible to manage in class. He would not sit in his seat for more than 5 minutes and often got up and ran around the room picking up objects at random. When she told him to sit down he would not pay attention to her or yelled "no" and ran in the other direction. During those times when he did sit down he had great difficulty working on the class assignment for more than a few minutes. As a result his academic performance was significantly below that of his peers and the level expected for his age. He was unable to learn the alphabet or write simple letters.

Andy also had great difficulty with impulse control and frequently yelled out incorrect answers to questions addressed to other children. He talked constantly and distracted his classmates in their work. At other times he provoked them by his intrusive behavior and comments. He was unable to wait his turn in games and often pushed to the front of the line. As a result he became quite unpopular and was eventually given the nickname "Dumbo" by the other students. Parents of some of the other children complained that their children felt intimidated by Andy and could not perform well in school because of his behavior.

Andy felt the ostracization of the other children even though he did not seem to understand why it was happening. Periodically he would comment to the teacher, "I'm stupid, I'm stupid, stupid Andy,170 and then run off again. The teacher expressed her concern that Andy was mentally retarded. She and the school counselor suggested that he be developmentally evaluated. Andy's parents had difficulty accepting the teacher's recommendations. They responded that the school was responsible for managing him in class and providing the help that he needed to learn.

After several meetings with the school counselor, during which Andy's parents described their feelings of guilt and helplessness, they agreed to have him evaluated. During the evaluation, Andy acted much the same as he did at home and at school. He had difficulty sitting still and concentrating on the tests. The preliminary test results indicated that he had normal motor development and an IQ of 97.

Vignette 2: Mommy, Don't Leave Me

John is a 7-year-old boy who was brought to see a child psychiatrist by his mother, who stated, "John won't let me out of his sight." John is the oldest of two children and the only boy. His mother reported that he was born after a normal pregnancy, labor, and delivery. He developed normally during his first 3 years. He walked at 1 year, began to talk in his second year, and was able to construct simple sentences in his third year. His mother describes John as a cuddly child who liked to climb in her lap and hug her before going off to play in another part of the house.

When John was 5½ his mother became pregnant again. The pregnancy was difficult from the beginning. She had severe morning sickness that was much worse than what she had experienced during her first pregnancy with John. She also had some bleeding in the first trimester. Early in her third trimester she began experiencing premature labor pains and was ordered to stay in bed. During that time John began to demand more attention and constantly come into her room to check on her. Toward the end of her pregnancy John became so demanding that his parents decided to send him to stay with his maternal grandparents. He was told, "You are going to visit Grandma and Grandpa for a little while until Mommy has her new baby. Then we will come and get you with the new baby." John was very unhappy about leaving. He later described his grandparents to the psychiatrist: "They were creepy. They lived in this big, old spooky house. It was all dark and scary."

John's mother continued to have problems with her pregnancy. She finally went into premature labor and delivered a little girl 4 weeks premature. During the delivery the infant required resuscitation and the mother lost a significant amount of blood. She stayed in the hospital for 2 weeks recovering, and the new baby stayed in the hospital for 6 weeks. John's parents went to get him from his grandparents more than 2 months after they had taken him there.

John seemed somewhat withdrawn when his parents first brought him home. During the next few days he watched his mother and the new baby closely, keeping his distance. Then he again began climbing in his mother's lap and hugging her. His mother reported that his hugging now had a frantic, clinging quality to it. John soon developed other problems. He became extremely worried that something might happen to his parents. He repeatedly asked, "Is Mommy going to have another baby? I'll be good. You don't have to send me to Grandma's again." His parents reassured him but he continued to be fearful. He began to worry that someone might come and kidnap him. He would not go out to play with other children because he was fearful that something might happen to him or his parents while he was playing.

One evening, a few weeks later, his parents were leaving to go out to dinner and John began crying and begging them not to leave. He ran to his mother, grabbed her, and would not let go. When she refused to stay home he ran halfway up the stairs and vomited on the carpet. The episodes of vomiting occurred several more times over the next few weeks when his parents tried to go out in the evening.

Core Concept of the Diagnostic Group

The group of Disorders Usually First Diagnosed in Infancy, Childhood, or Adolescence differs from all of the other diagnostic groups in DSM-IV because they are primarily categorized by their time of onset rather than their phenomenology and they are predominantly disorders of abnormal development and maturation. Within that larger organizing structure, specific subcategories reflect many of the diagnostic categories in the remainder of DSM-IV including: Psychotic Disorders, cognitive impairment disorders, Personality Disorders, Anxiety Disorders, and Eating Disorders. However, the emphasis remains on the inability of the individual to attain certain normal developmental milestones and the functions, capabilities, and behavior associated with those levels.

Unfortunately, the lack of a central phenomenological theme makes it difficult to conceptualize the disorders of childhood as a unified whole. In one sense each of the subcategories is comparable to a separate adult diagnostic group such as Adjustment Disorders or Dissociative Disorders. However, unlike other diagnostic groups, it is common for individuals in this group to have comorbid disorders. For example, many children with Autistic Disorder also have Mental Retardation.

Definitions

coprolalia   The involuntary utterance of socially unacceptable or obscene words.

dyslexia   A disorder of reading characterized by difficulty learning to read despite routine instruction, normal intelligence, and adequate opportunity to read.

echolalia   A repetition of a recently heard sound or phrase. Often the patient repeats the last words spoken by the interviewer.

hyperactivity   Excessive motor activity that is seen in Attention-Deficit/Hyperactivity Disorder.

phoneme   The smallest identifiable unit of speech sound (e.g., r, sh, th, ch, dg, j, f).

stereotyped movements   Motor activity that is persistent and mechanically repetitive, such as rapidly flapping or moving the hands back and forth or repeating the same sounds. Stereotyped movements are generally voluntary.

tic   An involuntary, intermittent, rapid, spasmodic, stereotyped motor movement or vocalization. Tics may be simple or complex. Simple motor tics include eyelid and eyebrow twitches, blinking, abrupt head jerks or shoulder-shrugging, and grimaces or twitches of the mouth or face. Simple vocal tics include barks, coughs, grunts, and snorts. Complex motor tics include grooming behavior such as smoothing the hair, touching or hitting various parts of the body or other objects, and foot stamping. Complex vocal tics include echolalia, coprolalia, and the repetition of words or phrases out of context.

Synopses and Diagnostic Prototypes
of the Individual Disorders

There are 10 subgroups or subcategories of diagnoses in the Disorders Usually First Diagnosed in Infancy, Childhood, or Adolescence group.

 1. Mental Retardation
 2. Learning Disorders
 3. Motor Skills Disorders
 4. Communication Disorders
 5. Pervasive Developmental Disorders
 6. Attention-Deficit Disorders and Disruptive Behavior Disorders
 7. Feeding and Eating Disorders of Infancy and Early Childhood
 8. Tic Disorders
 9. Elimination Disorders
10. Other Disorders of Infancy, Childhood, or Adolescence

Each of the first nine subcategories is organized around a specific theme or core group of impairments. For example, in the Pervasive Developmental Disorders, the theme is a broad-based developmental impairment of social interaction and communication associated with stereotypic behavior. Similarly, the diagnoses in the Communication Disorders subcategory cluster around impairments of language development, articulation, and speech. The individual disorders in each subcategory are further differentiated by criteria that either delineate the symptoms in finer detail or stratify the diagnoses by time of onset. The tenth subcategory is a residual group for disorders that do not fit any of the more specific subcategories.

The phenomenological diversity of the diagnoses in the disorders of infancy, childhood, or adolescence category makes a systematic approach to diagnosis difficult. However, the diagnostic process can be simplified by rearranging the subcategories into the four groups shown in Table 2–1 based on the patient's predominant symptoms or deficits. Each of the four groups contain one or more of the first nine subcategories above. The diagnoses in the tenth subcategory (Other Disorders of Infancy, Childhood, or Adolescence) are distributed to the appropriate group based on their clinical phenomenology. A final diagnosis, Disorders of Infancy, Childhood, or Adolescence Not Otherwise Specified, serves

Table 2–1	Disorders of infancy, childhood, or adolescence grouped by predominant symptoms or deficits
Disorder groups	**Diagnoses**
Intellectual and cognitive impairment	All Mental Retardation All Learning Disorders
Motor function impairment	All Motor Skills Disorders All Tic Disorders subcategories Stereotypic Movement Disorder

Disruptive or self-injurious behavior	All Attention-Deficit Disorders and
	   Disruptive Behavior
	 All Feeding and Eating Disorders of
	   Infancy or Early Childhood
	 All Elimination Disorders
	 Separation Anxiety Disorder
	 Reactive Attachment Disorder of
	   Infancy and Early Childhood

Information exchange	All Pervasive Developmental Disorders All Communication Disorders Selective Mutism

as a residual diagnosis for disorders with onset in infancy, childhood, or adolescence that do not meet the criteria for any specific disorder.

The arrangement of the disorders diagnosed in infancy, childhood, or adolescence into these four groups is not a part of DSM-IV. However, it provides a useful way of approaching the diagnosis of these disorders based on their predominant clinical presentation. Because the boundaries between the four groups are not fixed, there is substantial overlap between groups. For example, abnormal behavior may be present in many disorders other than those in the group of disruptive and self-injurious behaviors. Children with Autistic Disorder have inappropriate and disruptive behavior that is manifested by poor social interaction. However, even this abnormal behavior can be conceptualized as primarily an information-exchange disorder because it involves impairment of the verbal and nonverbal communications that occur in normal social interactions. Similarly, children who are mentally retarded may have disruptive behavior or abnormal motor activity, but their predominant symptom is an impairment of intellectual functions. Despite these imperfections, the division of the disorders of infancy, childhood, and adolescence into four groups characterized by their predominant clinical symptoms can be a useful model for the differential diagnosis of these disorders, especially for clinicians who are not trained in child psychiatry.

The common core concept for each of the groups and diagnostic subcategories is presented below. This is followed by a list of the specific diagnoses in the subcategory and a brief synopsis of the specific requirements or criteria that must be fulfilled for each diagnosis. For at least one diagnosis from each subgroup, usually the most representative, a vignette is provided that gives a brief clinical example of that diagnosis. Each vignette is a prototype in the sense that it represents a typical patient with that specific diagnosis. The prototypes provide a more lifelike portrayal of the diagnosis than the criteria alone. They also provide a clinical baseline that can be used in the discussion of problems associated with the diagnosis of these disorders and as a standard for comparison, even if they do not exhaust all the possibilities for the clinical presentation of a specific diagnosis.

Intellectual and Cognitive Function Disorders

The disorders in this group are predominantly characterized by impaired intellectual functioning and specific learning problems.

Mental Retardation

Mental Retardation is characterized by an IQ significantly below average and accompanying deficits in adaptive functioning. The adaptive functioning does not necessarily follow the IQ. For example, an individual with a tested IQ of 52 might function at a higher adaptive level than a person with an IQ of 68. The criteria for Mental Retardation include:

A. Significantly subaverage intellectual functioning: an IQ of approximately 70 or below on an individually administered IQ test (for infants, a clinical judgment of significantly subaverage intellectual functioning).

B. Concurrent deficits or impairments in present adaptive functioning (i.e., the person's effectiveness in meeting the standards expected for his or her age by his or her cultural group) in at least two of the following areas: communication, self-care, home living, social/interpersonal skills, use of community resources, self-direction, functional academic skills, work, leisure, health, and safety.

C. The onset is before age 18 years.

317   Mild Mental Retardation.   Individuals with this disorder fulfill the general criteria for Mental Retardation presented above and have an IQ level from 50–55 to approximately 70.

Mary was born to parents in their late 30s who had two other daughters and a son. Her parents reported that she was a friendly baby who seemed to smile, make eye contact, and interact with them normally. Her mother observed that she seemed to sit, stand, and talk later than her sisters. Mary began school at a regular age. She did poorly in elementary school and had difficulty learning to read and understanding her schoolwork. In class she blurted out nonsensical comments, made silly expressions, and generally disrupted the class. She would not obey the teacher, and her parents were called to the school several times for conferences about her behavior and schoolwork. The other children began making fun of her, calling her "Mary the baby." Mary spent her time outside of school playing with younger children who seemed to tolerate her better than the children her own age did.

By the time Mary was 8 years old, she had fallen significantly behind her classmates in academic achievement. The school informed her parents that she would not be promoted to the fourth grade. Mary was tested and found to have an IQ of 65. The school recommended that she be transferred to a school for students with developmental disabilities. At first her parents protested and took Mary to a child psychiatrist, hoping that her problem was emotional and could be treated. The psychiatrist concurred with the schools' assessment and also recommended that Mary be placed in a special educational environment. At the beginning of the next academic year Mary was transferred to a special school.

Gradually over the next 5 years, her reading, writing, and mathematics skills increased to about the sixth grade level. Mary was always aware that she was different from her sisters. At age 14 she told her parents that she felt bad as she watched her sisters dating but no boys asked her out. Mary became withdrawn, lost weight, and complained of difficulty sleeping. Her parents took her to a psychiatrist, who diagnosed a Major Depressive Disorder, Single Episode, and started her in treatment.

318.0   Moderate Mental Retardation.   Individuals with this disorder fulfill the general criteria for Mental Retardation presented above and have an IQ level of 35–40 to 50–55.

318.1   Severe Mental Retardation.   Individuals with this disorder fulfill the general criteria for Mental Retardation presented above and have an IQ level of 20–25 to 35–40.

318.2   Profound Mental Retardation.   Individuals with this disorder fulfill the general criteria for Mental Retardation presented above and have an IQ level below 20 or 25.

319   Mental Retardation, Severity Unspecified.   There is a strong presumption of Mental Retardation but the person is untestable by standard intelligence tests.

Learning Disorders (Academic Skills Disorders)
The Learning Disorders are characterized by inadequate development of specific academic skills (i.e., reading, mathematics and written expression) that are

not due to demonstrable physical or neurological disorders, Mental Retardation, or Pervasive Developmental Disorders.

315.00   Reading Disorder.   Individuals with this disorder have a tested reading achievement that is substantially below that expected of someone of their age, intelligence, and education. The disturbance significantly interferes with all aspects of their life that require reading and cannot be solely explained by a sensory deficit if one is present.

> Steven was born 5 weeks prematurely and remained hospitalized for the first several weeks of his life. During that time he developed repeated infections and had difficulty gaining weight. He was finally discharged after two months in the hospital and appeared to do well for the first two years. His mother reported that he was alert and responsive to her. Steven frequently laughed and played with his siblings and father. He walked at age 1 year and was soon toddling around exploring the house. However, Steven did not begin speaking until well into his second year. He did not use simple sentences until late in his third year although he clearly seemed to understand what his parents and siblings said to him.
>
> Steven's difficulties in reading first became apparent when he was 4 or 5 because he was unable to recognize simple letters and numbers. In kindergarten he continued to have trouble reading. He did not learn the alphabet, could not read or write his name, and was unable to recognize simple words that his peers could easily read. In first and second grade he was given remedial training in reading and his reading skills began to improve. Reading tests indicated that he had significant difficulty recognizing words and comprehending text. Steven frequently transposed words and had great difficulty with spelling.
>
> The remedial education continued through fifth grade. At that time additional standardized testing showed that Steven had an above-average IQ of 110 and normal mathematical abilities. The testing again verified that he had a significant reading impairment but showed some improvement in his word recognition and reading comprehension skills. With additional training Steven began to compensate for his impairment and progressed into high school with little obvious impairment to the casual observer. However, he found it very difficult to spontaneously read out loud and became very anxious if asked to do so in class.

315.1   Mathematics Disorder.   Individuals with this disorder have a tested mathematical ability that is substantially below that expected of someone of their age, intelligence, and education. The disturbance significantly interferes with all aspects of their life that require mathematical ability and cannot be solely explained by a sensory deficit if one is present.

315.2   Disorder of Written Expression.   Individuals with this disorder have writing skills that are substantially below that expected of someone of their age, intelligence, and education. The disturbance significantly interferes with all aspects of their life that require basic writing skills (e.g., grammar, communication of organized thoughts) and cannot be solely explained by a sensory deficit if one is present.

315.9   Learning Disorder Not Otherwise Specified.   Individuals with this disorder have disorders in learning (e.g., an impairment in spelling skills) that do not meet the criteria for any specific learning disorder.

Motor Function Disorders

The motor functions disorders are predominantly characterized by problems in motor coordination, abnormal involuntary movement, and stereotypic movements that interfere with the patient's usual activities.

Motor Skills Disorder

315.4   Developmental Coordination Disorder.   Individuals with this disorder have substantial impairments in motor coordination that significantly interfere with academic achievement or daily activities and are not due to a general medical condition. These may be manifested by marked delays in achieving normal motor milestones (e.g., sitting, crawling, walking), "clumsiness," poor performance in sports, or poor handwriting.

Tic Disorders
Tic Disorders are characterized by involuntary, sudden, rapid, nonrhythmic, stereotyped motor movements or vocalizations. The tics must be differentiated from the abnormal movements caused by substances (e.g., stimulants) and those associated with neurological diseases.

307.23   Tourette's Disorder.   Patients with this disorder have multiple motor tics and one or more vocal tics that occur many times a day, nearly every day, or intermittently for more than 1 year. The patient is never without tics for more than 3 months.

> Billy is a 12-year-old boy who was first evaluated when he was 8 years old for repeated eye blinking, head jerking, and shrugging. At that time the motor tics were periodic. Gradually over the next 2 years, the number, quality, and intensity of the tics increased. Billy began to have severe facial grimaces and wild arm thrusts. He became so embarrassed about these tics that he stopped going out with his friends. Some of his friends, who did not understand Billy's problem, began making fun of him in school.
>
> Approximately 1 year ago Billy began to produce involuntary sounds. These started as slight grunts and squeaks but progressed to loud barks. They frequently occurred in nonstop bursts that he was unable to control. A few months ago he began

yelling obscenities such as "fuck," "shit," and "bitch." The outbursts disrupted his classes, and the school called Billy's parents to discuss his problems. They suggested that he might not be able to continue in school if his outbursts could not be controlled by medical treatment.

307.22   Chronic Motor or Vocal Tic Disorder.   Patients with this disorder have *either* vocal or motor tics but *not both*. The tics occur many times a day, almost every day or intermittently for more than one year. The onset is before age 18 and the patient is never without tics for more than 3 consecutive months for more than 1 year.

307.21   Transient Tic Disorder.   Patients with this disorder have single or multiple motor and/or vocal tics that occur many times a day, nearly every day for at least 4 weeks, for no longer than 12 consecutive months. The onset is before age 18.

307.20   Tic Disorder Not Otherwise Specified.   This is a residual diagnosis for patients who have tics that do not meet the criteria for a specific Tic Disorder.

Other Disorders of Infancy, Childhood, or Adolescence
Other Disorders of Infancy, Childhood, or Adolescence contains five diverse disorders, of which one is in this group of motor function disorders.

307.3   Stereotypic Movement Disorder (Stereotypic/Habit Disorder).   Patients with this disorder have repetitive, seemingly driven, nonfunctional motor behavior (stereotyped movements) that interfere with usual activities or result in bodily injury. If Mental Retardation is present, the stereotypic or self-injurious behavior is of sufficient severity to become a focus of treatment.

Disruptive and Self-Injurious Behavior Disorders

The disruptive and self-injurious behavior disorders are predominantly characterized by behaviors that are socially unacceptable or potentially harmful to the individual. They include hyperactive, impulsive, inattentive, oppositional, defiant, impulsive, and disruptive behavior, as well as abnormalities of eating and elimination.

Attention-Deficit and Disruptive Behavior Disorders
The Attention-Deficit and Disruptive Behavior Disorders contains two groups of disorders characterized by irritating, impulsive, disruptive, defiant, or antisocial behavior that is contrary to acceptable social norms. Individuals with these disorders are generally considered "management problems."

Attention-Deficit Disorders
Attention-Deficit/Hyperactivity Disorder is a composite disorder that includes two major syndromes, inattention and hyperactivity-impulsivity. The two syndromes may occur independently or together. The symptoms begin before the age of 7 years and cause some impairments in two or more settings. The criteria for the diagnosis include:

A. Either (1) or (2):

  (1) *inattention:* six (or more) of the following symptoms of inattention have persisted for at least 6 months to a degree that is maladaptive and inconsistent with developmental level:

  (a) often fails to give close attention to details or makes careless mistakes in schoolwork, work, or other activities
  (b) often has difficulty sustaining attention in tasks or play activities
  (c) often does not seem to listen when spoken to directly
  (d) often does not follow through on instructions and fails to finish schoolwork, chores, or duties in the workplace (not due to oppositional behavior or failure to understand instructions)
  (e) often has difficulty organizing tasks and activities
  (f) often avoids, dislikes, or is reluctant to engage in tasks that require sustained mental effort (such as schoolwork or homework)
  (g) often loses things necessary for tasks or activities (e.g., toys, school assignments, pencils, books, or tools)
  (h) is often easily distracted by extraneous stimuli
  (i) is often forgetful in daily activities

  (2) *hyperactivity-impulsivity:* six (or more) of the following symptoms of hyperactivity-impulsivity have persisted for at least 6 months to a degree that is maladaptive and inconsistent with developmental level:

  Hyperactivity

  (a) often fidgets with hands or feet or squirms in seat
  (b) often leaves seat in classroom or in other situations in which remaining seated is expected
  (c) often runs about or climbs excessively in situations where it is inappropriate (in adolescents or adults, may be limited to subjective feelings of restlessness)
  (d) often has difficulty playing or engaging in leisure activities quietly
  (e) is often "on the go" or often acts as if "driven by a motor"
  (f) often talks excessively

  Impulsivity

  (g) often blurts out answers before questions have been completed

    (h) often has difficulty awaiting turn

    (i) often interrupts or intrudes on others (e.g., butts into conversations or games)

314.00   Attention-Deficit/Hyperactivity Disorder, Predominantly Inattentive Type.   Individuals with this disorder fulfill Criterion A,1 but not Criterion A,2 for the past 6 months.

314.01   Attention-Deficit/Hyperactivity Disorder, Predominantly Hyperactive-Impulsive Type.   Individuals with this disorder fulfill Criterion A,2 but not criterion A,1 for the past 6 months.

314.01   Attention-Deficit/Hyperactivity Disorder, Combined Type.
Individuals with this disorder fulfill both Criteria A,1 and A,2 for the past 6 months

314.9   Attention-Deficit/Hyperactivity Disorder Not Otherwise Specified.
Individuals with this disorder have prominent symptoms of attention deficit or hyperactivity-impulsivity that do not meet the criteria for a specific Attention-Deficit/Hyperactivity Disorder.

Disruptive Behavior Disorders

312.8   Conduct Disorder.

A. A repetitive and persistent pattern of behavior in which the basic rights of others or major age-appropriate societal norms or rules are violated, as manifested by the presence of three (or more) of the following criteria in the past 12 months, with at least one criterion present in the past 6 months:

Aggression to People and Animals

    (1) often bullies, threatens, or intimidates others
    (2) often initiates physical fights
    (3) has used a weapon that can cause serious physical harm to others (e.g., a bat, brick, broken bottle, knife, gun)
    (4) has been physically cruel to people
    (5) has been physically cruel to animals
    (6) has stolen while confronting a victim (e.g., mugging, purse snatching, extortion, armed robbery)
    (7) has forced someone into sexual activity

Destruction of Property

    (8) has deliberately engaged in fire setting with the intention of causing serious damage
    (9) has deliberately destroyed others' property (other than by fire setting)

Deceitfulness or Theft

(10) has broken into someone else's house, building, or car
(11) often lies to obtain goods or favors or to avoid obligations (i.e., "cons" others)
(12) has stolen items of nontrivial value without confronting a victim (e.g., shoplifting, forgery, but without breaking and entering)

Serious Violations of Rules

(13) often stays out at night despite parental prohibitions, beginning before age 13 years
(14) has run away from home overnight at least twice while living in parental or parental surrogate home (or once without returning for a lengthy period)
(15) often truant from school, beginning before age 13 years

Joe is a 15-year-old boy who was recently accused by a female classmate of forcing her to have sex with him. He replied that she agreed to have sex with him and then got angry because he went out with other girls. Joe is known as a bully and often fights with other students. He was removed from his biological mother's home when he was 4 years old because she stood by while he was repeatedly abused by her boyfriend. Joe was adopted by his current parents when he was 7 years old after he had lived in a series of foster homes. He was an attractive little boy who knew how to be charming. Despite his charm, he had difficulty controlling his temper and seemed to delight in being cruel to other children and animals.

   During the next few years Joe's adoptive parents tried to help him. They worked with the school to help him control his temper and provided him with therapy. However, his behavior became increasingly difficult to manage. He frequently lied and sometimes stole money from his mother. He began to spend time with other adolescents who were known to use drugs. His school performance, which had never been satisfactory, deteriorated even further. Soon after he was accused of the sexual assault, he ran away from home but was caught by the police and arrested.

313.81 Oppositional Defiant Disorder.   Individuals with this disorder persistently display a pattern of negativistic, hostile, and defiant behavior for a period of at least 6 months during which at least four of the following behaviors are present.

1. Often loses temper
2. Often argues with adults
3. Often actively defies or refuses to comply with adults' requests or rules
4. Often deliberately annoys people
5. Often blames others for his or her mistakes or misbehavior
6. Is often touchy or easily annoyed by others

7. Is often angry and resentful
8. Is often spiteful or vindictive

312.9   Disruptive Behavior Disorder Not Otherwise Specified.   Individuals with this disorder have conduct or oppositional-defiant behaviors that do not fulfill the criteria for Conduct Disorder or Oppositional Defiant Disorder.

Feeding and Eating Disorders of Infancy or Early Childhood
The Feeding and Eating Disorders of Infancy and Early Childhood are characterized by disturbances of eating, which include eating substances that have no nutritive value, repeated regurgitation of food, and failure or refusal to eat.

307.52   Pica.   Individuals with this disorder repeatedly eat nonnutritive substances for at least 1 month beyond the developmental age in which it is considered appropriate.

> Jane is a 5-year-old girl who recently began attending kindergarten. Her family is poor but she always appears to be well groomed and wears a worn but clean dress. Jane plays well with the other children and seems to be interested in the school activities. Recently the teacher has noticed that most of the library paste jars in the art room were empty. She asked some of the children if they knew what had happened to the paste. One child replied, "Jane ate it. She always eats paste."
>
> The teacher spoke with Jane, who seemed fearful. When the teacher reassured her that she would not be punished, she reluctantly admitted that she had been eating paste. Her mother confirmed that Jane sometimes ate paste and glue at home.

307.53   Rumination Disorder.   Individuals with this disorder frequently regurgitate and then rechew their food.

307.59   Feeding Disorder of Infancy or Early Childhood.   Children with this disorder persistently fail to gain weight or lose a significant amount of weight over a period of 1 month because they do not eat adequately. The onset is before age 6 years.

Elimination Disorders
The Elimination Disorders are characterized by the involuntary or voluntary passage of feces or urine in developmentally inappropriate places.

307.7   Encopresis.   Children with this disorder pass feces into inappropriate places at least once a month for three months. The child must be at least age 4 years.

307.6   Enuresis.   Children with this disorder repeatedly urinate into their beds or clothes. The behavior either occurs twice a week for 3 consecutive months or produces clinically significant distress or impairment. The child must be at least age 5 years.

Other Disorders of Infancy, Childhood, or Adolescence
The Other Disorders of Infancy, Childhood, or Adolescence subcategory contains five diverse disorders, of which two are in this group of disruptive and self-injurious behavior disorders.

309.21   Separation Anxiety Disorder.   Patients with this disorder have inappropriate or excessive anxiety about separation from home or from those to whom the child is attached as evidenced by at least three of the following for at least 4 weeks. The onset is before age 18 years.

1. Recurrent excessive distress when separation from home or major attachment figures occurs or is anticipated
2. Persistent and excessive worry about losing, or possible harm befalling, major attachment figures
3. Persistent and excessive worry that an untoward event will lead to separation from a major attachment figure (e.g., getting lost or being kidnapped)
4. Persistent reluctance or refusal to go to school or elsewhere because of fear of separation
5. Persistently and excessively fearful or reluctant to be alone or without major attachment figures at home or without significant adults in other settings
6. Persistent reluctance or refusal to go to sleep without being near a major attachment figure or to sleep away from home
7. Repeated nightmares involving the theme of separation
8. Repeated complaints of physical symptoms (such as headaches, stomachaches, nausea, or vomiting) when separation from major attachment figures occurs or is anticipated

313.89   Reactive Attachment Disorder of Infancy or Early Childhood.   Children with this disorder have either excessively inhibited, hypervigilant, or ambivalent and contradictory responses to most social interactions or diffuse, indiscriminate attachments to other people. The presumed cause is pathogenic care evidenced by at least one of the following: 1) disregard for the child's emotional needs, 2) disregard for the child's physical needs, or 3) repeated change of primary caregiver.

Information-Exchange Disorders

Information-Exchange Disorders are predominantly characterized by difficulties in social and interpersonal communication.

Pervasive Developmental Disorders
The Pervasive Developmental Disorders are characterized by a broad-based impairment or loss of the functions that would be expected for a child's age. These include three components: impairment in social interactions; impairment in

communication; and the appearance of restricted, repetitive, and stereotyped patterns of behavior, interests, and activities. The prototypic syndrome for this group of disorders is Autistic Disorder.

299.00 Autistic Disorder. Individuals with this disorder have abnormal functioning in at least one of the following areas, with onset before age 3 years: 1) social interaction, 2) language as used in social communication, or 3) symbolic or imaginative play. The diagnosis also requires:

A. A total of six (or more) items from (1), (2), and (3), with at least two from (1), and one each from (2) and (3):

   (1) qualitative impairment in social interaction, as manifested by at least two of the following:

       (a) marked impairment in the use of multiple nonverbal behaviors such as eye-to-eye gaze, facial expression, body postures, and gestures to regulate social interaction
       (b) failure to develop peer relationships appropriate to developmental level
       (c) a lack of spontaneous seeking to share enjoyment, interests, or achievements with other people (e.g., by a lack of showing, bringing, or pointing out objects of interest)
       (d) lack of social or emotional reciprocity

   (2) qualitative impairments in communication as manifested by at least one of the following:

       (a) delay in, or total lack of, the development of spoken language (not accompanied by an attempt to compensate through alternative modes of communication such as gesture or mime)
       (b) in individuals with adequate speech, marked impairment in the ability to initiate or sustain a conversation with others
       (c) stereotyped and repetitive use of language or idiosyncratic language
       (d) lack of varied, spontaneous make-believe play or social imitative play appropriate to developmental level

   (3) restricted repetitive and stereotyped patterns of behavior, interests, and activities, as manifested by at least one of the following:

       (a) encompassing preoccupation with one or more stereotyped and restricted patterns of interest that is abnormal either in intensity or focus
       (b) apparently inflexible adherence to specific, nonfunctional routines or rituals
       (c) stereotyped and repetitive motor mannerisms (e.g., hand or finger flapping or twisting, or complex whole body movements)
       (d) persistent preoccupation with parts of objects

George was the third of three children born to a professional couple after an uneventful pregnancy and delivery. His development appeared normal for the first few months. He turned over, sat up, and crawled at appropriate times during his first year. However, his mother became concerned about other aspects of his development. A few weeks after he was born she noticed that he seemed different than his brother had at the same age. George rarely made eye contact with her and could not be soothed by being held when he was upset. His lack of interest in other people continued during his first 2 years. He did not interact with his parents or siblings when they were around or follow them when they left the room. Instead, he became extremely attached to a large plastic serving spoon that he played with endlessly, spinning it round and round in his hands.

In the middle of his second year George's parents became increasingly concerned because he had not started to speak. Initially they thought that he might have difficulty hearing because he did not respond when his name was called or members of the family spoke to him. However, they noticed that he did respond to the sound of the washing machine and cars honking their horns in the street outside the house. When they mentioned their concerns to the family pediatrician, they were told, "George is probably a late talker. Don't worry, some kids take longer." However, George's lack of social interaction and communication with the people around him continued. His play was also unusual. He appeared unable to grasp the concept of various toys. He examined them in detail, but could not use them appropriately.

At the beginning of his third year George was referred for a developmental evaluation. The tests showed that his motor skills were near normal, his nonverbal skills were mild to moderately impaired, and his language and social skills were severely impaired. George began receiving remedial education, and gradually his social skills and language began to improve. He developed some recognition of his parents and appeared able to differentiate between them. His speech was clearly abnormal and sounded stilted and artificial. He was able to communicate concrete needs but unable to engage in a social conversation.

Subsequent testing when George was age 9 years showed that he was mildly mentally retarded with an IQ of 53. George continued to receive special education through adolescence. At age 15 he developed a seizure disorder. Despite this he began to gain some self-sufficiency and a limited ability to relate to other people.

299.80   Rett's Disorder.   Individuals with this disorder develop normally for the first 5 months of life, followed by a deceleration of head growth (between 5 and 48 months), loss of previously acquired purposeful hand movement (between 5 and 30 months), loss of social engagement, development of poorly coordinated gait or trunk movements, and severely impaired expressive and receptive language development with severe psychomotor retardation.

299.10   Childhood Disintegrative Disorder.   Individuals with this disorder develop normally for the first 2 years and then demonstrate a significant loss of previously acquired skills in two of the following areas: expressive or receptive language, social skills, bowel or bladder control, play, or motor skills. They also have abnormalities of functioning in two of the following: social interaction; communication; and restricted, repetitive, and stereotyped patterns of behavior, interests, and activities such as those described in the criteria for Autistic Disorder.

299.80   Asperger's Disorder.   Individuals with this disorder fulfill Criteria A and B below but lack any clinically significant delay in language or cognitive development.

A. Qualitative impairment in social interaction, as manifested by at least two of the following:

    (1)   marked impairment in the use of multiple nonverbal behaviors such as eye-to-eye gaze, facial expression, body postures, and gestures to regulate social interaction

    (2)   failure to develop peer relationships appropriate to developmental level

    (3)   a lack of spontaneous seeking to share enjoyment, interests, or achievements with other people (e.g., by a lack of showing, bringing, or pointing out objects of interest to other people)

    (4)   lack of social or emotional reciprocity

B. Restricted repetitive and stereotyped patterns of behavior, interests, and activities, as manifested by at least one of the following:

    (1)   encompassing preoccupation with one or more stereotyped and restricted patterns of interest that is abnormal either in intensity or focus

    (2)   apparently inflexible adherence to specific, nonfunctional routines or rituals

    (3)   stereotyped and repetitive motor mannerisms (e.g., hand or finger flapping or twisting, or complex whole-body movements)

    (4)   persistent preoccupation with parts of objects

299.80   Pervasive Developmental Disorder Not Otherwise Specified.
Individuals with this disorder may have severe and pervasive impairments in reciprocal social interactions and communication skills or may develop stereotyped behavior, interests, or activities, but the criteria for a specific Pervasive Developmental Disorder are not met.

Communication Disorders
The Communication Disorders are characterized by difficulty expressing or understanding verbal or sign language and difficulty articulating speech sounds or speaking with the age-appropriate fluency or rhythm.

315.31   Expressive Language Disorder.   Patients with this disorder have developmental impairments in the capacity to express their thoughts and ideas with language (e.g., limited vocabulary, errors in tense, cannot recall words, cannot produce sentences of appropriate length and complexity).

> Liz is a 7-year-old girl who has problems speaking. Her mother reports that Liz began speaking much later than her sister. By age 18 months she still was not speaking simple words like "mama" although she was interacting otherwise normally with her parents. She gradually started using single words and then simple phrases by the time she was age 4 years. However, she had some difficulty with articulation and her vocabulary was markedly diminished.
>
> By age 6 years her impairment was more obvious. Liz often forgot words she had previously known and had difficulty finding the correct name for objects. When this occurred she frequently substituted incorrect but related words. For example, when she could not remember the word for "sock" she used the word "shoe" or the phrase "shoe on." Her use of grammar was also impaired, and she frequently used incorrect word order (e.g., "Food, Liz eat"). Although Liz had difficulty speaking, she had no difficulty understanding what was said to her. She responded appropriately when asked to perform various simple tasks.
>
> When Liz was 6½ years old, she underwent formal testing to evaluate her disability. The standardized measures showed that she had a significant impairment of expressive language but that her receptive language was intact and age appropriate.

315.31   Mixed Receptive-Expressive Language Disorder.   Patients with this disorder have developmental impairments in the capacity to understand language and to express their thoughts and ideas with language. Symptoms include those for Expressive Language Disorder as well as difficulty understanding words, sentences, or specific types of words such as spatial terms.

315.39   Phonological Disorder.   Patients with this disorder have difficulty articulating normal speech sounds.

307.0   Stuttering.   Patients with this disorder have difficulty producing speech with normal fluency and time patterning. Their speech is characterized by one or more of the following.

1. Sound and syllable repetitions
2. Sound prolongations
3. Interjections
4. Broken words (e.g., pauses within a word)
5. Audible or silent blocking (filled or unfilled pauses in speech)
6. Circumlocutions (word substitutions to avoid problematic words)
7. Words produced with an excess of physical tension
8. Monosyllabic whole word repetitions (e.g., "I-I-I-I-see him.")

307.9 Communication Disorder Not Otherwise Specified. Patients with this disorder have a deficit in communication that does not meet the criteria for a specific Communication Disorder.

Other Disorders of Infancy, Childhood, or Adolescence
The Other Disorders of Infancy, Childhood, or Adolescence contains five diverse disorders of which one is in this group of information-exchange disorders.

313.23 Selective Mutism. Patients with this disorder fail to speak in specific social situations in which there is an expectation of speaking (e.g., at school) despite speaking in other situations (e.g., at home). The failure to speak is not due to a lack of knowledge or comfort with the spoken language and lasts at least one month.

313.9 Disorder of Infancy, Childhood, or Adolescence Not Otherwise Specified. This is a residual category for disorders with onset in infancy, childhood, or adolescence that do not meet criteria for any specific disorder in the classification.

Necessary Clinical Information

* Times of developmental milestones (i.e., walking, talking)

* Capacity to communicate with other people

* Language impairment (expressive, receptive, and articulation)

* Capacity for human relationships

* Quality of social interaction

* Abnormal motor movements (e.g., tics, clumsiness)

* Hyperactivity, inattention, or poor impulse control

* Abnormal behaviors (e.g., fire setting, cruelty to animals)

* Enuresis or encopresis

Making a Diagnosis

The disorders of infancy, childhood, or adolescence differ from those in other categories in DSM-IV because they are primarily categorized by their time of onset and only then by their phenomenology. Some disorders, such as Feeding Disorder of Infancy or Early Childhood, can only occur during childhood. Other childhood disorders have symptoms that can also be found in adult disorders.

When these symptoms occur in adults, the diagnosis is usually different. For example, adult patients who have many of the symptoms of Autistic Disorder would probably receive a diagnosis of Schizophrenia, adults who have the cognitive and adaptational impairment of Mental Retardation would receive a diagnosis of Dementia or other cognitive disorder, and adults with symptoms meeting the criteria for Conduct Disorder would receive a diagnoses of Antisocial Personality Disorder.

Even within a specific subcategory, the disorders of infancy, childhood, or adolescence are often characterized by their time of onset. For example, Autistic Disorder is differentiated from Rett's Disorder and Childhood Disintegrative Disorder because the appearance of symptoms of Autistic Disorder are usually evident early in the first year of life, whereas the other two disorders have an onset after the sixth month and second year, respectively, after a period of normal development.

The diagnosis of childhood disorders also differs from that of adult disorders in their rules of diagnostic precedence and comorbidity. Although it is possible to make a diagnosis of Major Depressive Episode superimposed on an episode of Schizophrenia, the co-occurrence of the two syndromes often leads to a diagnosis of Schizoaffective Disorder or Major Depressive Disorder With Mood-Incongruent Psychotic Features. However, it is not at all unusual to make a diagnosis of Mental Retardation and a comorbid diagnosis of Attention-Deficit/Hyperactivity Disorder. Similarly, a child may receive a diagnosis of Attention-Deficit/Hyperactivity Disorder and Oppositional Defiant Disorder.

The diversity and lack of a consistent phenomenological theme between the various subcategories of the disorders of infancy, childhood, and adolescence sometimes makes the differential diagnosis easier than in other DSM-IV diagnostic groups. For example, the differentiation of Feeding and Eating Disorders from Elimination Disorders or Tic Disorders is reasonably straightforward. Patients either have the cardinal symptoms of the subcategory, such as enuresis, encopresis, tics, and failure to eat, or they do not. However, the distinction between subcategories may not always be so simple. For example, it may be difficult to distinguish whether a person with a language impairment has Pervasive Developmental Disorder or Communication Disorder. The differential diagnosis within a subcategory can also be difficult. For example, the distinction between the various Disruptive Behavior and Attention-Deficit Disorders may be difficult, especially in older children.

The questions in this section provide guidelines for processing the clinical information necessary to make the diagnosis of a disorder of infancy, childhood, or adolescence. The first step in diagnosis is determining which one or more of the four groups discussed above best describes the person's predominant presenting symptoms. Once this has been established, the individual subcategories and diagnoses can be verified or excluded. For each of the following questions, it is assumed that the individual is an infant, child, or adolescent under age 18 years.

1. Is the child's predominant symptom an impairment of learning or intellectual functioning?

* If the patient has significantly subaverage intellectual functioning in all areas, the diagnosis is Mental Retardation. The patient must have an IQ of less than 70 verified by a standardized test. In infants the decision is made by clinical judgment. The patient must also have an impairment in two areas of adaptive functioning. These impairments may be mild or profound and are generally assessed subjectively. Many patients with a diagnosis of Mental Retardation are quite able to communicate and establish relationships with other people. These patients may have impairments in other areas of adaptive functioning that relate more to the skills of daily life.

* If the patient has a deficit or impairment in one or two specific academic areas, the diagnosis is Learning Disorder. The deficits must be verified by a standardized test. The diagnosis of a specific Learning Disorder is inappropriate if the patient has a broad deficit in intellectual functioning that meets the criteria for Mental Retardation. The deficits may be in reading achievement (Reading Disorder), mathematical ability (Mathematics Disorder), or writing skills (Disorders of Written Expression). If the patient has a learning disorder that does not meet the criteria for any of the three disorders above, the diagnosis is Learning Disorder Not Otherwise Specified.

2. Is the child's predominant symptom abnormal motor activity?

The differential diagnosis of abnormal motor activity is based on distinguishing between poor coordination, motor tics, vocal tics, and stereotypic movements.

* If the patient has poor motor coordination that is substantially below that expected for his or her age, the diagnosis is Developmental Coordination Disorder.

* If the patient has motor or vocal tics, the diagnosis depends on the type of tic and length of time the patient has had the tics. 1) If the patient has motor *and* vocal tics for more than 1 year, the diagnosis is Tourette's Disorder. 2) If the patient has either motor *or* vocal tics, but not both, for more than 1 year, the diagnosis is Chronic Motor or Vocal Tic Disorder. 3) If the patient has single or multiple motor or vocal tics for at least 4 weeks and no longer than 12 months, the diagnosis is Transient Tic Disorder. 4) If the patient has tics that do not fulfill the criteria for a specific Tic Disorder, the diagnosis is Tic Disorder Not Otherwise Specified.

* If the patient has stereotyped movements (i.e., persistent, repetitive, seemingly driven, and nonfunctional motor behavior) such as hand shaking, head bang-

ing, body rocking, self-hitting, self-biting, or other similar behaviors, the diagnosis is Stereotypic Movement Disorder.

3. Is the child's predominant symptom socially inappropriate or self-injurious behavior?

The disorders in this group are primarily characterized by behavior that is socially inappropriate or self-injurious. Several other disorders of infancy, childhood, or adolescence include abnormal behavior, but that behavior is not the predominant or defining feature of those disorders in the same way that it is in this group.

* If the patient has abnormal eating behavior, the diagnosis is included in the Feeding and Eating Disorders of Infancy or Early Childhood subcategory. If the child persistently fails to eat and loses weight, the diagnosis is Feeding Disorder of Infancy or Early Childhood. If the child repeatedly regurgitates and rechews food, the diagnosis is Rumination Disorder. If the child persistently and inappropriately eats nonnutritive substances, the diagnosis is Pica.

* If the child passes urine or feces into inappropriate places, the diagnosis is located in the Elimination Disorders subcategory. If the child urinates into bed or clothes after the age 5 years, the diagnosis is Enuresis. If the child passes feces into inappropriate places (e.g., clothes, floor) after the age 4 years, the diagnosis is Encopresis.

* If the child's predominant abnormal behavior is difficulty separating from home and major attachment figures as evidenced by anxiety, fear, nightmares, refusal to go to school, and other symptoms, the diagnosis is Separation Anxiety Disorder.

* If a child's predominant abnormal behavior is persistent violation of the rights of others or of generally accepted social rules, the diagnosis is Conduct Disorder. The core feature of this disorder is a violation of the rights of other people, not merely a defiance or opposition to social or parental authority. However, it is possible to fulfill the criteria if the child or adolescent seriously violates social and parental norms.

* If a child's predominant abnormal behavior is defiance of adult authority accompanied by a negative, hostile attitude and there is no persistent violation of the rights of other people, the diagnosis is Oppositional Defiant Disorder.

* Reactive Attachment Disorder of Infancy or Early Childhood can be distinguished from Pervasive Developmental Disorders because the capacity and motivation to communicate with other people remain intact in the former. This disorder can be distinguished from the Communication Disorders because expressive and receptive language are usually intact.

- Attention-Deficit/Hyperactivity Disorder can be distinguished from Conduct Disorder and Oppositional Defiant Disorder because the disruptive behavior associated with the former diagnosis is not hostile nor is it a conscious effort to defy authority or violate the rights of other people.

4. Is the child's predominant symptom an impairment in the ability to communicate or exchange meaningful information with other people?

Patients with these disorders either do not communicate or communicate poorly with other people. The deficit may be due to a broad impairment in all communication associated with social interaction or it may be due to an impairment in the capacity to understand or express spoken language.

- If a patient's predominant abnormal behavior is an inability to verbally communicate with other people despite evidence of a desire to do so, Autistic Disorder and other Pervasive Developmental Disorders are excluded.

- If a patient's predominant abnormal behavior is an inability and disinterest in communicating with other people associated with a deficit in social interaction and a preoccupation with stereotyped patterns of behavior, interests, and activities, the diagnosis is Pervasive Developmental Disorder. If the child did not experience at least an initial 6 months of normal development after birth, the diagnosis is Autistic Disorder.

- If the child has difficulty producing spoken language (e.g., problems recalling words, limited vocabulary, improper use of tense, and inability to produce sentences of developmentally appropriate length and complexity) and no difficulty understanding language, the diagnosis is Expressive Language Disorder.

- If the patient has difficulty producing spoken language (e.g., problems recalling words, limited vocabulary, improper use of tense, and inability to produce sentences of developmentally appropriate length and complexity) as well as understanding language (e.g., understanding most words, specific types of words, or sentences), the diagnosis is Mixed Receptive-Expressive Language Disorder.

- If the patient produces and understands language normally but is unable to articulate speech sounds at the developmentally expected level (e.g., distorts, substitutes, or omits the affected speech sounds or phonemes), the diagnosis is Phonological Disorder. This disorder may be referred to as "baby talk."

- If the patient understands and expresses language normally but has a disturbance in the normal fluency and pattern of speech (e.g., sound and word repetitions, sound prolongations, abnormal pauses, word blocking, word substitutions to avoid problem words), the diagnosis is Stuttering.

- If the child speaks normally in some social situations but does not speak in other specific situations, the problem is not a language disorder or Pervasive Developmental Disorder. The decision not to speak in specific social situations, such as school, is a voluntary decision. The diagnosis is Selective Mutism.

Common Problems in Making a Diagnosis

There are three main problem areas in the differential diagnosis of disorders of infancy, childhood, or adolescence.

1. Some individuals have symptoms that initially come close but do not actually fulfill the criteria for a specific diagnosis. More information or a further consideration of the diagnostic criteria may or may not resolve the problem.
2. Some individuals have symptoms that fulfill the diagnostic criteria for more than one childhood disorder. The clinician must decide whether the disorders are mutually exclusive or comorbid.
3. Some individuals have symptoms that fulfill the criteria for a childhood disorder and also have physical or psychiatric symptoms of nonchildhood disorders.

The clinician must decide whether one disorder takes precedence over the other, the disorders are mutually exclusive, or they are comorbid. In other cases, patients may have psychiatric symptoms that are not included in the disorders of infancy, childhood, or adolescence group but may be confused with one of these disorders.

Patients Who Almost Fulfill the Diagnostic Criteria

Problems in the diagnosis of childhood disorders commonly occur when a patient fulfills some but not all of the criteria for a diagnosis. A patient might not quite meet the age requirement for a specific disorder or the required number of symptoms. For example, a hostile adolescent may fulfill only three of the four required symptoms for the diagnosis of Oppositional Defiant Disorder. In another case it may be difficult to determine if a child with impairments in communication, social interaction, and stereotypic activities actually had a period of normal development before the symptoms appeared.

Sometimes further inquiry will reveal the presence or absence of the necessary information. At other times it may be impossible to determine if the child had a period of normal development because the parents are poor historians or the child was neglected. In these circumstances the diagnostician is forced to make the best possible decision using his or her clinical judgment and the available information. The following examples present similar problems in the diagnosis of patients who almost fulfill criteria for a specific disorder.

Example 1

A boy, 3 years and 9 months old, who is unusually verbal and intelligent for his age, persistently defecates in the middle of his parent's bed or on the floor of their bedroom. He carefully removes his clothes before defecating. The patient's parents have tried various methods of toilet training him including behavioral modification. Nothing has been successful. What is the patient's diagnosis?

The diagnosis of Encopresis requires that the child be age 4 years or at an equivalent developmental level. Although this child is chronologically younger than 4 years, his verbal skills and intelligence are more advanced. In addition, his deliberate choice of the site for defecation and care for his clothes suggests that he has mastery over his bowel movements and the defecation is more a voluntary than involuntary act. Given these circumstances, the diagnosis of Encopresis for this patient seems justifiable.

Example 2

A 10-year-old boy has been doing poorly in school. His teachers describe him as a slow learner. He also has difficulty communicating with his fellow students. Formal IQ testing revealed that he has an IQ of 73. What is the patient's diagnosis(es)?

The patient has impairments in two areas of adaptive functioning— communication and academic skills. However, his IQ is on the borderline between low normal and Mild Mental Retardation, which requires an IQ level of between 50 and 55 to approximately 70. The clinician could interpret the upper limit of approximately 70 as including the patient's score of 73 and make a diagnosis of Mild Mental Retardation. On the other hand, the clinician might suggest that the patient receive tutoring to improve his academic performance and counseling for his difficulty communicating with his peers. A repeat IQ test a year later might also be useful in resolving the patient's borderline score. If his adaptive functions improve, the diagnosis of Mental Retardation with an IQ of 73 would not be warranted.

Example 3

Joan is a 9-year-old girl whose parents were called to school to meet with their daughter's teacher. The teacher explained that she was concerned with the child's academic performance. She reported that Joan often made careless mistakes in her schoolwork, had difficulty paying attention to the work, and usually did not listen to what was being said to her. Joan apparently disliked and tried to avoid any work that required her to concentrate on a problem for an extended period of time. In addition, she continually misplaced or lost books, pencils, art supplies, and other paraphernalia necessary for her work. Joan's parents acknowledged that she had similar problems at home. What is Joan's diagnosis(es)?

Joan's main problem appears to be difficulty paying attention to her work or other activities for an extended period of time. She fulfills five of the six necessary criteria for the diagnosis of Attention-Deficit/Hyperactivity Disorder, Predominantly Inattentive Type. The clinician should inquire further to see if the patient fulfills at least one more of the four remaining criteria. Many of the criteria in this diagnosis are related. For example, if a patient is easily distracted by extraneous stimuli, it is probably difficult for her to maintain attention in her school tasks. Similarly, if the patient is often forgetful, it would not be surprising if she had difficulty organizing tasks and activities. If the patient fulfills a sixth criterion for inattention, the diagnosis is Attention-Deficit/Hyperactivity Disorder, Predominantly Inattentive Type. If she does not completely fulfill the criteria, the diagnosis is Attention-Deficit/Hyperactivity Disorder Not Otherwise Specified.

Example 4

A 5-year-old boy, who has been physically and emotionally neglected, does not interact with his peers or adults. He makes no eye contact with other people and does not acknowledge their presence. He showed no anxiety when he was left for evaluation in a childrens' clinic. The patient has poor language skills and his speech is filled with distortions, repeated phrases, and grammatical inaccuracies. What is the patient's diagnosis(es)?

The main differential diagnosis for this patient would include Reactive Attachment Disorder of Infancy or Early Childhood, Autistic Disorder, or Communication Disorder. The first disorder requires grossly pathogenic care and significant problems with social interactions. The second includes impairments of social interaction, impairments in communication, and stereotyped patterns of behavior attitudes and activities. The patient has a significant impairment of social interaction and severe language deficits. However, there is no evidence of stereotypic behavior or activities. Therefore, the patient does not meet the criteria for Autistic Disorder. He does fulfill the criteria for Pervasive Developmental Disorder Not Otherwise Specified.

His behavior could be secondary to his pathogenic care. If this is the case, the diagnosis of Reactive Attachment Disorder of Infancy or Early Childhood might be appropriate. However, this disorder does not usually include a language deficit. Therefore, unless there is an associated Communication Disorder, the most likely diagnosis is Pervasive Developmental Disorder Not Otherwise Specified. If he begins to improve significantly in an enriched and supportive environment, the diagnosis can be revised to Reactive Attachment Disorder of Infancy or Early Childhood at a later time.

Patients Who Fulfill Diagnostic Criteria for More Than One Childhood Disorder

The disorders of infancy, childhood, or adolescence are gathered in a diverse group of 10 subcategories that are defined in more detail above (see Synopses and Diagnostic Prototypes of the Individual Disorders). Despite their diversity, it is not unusual to see symptoms from one subcategory appear in patients whose symptoms fulfill the criteria for a diagnosis from another subcategory. For example, a patient with a diagnosis of Mental Retardation may have symptoms of inattention or hyperactivity-impulsivity. These symptoms may or may not be sufficient for a comorbid diagnosis of Attention-Deficit/Hyperactivity Disorder. The examples in this section explore the diagnosis of patients who appear to have symptoms from more than one diagnostic subcategory in the childhood disorders.

Example 5

A 6-year-old girl is severely intellectually impaired and has an IQ of 34. She has few social skills, communicates little, if at all, with other people, and repeatedly bangs her head against the wall. What is the patient's diagnosis(es)?

The patient's symptoms meet the criteria for a diagnosis of Severe Mental Retardation because her IQ is below the range of 35–40 and she has significant deficits in communication and interpersonal skills. However, her impairments in communication and social interaction, in conjunction with stereotypic head banging, also meet the criteria for Autistic Disorder. Therefore, the patient should receive both diagnoses.

Example 6

A 9-year-old girl has difficulty sitting still in class and at home and often runs around the room or climbs on the furniture. She constantly squirms and fidgets when she is forced to sit in a chair and has difficulty waiting her turn when playing with other children. The patient's hyperactivity has made it difficult for her to concentrate on her schoolwork, and tests of her mathematics skills are significantly below what would be expected for a child her age. What diagnosis(es) should the child receive?

The patient fulfills the criteria for a diagnosis of Attention-Deficit/Hyperactivity Disorder, Predominantly Hyperactive-Impulsive Type. She also meets the criteria for Mathematics Disorder. In this case, neither diagnosis takes precedence over the other and the patient can receive both diagnoses as comorbid disorders.

Example 7

A 13-year-old boy has an IQ of 61 and academic problems in school as well as problems with his interpersonal skills. The patient is easily annoyed by other people and frequently becomes angry and has a temper tantrum. When he is asked, by his parents, to do a simple chore he refuses to comply or cooperate. What is the patient's diagnosis(es)?

The patient meets the criteria for the diagnosis of Mild Mental Retardation. When severe and pervasive oppositional and defiant behavior occurs in the presence of Mental Retardation and becomes a focus of treatment, it is appropriate to also give the patient a diagnosis of Oppositional Defiant Disorder.

Example 8

A 7-year-old boy has markedly impaired social interactions with other people and severely impaired language skills. The patient also picks at his skin and lips and repeatedly bites himself. This behavior has led to numerous infections and scarring and has become the main focus of the patient's current treatment. What is the patient's diagnosis(es)?

The patient's impairment of social interactions, communication, and repetitious self-mutilating behavior meets the criteria for Autistic Disorder. Because his stereotypic behavior is severe and has become the focus of treatment, the additional diagnosis of Stereotypic Movement Disorder is also appropriate.

Example 9

A 13-year-old boy continually defies adult rules by running away from home, repeatedly skipping school, and staying out late at night. He constantly argues with his parents, frequently loses his temper, and is usually angry and resentful. What is the diagnosis(es)?

This adolescent's behavior meets the criteria for both Conduct Disorder and Oppositional Defiant Disorder. However, the diagnosis of Conduct Disorder takes precedence over the diagnosis of Oppositional Defiant Disorder.

Other Symptoms Seen With Disorders of Infancy, Childhood, or Adolescence

Children also have many of the same psychiatric illnesses that afflict adults, including disorders of anxiety, mood, thought, perception, and others. The diagnosis of these disorders in children requires fulfillment of the same, or almost the same, criteria as are required in the adult diagnosis. The modifications of the criteria for application to children are minimal. For example, children and adolescents may have many symptoms that fulfill the criteria for Major Depressive Episode with an irritable mood rather than a depressed mood. Furthermore, mood, anxiety, and other psychiatric disorders can be comorbid with many, but not all, of the childhood disorders. Patients with a diagnosis of Mental Retardation can also have Major Depressive Episode. However, the diagnosis of Attention-Deficit/Hyperactivity Disorder cannot be made if the symptoms are better accounted for by Mood Disorder.

Example 10

Jean is a 10-year-old girl who had a normal infancy, interacting and communicating well with her family and friends. She began having some academic problems when she started school. In second grade she was diagnosed with Reading Disorder based on standardized tests. Her reading appeared to improve with special education. Approximately 7 months ago her teacher noticed a gradual change in Jean's behavior. She became more withdrawn, interacted less, and her thoughts seemed jumbled when she spoke. In addition, her reading skills began to deteriorate. Approximately 1 month ago she reported hearing several voices telling her that she is a bad child. What is Jean's diagnosis(es)?

Jean's normal development for the first several years of life exclude the diagnosis of Autistic Disorder or any other Pervasive Developmental Disorder. Her Reading Disorder seems independent of her later withdrawal and decompensation with the exception of a deterioration of the progress she had made overcoming her reading deficits. The patient has had a thought disorder and deteriorated behavior for the last 7 months. During the last month she has reported auditory hallucinations. These symptoms fulfill the criteria for the diagnosis of Schizophrenia. In this case the Schizophrenia is comorbid with the Reading Disorder.

Example 11

A 6-year-old boy has been experiencing academic difficulties in school. Recent testing has demonstrated that he has a mild impairment of reading skills and a moderate hearing impairment. What diagnosis(es) should the child receive?

The criteria for the diagnosis of Reading Disorder requires that the patient's reading skills, determined by standardized testing, be substantially below that expected for his age and intelligence. If a sensory deficit is present, the learning difficulties must be in excess of those that are usually associated with it. In this case, the patient has a mild reading impairment and a moderate hearing loss. The diagnostician must use his or her clinical judgment to decide whether the moderate hearing loss is sufficient to account for the patient's reading impairment. It would appear that it is sufficient. Therefore, the patient should not receive a diagnosis of Reading Disorder.

Example 12

A 14-year-old girl has a tested IQ of 56 and complains of feeling bad. She is irritable, sleeps poorly, eats little, and has lost 10 pounds in the last few months. She appears disinterested in many of the activities she previously enjoyed, such as going shopping with her mother. Instead she lies around the house, communicates little with her family, and appears to have little energy or self-direction. What diagnosis(es) should this patient receive?

The patient's IQ of 56 meets the criteria for a diagnosis of Mild Mental Retardation if the patient also has impairments in two areas of adaptive functioning. The patient's additional symptoms appear to be a change from her previous behavior. In the past she has enjoyed shopping with her mother. Currently she describes feeling bad. The symptoms associated with this feeling (e.g., sleep disturbance, anorexia, weight loss, irritability) suggest that she is actually depressed. The length of time that she has had these symptoms is unclear. If she has had them for at least 2 weeks she has met the criteria for the diagnosis of Major Depressive Episode. If this is her first experience with severe depression, it would be appropriate to give the patient a diagnosis of Major Depressive Disorder, Single Episode.

Precedence of Diagnosis

Some of the cases in preceding sections discuss diagnostic dilemmas that arise when patients have symptoms consistent with more than one diagnosis. The diagnoses may belong to the same diagnostic group (e.g., Disorders of Infancy, Childhood, or Adolescence) or other groups (e.g., Mood Disorders, Schizophrenia, and Other Psychotic Disorders), as well as Disorders of Infancy, Childhood, or Adolescence. When these conflicts occur, they are often resolved using the rules of diagnostic precedence that are included in the criteria for many diagnoses (Table 2–2). However, these rules are not infallible, and, in some circumstances, they are mutually exclusive. Therefore, the rules of diagnostic precedence, rather than taken as hard and firm, should be seen as guidelines.

Table 2–2 Precedence of diagnosis for infancy, childhood, and adolescent disorders	
Infancy, childhood, or adolescent disorder	**Disorders taking precedence**
Mental Retardation	None
Reading Disorder Mathematics Disorder Disorder of Written Expression Learning Disorder NOS	Not better accounted for by a sensory deficit (e.g., deafness, blindness)
Developmental Coordination Disorder	Not due to a general medical condition
Autistic Disorder	Not better accounted for by Rett's Disorder, or Childhood Disintegrative Disorder
Rett's Disorder	None
Childhood Disintegrative Disorder	Not better accounted for by another specific Pervasive Developmental Disorder or Schizophrenia
Pervasive Developmental Disorder NOS	Does not meet the criteria for a specific Pervasive Developmental Disorder
Attention-Deficit/Hyperactivity Disorders	Does not occur exclusively during Pervasive Developmental Disorder, Schizophrenia, or other Psychotic Disorder Not better accounted for by Mood Disorder, Anxiety Disorder, Dissociative Disorder, or Personality Disorder
Conduct Disorder	Does not meet criteria for Antisocial Personality Disorder (if 18 or older)
Oppositional Defiant Disorder	Does not meet criteria for Conduct Disorder, Antisocial Personality Disorder (if 18 or older) Does not occur exclusively during Psychotic Disorder or Mood Disorder
Disruptive Behavior NOS	Does not meet criteria for a specific Attention-Deficit/Hyperactivity Disorder
Pica	Not better accounted for by a culturally sanctioned practice
Rumination Disorder	Not due to a general medical condition Does not occur exclusively during Anorexia Nervosa or Bulimia Nervosa

(continued)

Table 2–2 Precedence of diagnosis for infancy, childhood, and adolescent disorders *(continued)*

Infancy, childhood, or adolescent disorder	Disorders taking precedence
Feeding Disorder of Infancy or Early Childhood	Not better accounted for by another mental disorder Not due to the direct effects of a substance or general medical condition
Tourette's Disorder	Not due to effects of a substance or general medical condition
Chronic Motor or Vocal Tic Disorder	Has never met criteria for Tourette's Disorder Not due to effects of a substance or general medical condition
Transient Tic Disorder	Has never met criteria for Tourette's Disorder, Chronic Motor, or Vocal Tic Disorder Not due to effects of a substance or general medical condition
Tic Disorder NOS	Not better accounted for by a specific Tic Disorder
Expressive Language Disorder	Does not meet criteria for Mixed Receptive/Expressive Language Disorder, or Pervasive Developmental Disorder Not better accounted for by Mental Retardation, speech-motor or sensory-motor deficit, or environmental deprivation
Mixed Receptive/Expressive Language Disorder	Does not meet criteria for Pervasive Developmental Disorder Not better accounted for by Mental Retardation, speech-motor or sensory-motor deficit, or environmental deprivation
Phonological Disorder	Not better accounted for by Mental Retardation, speech-motor or sensory-motor deficit, or environmental deprivation
Stuttering	Not better accounted for by speech-motor or sensory-motor deficit

Table 2–2	Precedence of diagnosis for infancy, childhood, and adolescent disorders *(continued)*
Infancy, childhood, or adolescent disorder	**Disorders taking precedence**
Communication Disorder NOS	Not better accounted for by a specific Communication Disorder
Encopresis Enuresis	Not due to effects of a general medical condition
Separation Anxiety Disorder	Does not occur exclusively during Pervasive Developmental Disorder, Schizophrenia, or Other Psychotic Disorder
Selective Mutism	Not better accounted for by Communication Disorder
Reactive Attachment Disorder of Infancy or Early Childhood	Does not meet criteria for Pervasive Developmental Disorder Not better accounted for by developmental delay
Stereotypic Movement Disorder	Not better accounted for by Obsessive-Compulsive Disorder, Tic Disorder, or Trichotillomania
Disorder of Infancy, Childhood, or Adolescence NOS	Not better accounted for by any other specific infancy, childhood, or adolescent disorder

Note. NOS = Not Otherwise Specified.

They suggest the other diagnoses that should be considered before a specific diagnosis is made, and they indicate the circumstances under which the diagnosis in question may be excluded if the patient's symptoms fulfill the criteria for other diagnoses.

Discussion of Clinical Vignettes

Vignette 1: Sit in Your Seat

Andy is a 6-year-old boy who is unable to control himself. His mother is barely able to tolerate his behavior. His teacher, other children, and their parents are completely unwilling to accept his behavior. Andy has problems at home and at school. He is unable to sit still in either setting. He fidgets and runs from place to place. This has become a major problem at school because he disrupts the class and makes it difficult for the other students to concentrate on their studies. He repeatedly tries to get attention by making extraneous and inappropriate comments in class.

Andy's academic performance is poor and his teacher has suggested that he may be mentally retarded. The diagnosis of Mental Retardation requires an IQ of 70 or below and deficits or impairments in two skill areas including communication, social/interpersonal, functional academic, etc. Andy's poor academic performance and difficulty interacting with other children fulfills this part of the criteria. However, his IQ is 97. This excludes the diagnosis of Mental Retardation.

Andy's symptoms are mainly examples of hyperactive and impulsive behavior. He fidgets, leaves his seat in class, runs about, has difficulty playing quietly, and blurts out answers to questions before other children have a chance to respond. These symptoms fulfill the criteria for Attention-Deficit/Hyperactivity Disorder, Predominantly Hyperactive-Impulsive Type.

Vignette 2: Mommy, Don't Leave Me

John's main symptoms revolve around fears of abandonment presumably stimulated or reinforced by his unfortunate lengthy stay with his grandparents when his sister was born. Since returning he has been excessively anxious, clinging, and fearful that something might happen to his parents or that he might be sent away again because he was not behaving properly. He recently developed physical symptoms (i.e., vomiting) that occur when he is about to experience a brief separation from his parents. These symptoms have lasted for several weeks and markedly interfere with John's ability to play with his friends.

The diagnosis of Separation Anxiety Disorder requires that the patient have three of eight possible symptoms that involve fear about loss or separation from important attachment figures or the potential for a loss or separation. The anxiety can also be manifest in nightmares or physical complaints. John's worries that something might happen to his parents, his fears that he might be kidnapped, and his physical symptoms (i.e., vomiting) at the threat of brief separation fulfill the criteria for the diagnosis of Separation Anxiety Disorder.

Key Diagnostic Points

- Patients with Mental Retardation have delays in development in many areas. Patients with Learning Disorders have a delay or failure of development in one or a few specific areas (e.g., reading, mathematics).

- The diagnosis of Conduct Disorder requires that the patient violate the basic rights of others or age-appropriate social rules. The behaviors are generally

more serious and socially inappropriate than those associated with Oppositional Defiant Disorder.

- The core symptoms of Autistic Disorder are impairments in social interaction;
impairments in communication; and stereotyped and repetitive patterns of behavior, interests, and activities.

Common Questions in Making a Diagnosis

1. Joey is a 14-year-old boy with an IQ of 61 who has had academic difficulty
in school and is currently reading and writing at a fifth-grade level. He has
also had some difficulty making friends and fitting in with his peer group.
Over the last 2 months Joey has become unusually irritable and his school
work has begun to deteriorate. He has difficulty sleeping, has little appetite,
and no longer enjoys playing ball or sharing other activities with his father.
Recently, his younger sister started teasing him at the dinner table saying,
"Joey's in love, Joey's in love." Joey exploded and began screaming, "You
think I'm just dumb and no one likes me!" and ran out of the room. A few
minutes later his mother tried to talk with him. In response to her repeated
questions Joey replied, "Everyone knows I'm dumb. None of the girls talk
with me like they do with the other guys. I'm not worth anything. I wish I
was dead." His mother became alarmed and called Joey's therapist. What is
Joey's diagnosis(es)?

   Answer: Joey's IQ of 61 and his difficulty with academic work and social
relationships fulfill the criteria for a diagnosis of Mild Mental Retardation.
However, his recent behavior changes, including irritability, insomnia, anorexia, anhedonia, and a sense of worthlessness suggest that he has also become depressed. These symptoms fulfill the criteria for a diagnosis of Major
Depressive Disorder, Single Episode. Joey's sensitivity to his sister's taunts
and his concerns about talking with girls suggest that he is having difficulty
adjusting to adolescent changes in sexual feelings and to the increasing
awareness that he is different from other boys his age.

2. Sally is a 4-year-old girl who is the second of three children born to middle-
class parents. Her mother's pregnancy, labor, and delivery were normal.
Sally appeared to be developing well through her second year. She began to
walk at 12 months and to talk at 15 months. By 24 months she was speaking
simple sentences. Sally interacted well with her parents and her older sister
who was 18 months older. In the middle of her third year, Sally's mother
began to notice some changes in her behavior. Sally began talking less rather
than more. Her speech changed, and she started repeating the same words
over and over, and using words and phrases that made no sense. There were

also changes in her play. For example, she no longer held her toy telephone to her ear to imitate her mother speaking on the telephone. Instead, she used it to bang on the floor and make noise. Although she had previously been quite responsive, she no longer smiled at her mother or met her gaze. What is the patient's diagnosis(es)?

Answer: Sally's normal development for the first 2½ years rules out the diagnosis of Autistic Disorder. In the middle of her third year she had a deterioration of her previously normal verbal skills, social interaction, and play. These symptoms fulfill the criteria for the diagnosis of Childhood Disintegrative Disorder.

3. Steven is a 13-year-old boy who is known as a chronic bully in his neighborhood. He delights in fighting with other adolescents and hurting them. He continually defies his parents and refuses to follow school rules. Steve has been suspended from school twice in the past for fighting and hurting another student. When Steve wants something he can be exceedingly charming until he gets it. He has no compunctions about lying to friends or his parents. What is his diagnosis(es)?

Answer: The differential diagnosis here is between Oppositional Defiant Disorder and Conduct Disorder. Steve's behavior is hostile and defiant and therefore consistent with the former diagnosis. However, his predominant behavior consists of repeated violations of the rights of other people. His physical cruelty to other people, bullying, and lying fulfill the criteria for Conduct Disorder. Even if he did meet the requirements for the diagnosis of Oppositional Defiant Disorder, the diagnosis of Conduct Disorder would take precedence over that disorder.

4. A 7-year-old boy with a mild to moderate speech deficit was tested and found to have an IQ of 57. A subsequent examination demonstrated that he has a moderate hearing impairment. What is the best diagnosis for the patient?

Answer: IQ cannot be adequately determined in the presence of a sensory deficit such as deafness unless compensation is made for the deficit. This child's deafness was not discovered until after the IQ testing and therefore was probably not taken into account during the testing. The diagnosis of Mental Retardation cannot be made under these circumstances.

5. A severely physically and emotionally neglected 4-year-old girl does not communicate with examiners and demonstrates no social interaction with peers or adults. She spends most of her time picking at her fingers. What is the child's diagnosis(es)?

Answer: It is difficult to make a definitive diagnosis in a child who has had severe physical and emotional abuse until the child has been placed in a supportive and enriched environment and given a chance to respond. An appropriate tentative diagnosis would be Reactive Attachment Disorder of Infancy or Early Childhood.

6. Jeffrey is an 8-year-old boy who was brought to see the family pediatrician by his mother, who states, "Jeffrey has been acting strange for a several weeks. He makes funny faces at me, his teachers, and the other members of the family." The physician noted that Jeffrey periodically grimaced, winked, and bit his lips. When he asked the child about this behavior, Jeffrey replied, "It just happens. I don't do anything." Jeffrey has no other medical problems. What diagnosis(es), if any, should Jeffrey receive?

   Answer: Jeffrey is experiencing motor tics. Because the tics have only oc-curred for approximately 1 month, the diagnoses of Tourette's Disorder and Chronic Motor or Vocal Tic Disorder are excluded. The diagnosis of Tourette's Disorder requires the presence of vocal tics and motor tics. The patient's symptoms fulfill the criteria for Transient Tic Disorder. If the tics continue for at least a year with or without vocal tics, the diagnosis can be revised to the two Tic Disorders mentioned first.

7. Benjie is a 6-year-old boy who talks "baby talk." He refers to his thumb as "my fum" and to the family car as "Daddy's ka." His parents think that Benjie's speech is adorable. Some of the other children make fun of Benjie. What diagnosis(es), if any, should he receive?

   Answer: Benjie's hearing should be evaluated initially to determine if he has a sensory deficit that might explain his inability to pronounce simple phonemes. If his hearing is intact and he has difficulty pronouncing other phonemes (e.g., r, sh, th, f, z, l, and ch), or substitutes sounds such as "f" for "th" in "thumb," the diagnosis is Phonological Disorder.

8. Jimmy is a 4-year-old boy who repeatedly urinates in his clothes during the day and in his bed at night. His parents have tried various means of toilet training and behavioral techniques to help Jimmy control his bladder func-tion to no avail. What is his diagnosis(es)?

   Answer: Although Jimmy does have problems controlling his bladder function, he must be 5 years old to receive a diagnosis of Enuresis. At present his lack of bladder control is still within the range of normal behavior.

9. Carly is a 5-year-old girl who interacts well socially but has difficulty com-municating. Her problems were apparent by the time she was 18 months old

at which point she had not uttered a single word. At that time she was able to understand simple commands and could point to common objects when they were named. Carly began using simple words by the time she was age 3 years and spoke simple phrases by age 4 years. However, her articulation was poor and she seemed to learn words more slowly than did other children. She sometimes had difficulty retrieving appropriate words and compensated by using incorrect or related words that did not convey the appropriate meaning. What is Carly's diagnosis(es)?

Answer: Carly's normal social interaction excludes the diagnosis of Pervasive Developmental Disorder. The differential diagnosis includes Expressive Language Disorder and Mixed Receptive-Expressive Language Disorder. Because she was able to understand simple verbal commands at age 18 months, the diagnosis of Mixed Receptive-Expressive Language Disorder is excluded. Therefore, the diagnosis is Expressive Language Disorder. Her problems with articulation may also meet the criteria for Phonological Disorder.

10. Jane is a shy 6-year-old girl who will not speak at school. When she is asked a question she responds by nodding or shaking her head. Jane talks normally at home. Her school problem has persisted for 3 months. What is Jane's diagnosis(es)?

   Answer: Because Jane can talk normally at home, the Pervasive Developmental Disorders and the Communication Disorders are excluded. The appropriate diagnosis is Selective Mutism.

Delirium, Dementia, and Amnestic and Other Cognitive Disorders

Clinical Vignettes

Vignette 1: Grandma Doesn't Know Me Anymore

Mary is a 72-year-old woman who currently lives with her daughter Sharon's family. She has always led an active life and was a high school mathematics teacher before retiring at the age of 62. Her husband died approximately 9 years ago, leaving her financially comfortable but not wealthy. Mary continued to live alone in the small apartment she had shared with her husband. Her two sons lived some distance away but her daughter lived in a nearby city and spoke with her frequently and visited her with the grandchildren every few weeks. Mary was particularly close to her daughter's two children, and enjoyed taking them out for ice cream when they visited her.

Approximately 5 years ago her daughter began to notice some subtle changes in her mother's behavior. Mary had always been a good housekeeper and prided herself on how clean she kept her apartment. During one visit Sharon noticed that the kitchen floor in her mother's apartment was dirty, the carpets had not been vacuumed recently, and there were dirty dishes in the sink. She suggested that her mother might want to have someone come in and help with the housework. Mary seemed irritated by the suggestion and replied, "I've always done my own house work. Why would I want someone to help me now?" She seemed indifferent to the dirty kitchen floor but was obsessed with cleaning the sink and toilet in the bathroom. Her daughter was concerned because this behavior seemed unlike her mother.

Sharon began to detect additional changes in her mother over the next 2 years.

Mary seemed increasingly forgetful. On one visit Sharon noticed that little notes were taped on the cabinets in her mother's kitchen. She asked her mother about the notes and was told, "They're just reminders dear. I have so much to do these days." A few months later the notes appeared all over the house. When she asked about them again her mother seemed offended and said, "Stop treating me like a child."

Additional problems appeared. Sharon noticed that some unopened mail had been sitting on the living room coffee table for several weeks. She opened the mail and discovered that one envelope contained a notice from her mother's bank indicating that she had overdrawn her checking account by $123.43. When Sharon asked her mother about the notice from the bank her mother was furious. Sharon pressed the issue and discovered that her mother's checkbook was filled with errors. She made an appointment for her mother with the family internist and explained her concerns to the doctor. He examined Mary and told Sharon, "I can't find anything wrong with your mother. She's as healthy as a horse and just as charming as ever. Everyone forgets things when they get older. Don't worry so much about her." Sharon was somewhat reassured but continued to have a nagging doubt about her mother's condition.

During the next few months Sharon's concerns increased again. Mary started calling her daughter every night complaining that someone had placed a computer in her bedroom. One day she began accusing Sharon of trying to steal her money. Two weeks later she got a call from her mother's neighbor who reported that two strange men had brought her mother home the day before. The men informed the neighbor that Mary had stopped her car and asked them for directions but didn't seem to understand how to follow them. Sharon became alarmed and took her youngest child with her to visit her mother. When they arrived Mary seemed glad to see them. She kissed her daughter, looked down at her 7-year-old granddaughter, Louise, and said, "What a darling child. What's her name?" Louise looked at her mother, began crying, and said, "Grandma doesn't know me anymore."

Vignette 2: I'm Fine, Let Me Go

Tom, a 19-year-old young man was riding his bike down the highway near his home one night. As he approached an intersection the traffic light turned yellow. Tom pedaled harder to get through but the light changed to red while he was in the middle of the intersection. Suddenly, a car approached from his right. Tom was hit, knocked off his bike, and thrown onto the ground next to the highway. Several cars stopped and the drivers came over to help. Tom was unconscious for a few minutes. When he regained consciousness he looked at the people around him and asked, "What happened?" One of the drivers knelt down beside him and said, "You were hit by a car. An ambulance is coming. How do you feel?" Tom looked around again and said, "I'm fine, let me go," and he began to get up. The driver tried to restrain him saying, "I think you ought to wait for the ambulance." Tom looked at him, lay down again and asked, "What happened?" The driver explained what had happened again but Tom didn't seem to understand. He repeated his question, "Where am I? What happened? I need to go home." When no one answered he stated, "I'm fine, let me go," and began to get up again.

The driver seemed uncertain what to do next. He tried to convince Tom to lie down again but Tom had become excited and began yelling, "I need to go home, I need to go home." He got to his feet and began wandering toward the highway. Two other observers tried to guide him away from the street. Suddenly, the ambulance and paramedics arrived. They ran over to Tom and asked him how he was feeling. Tom seemed bewildered. He looked at the two paramedics and asked, "What happened?" The two paramedics examined Tom, placed him on a stretcher, loaded him into the ambulance and took him to a nearby hospital emergency room. The next day one of the drivers called the hospital to find out Tom's condition. The hospital reported that he was currently unconscious in the intensive care unit as a result of the head trauma he had during the accident.

Core Concept of the Diagnostic Group

The core concept of the Delirium, Dementia, and Amnestic and Other Cognitive Disorders group is the presence of impairments in cognition (e.g., memory deficit, language disturbance, perceptual disturbance, impairment in the capacity to plan and organize, failure to recognize or identify objects) that appear to be caused by one or more substances and/or general medical conditions. In Delirium the patient also has a disturbance in consciousness. This diagnostic group can also be referred to as the Cognitive Disorders group.

Criteria Applicable to Multiple Disorders

The Cognitive Disorders group contains three specific sets of criteria that are applicable to multiple diagnoses. These criteria define the three core cognitive syndromes, Delirium, Dementia, and Amnestic Disorder.

Core Criteria for Deliriums

A delirium is distinguished by a disturbance of consciousness. It may be caused by a general medical condition, a substance, and/or multiple medical conditions and/or substances. The core criteria for deliriums remain the same for each of the etiologies. The criteria include:

1. Disturbance of consciousness (i.e., reduced clarity of awareness of the environment) with reduced ability to focus, sustain, or shift attention.
2. A change in cognition (such as memory deficit, disorientation, language disturbance) or the development of a perceptual disturbance that is not better accounted for by a preexisting, established, or evolving dementia.

3. The disturbance develops over a short period of time (usually hours to days) and tends to fluctuate during the course of the day.
4. There is evidence from the history, physical examination, or laboratory findings that the disturbance is caused by the direct physiological consequences of a substance or general medical condition.

Core Criteria for Dementia

Dementia is primarily distinguished by an impairment in memory with associated cognitive disturbances. It may be caused by a nonpsychiatric medical condition, a substance, or a mixture of the two problems. The core criteria for dementia remains the same for each etiology. The criteria include the following.

The development of multiple cognitive deficits manifested by both:

1. Memory impairment (inability to learn new information and to recall previously learned information)
2. One (or more) of the following cognitive disturbances:

   a. aphasia (language disturbance)
   b. apraxia (inability to carry out motor activities despite intact motor function)
   c. agnosia (failure to recognize or identify objects despite intact sensory function)
   d. disturbance in executive functioning (i.e., planning, organizing, sequencing, abstracting)

Core Criteria for Amnestic Syndrome

Amnestic Syndrome is an impairment of memory that may be caused by a nonpsychiatric medical condition, a substance, or a mixture of the two problems. The core criteria for Amnestic Disorder is the same for each etiology and includes one main element: the development of memory impairment as manifested by the inability to learn new information or the inability to recall previously learned information.

Definitions

agnosia   The inability to recognize objects despite intact sensory function. The individual receives the sensory impression of the object but is unable to interpret it.

aphasia   A disturbance in language that differs depending on the area of the brain that is affected. A Broca's aphasia is the loss of the ability to produce spoken, and often written, language without impairment in the comprehension of language. A Wernicke's aphasia is the loss of the ability to comprehend language coupled with an inability to produce coherent language.

apraxia The inability to carry out motor activities that the individual was previously able to perform. This deficit occurs in the presence of intact motor function.

executive functioning Higher cognitive functions such as planning for the future, organizing, abstracting from concrete examples using inductive reasoning, etc.

Synopses and Diagnostic Prototypes of the Individual Disorders

The brief synopses in this section include the specific requirements or criteria that must be fulfilled for each of the diagnostic categories. Following each synopsis is a vignette that provides a clinical example of the diagnoses. Each vignette is a prototype in the sense that it represents a typical patient from that specific diagnostic category. The prototypes provide a more lifelike portrayal of the diagnosis than the criteria alone. They also provide a clinical baseline that can be used in the discussion of problems associated with the diagnosis of these disorders and as a standard for comparison even if they do not exhaust all the possibilities for the clinical presentation of a specific diagnosis. Most of the diagnoses in this group are based on the three Cognitive Disorder syndromes: Delirium, Dementia, and Amnestic Syndrome. The specific diagnoses are differentiated according to the presumed etiology of the syndromes.

Deliriums

293.0 Delirium Due to a General Medical Condition. Individuals with this disorder fulfill the core criteria for Delirium and there is evidence (e.g., history, physical examination, laboratory) that the syndrome is caused by the direct physiological consequences of a general medical condition.

> Sandra is a 28-year-old woman with a seizure disorder that began after she was knocked unconscious in an automobile accident at the age of 16. Three months after the accident she had her first grand mal seizure. The seizures occurred approximately once a week but were gradually controlled with medication. Despite the medication she still occasionally experiences attacks of tonic-clonic seizures that occur with little warning and last for several seconds. Following the seizures she regains consciousness slowly and remains disoriented and unaware of her surroundings for up to an hour. During this postictal period she has difficulty responding to questions or speaking. The diagnosis is Delirium Due to Seizures.

29x.xx   Substance Intoxication Delirium.   Individuals with this disorder fulfill the core criteria for Delirium and there is evidence (e.g., history, physical examination, laboratory) that the symptoms developed during substance intoxication are etiologically related to medication use or toxin exposure.

The specific codes for intoxication delirium are determined by the specific substance: 291.0 alcohol; 292.81 amphetamines; cannabis; cocaine; hallucinogens; inhalants; opioids; phencyclidine; sedatives, hypnotics, anxiolytics; other (or unknown) substances (e.g., cimetidine, digitalis, benztropine).

> Matt is a 16-year-old adolescent who has been having problems with his academic work. Two days ago his mother knocked on Matt's bedroom door to tell him that dinner was ready. When he didn't respond she opened the door. Matt was lying on his bed, apparently asleep. There was a strong odor of paint in the room and a can of spray paint beside his bed. Matt's mother called him again and then went over to the bed and shook him. Matt mumbled something she could not understand, seemed irritated and hit his mother on the arm. She called his father and the couple stood by Matt's bed trying to talk to him. In a few minutes he began to wake up but seemed disoriented and had difficulty paying attention to what they said. He was fully alert 20 minutes later and admitted to his concerned parents that he had inhaled paint fumes to get "high." The diagnosis is Inhalant Intoxication Delirium.

29x.xx   Substance Withdrawal Delirium.   Individuals with this disorder fulfill the core criteria for Delirium and there is evidence (e.g., history, physical examination, laboratory) that the symptoms developed during, or within a month of, significant substance withdrawal.

The specific codes for withdrawal delirium are determined by the specific substance: 291.0 alcohol; 292.81 sedatives, hypnotics, anxiolytics; other (or unknown) substances.

> Jack is a 37-year-old man who is an alcoholic. He lives on the street, eats little, and generally drinks a pint or more of liquor a day. Five days ago Jack developed a viral syndrome, began vomiting, and was unable to eat or drink alcohol. Two days later he was found on the street by police and taken to the local emergency room where he was admitted to the hospital. The examination revealed a weak man with elevated blood pressure and heart rate, overactive reflexes, nausea, vomiting, and malnutrition. He also had a significant blood electrolyte disturbance due to his excessive vomiting. Jack was treated with intravenous fluids and medication to control his nausea and vomiting. He was encouraged to eat but ate little. On the third day of hospitalization Jack became agitated and began drifting in and out of consciousness. When Jack was conscious he was disoriented and made no sense when he spoke. His physician made a diagnosis of Alcohol Delirium with Onset During Withdrawal and started Jack on chlordiazepoxide and multivitamins. The diagnosis is Alcohol Withdrawal Delirium

29x.xx   Delirium Due to Multiple Etiologies.   Individuals with this disorder fulfill the core criteria for Delirium and there is evidence (e.g., history, physical examination, laboratory) that the symptoms have more than one etiology. The specific delirium and specific etiologies should be noted (e.g., 293.0 Delirium Due to Head Trauma, 291.0 Alcohol Intoxication Delirium).

> Jill is a 47-year-old woman who had surgery to remove a malignant brain tumor 3 days ago. She currently has an infection at the surgical wound site. The patient has received 10 mg of diazepam (Valium) twice a day to calm her down for the last 2 days. Her husband complains that his wife has become increasingly agitated since the surgery. When Jill's physicians examined her on morning rounds they found an agitated woman who was drifting in and out of consciousness. When conscious she was disoriented to person, place, and time. Jill periodically called out the names of her family members and waved her arms in the air as if she were trying to grab something. The diagnosis is Delirium Due to Multiple Etiologies

780.09   Delirium Not Otherwise Specified.   Individuals with this disorder fulfill the core criteria for Delirium but do not fit the criteria for any specific Delirium diagnosis.

> Nancy is a 71-year-old woman who had bilateral cataract surgery 3 days ago. She is recuperating at home with her husband who is 75 years old. Last night her husband called their son, David, to express his concern about Nancy's condition. He explained that his wife had become very confused. "David, your mother just isn't herself anymore. She doesn't recognize me and she talks to people who aren't there. I don't know what to do." David rushed over to his parent's house and found his mother lying awake in bed. When she spoke she didn't seem to know where she was. He became increasingly alarmed when she called him by his uncle's name and did not seem to be able to follow the conversation without wandering off on some tangent. The diagnosis is Delirium Not Otherwise Specified

Dementias

290.xx   Dementia of the Alzheimer's Type.   Individuals with this disorder fulfill the core criteria for Dementia. The course of their illness is characterized by gradual onset and continuing cognitive decline that is not produced by identifiable central nervous system conditions, general medical conditions, or substances that are known to cause progressive memory deficit or dementia.

Type of onset and predominant features of Alzheimer's Dementia	DSM-IV code for early onset: onset age 65 or less	DSM-IV code for late onset: onset after age 65
Uncomplicated	290.10	290.00
With Delirium	290.11	290.3
With Delusions	290.12	290.20
With Depressed Mood	290.13	290.21

Walter is a 69-year-old man who is active in a successful auto parts business that he runs with his two sons. Walter began the business 40 years ago after he was discharged from the army. He has a reputation for having an encyclopedic knowledge of parts for current American cars as well as those from the last 50 years. As a result his business has become a center for antique car hobbyists.

During the last 2 years his sons have noticed that their father was having increasing difficulty remembering details of the business and often couldn't recognize specific parts. Sometimes they joked about his mistakes, "The old memory isn't what it used to be, is it Dad?" Walter became increasingly irritated at these verbal jabs and responded, "I still know more about this business than you two boys ever will." At the same time he seemed more withdrawn and had considerable difficulty learning the new inventory. Walter's memory continued to deteriorate until his role in the business became mainly that of an observer. The decline in his abilities was painful for Walter and difficult for his sons to watch.

290.4x   Vascular Dementia.   Individuals with this disorder fulfill the core criteria for Dementia and have focal neurologic signs and symptoms or laboratory evidence indicative of cerebral vascular disease judged to be etiologically related to the disturbance.

Predominant features of Vascular Dementia	DSM-IV code
Uncomplicated	290.40
With Delirium	290.41
With Delusions	290.42
With Depressed Mood	290.43

George, a 67-year-old accountant, was admitted to the hospital for treatment of a duodenal ulcer and hypertension. He was taking medication for both disorders but his hypertension was not well controlled. At admission he was fully conscious, alert, and cooperative with the examiner but was noted to have some difficulty remembering his home address. Further examination demonstrated that, despite reasonably good vision, he was also unable to name some familiar objects such as table utensils.

George's wife reported that he was forced to stop working approximately 4 years before his admission because he was making an increasing number of mistakes. She also reported that he has had a few brief episodes, lasting several seconds, during which he appeared to be dazed and uncommunicative. The initial physical examination revealed that the patient had a significantly elevated blood pressure (i.e., 190/115) and some weakness in his left arm.

29x.xx   Dementia Due to Other General Medical Conditions.   Individuals with this disorder fulfill the core criteria for Dementia and have evidence from the history, physical examination, or laboratory findings of one of the conditions listed below that is judged to be etiologically related to the disturbance.

Medical condition etiologically related to the Dementia	DSM-IV code
Dementia Due to HIV Disease	294.9
Dementia Due to Head Trauma	294.1
Dementia Due to Parkinson's Disease	294.1
Dementia Due to Huntington's Disease	294.1
Dementia Due to Pick's Disease	290.10
Dementia Due to Creutzfeldt-Jakob Disease	290.10
Dementia Due to other general medical condition	294.1

Ted is a 32-year-old man who is a talented artist. He has been Human Immunodeficiency Virus (HIV)-positive for 8 years. Two of his close friends have died during the last year from active AIDS. Ted has had AIDS-related complex (ARC) with weight loss, fever, night sweats, fatigue, depression, and generalized lymphadenopathy for 2 years without other serious medical problems. Six months ago he developed pneumocystis carinii, which was treated successfully. Three months ago his lover, Randy, noted that Ted was becoming forgetful and had difficulty concentrating on his artwork. Gradually, his memory impairment worsened and he began to have problems painting. He described the problem to Randy, "I can't seem to make the brush go where I want it to go. My hands don't work right." Ted complained of a constant headache and depression. He became increasingly confused and finally, in frustration, stopped trying to paint. The diagnosis is Dementia Due to HIV Disease

29x.xx   Substance-Induced Persisting Dementia.   Individuals with this disorder fulfill the core criteria for Dementia and have evidence from the history, physical examination, or laboratory findings that the deficits are etiologically related to the persisting effects of substance use (e.g., drugs of abuse, medication, toxin exposure).

The specific codes for substance-induced persisting dementia are determined by the specific substance: 291.2 alcohol; 292.82 inhalants; sedatives,
hypnotics, anxiolytics; other (or unknown) substances.

John is a 42-year-old man who is the owner of the premier adult bookstore in his
city. He is also an alcoholic who drinks heavily every day, usually starting with a
drink in the morning before work when he feels shaky, followed by several cocktails
during lunch. At dinner he frequently drinks an entire bottle of wine. John has had
several medical problems associated with his alcoholism including gastric ulcers
and evidence of early liver disease. He has also experienced several blackouts.
These usually occurred during parties when he drank more than usual. He often
worried about what he did or said during the blackouts but the experience did not
upset him enough to make him stop drinking or get treatment for his alcoholism.
His physician confronted him about his drinking several times and advised him to
get help. John responded by periodically reducing the amount he drank but eventually resumed drinking at his previous high level.

During the past year his business began to deteriorate because John was frequently absent and didn't attend to the financial details of the business. Recently his
wife noticed that he was increasingly forgetful and had difficulty planning and organizing his daily routine. She took John to the family physician who hospitalized
him for observation and to stop his drinking. John was treated prophylactically with
benzodiazepines (Librium) and multivitamins to prevent acute alcohol withdrawal.
Despite the treatment his memory problems and difficulty making plans remained
unchanged for several weeks. There was no evidence that his cognitive deficits were
caused by any medical conditions or substances other than the alcohol. The diagnosis is Alcohol-Induced Persisting Dementia

29x.xx Dementia Due to Multiple Etiologies.   Individuals with this disorder
fulfill the core criteria for Dementia and have evidence from the history, physical
examination, or laboratory tests that the disturbance has more than one etiology.
The specific dementia and specific etiologies should be noted (e.g., 290.00 Dementia of the Alzheimer's Type, 290.40 Vascular Dementia).

An elderly man was found by the police lying unconscious in an alley. He was
brought to a nearby hospital and admitted for treatment. His wallet contained some
identification but no current home address. He had a record of two previous admis-
sions to the hospital for alcohol withdrawal over the last 2 years. Laboratory tests
showed a significant amount of alcohol in his blood and seriously impaired liver
functions. He also had a number of bruises on his head and body and apparently
had been beaten. A computerized axial tomography (CAT) scan of his head showed
a moderate-sized subdural hematoma. The patient was taken to surgery and the
hematoma evacuated.

A few days after the surgery the social worker tried to evaluate the patient's
social support system but he was unable to provide her with information about

family or friends. The psychiatrist was called to evaluate the patient's competence. She found the patient fully conscious and alert but with no memory of the incident leading to his admission. He also had an impairment of long-term memory, difficulty naming familiar objects, and difficulty following a logical sequence of thoughts. The diagnosis was subdural hematoma, liver cirrhosis, 305.00 Alcohol Abuse, and 291.2 Alcohol-Induced Persisting Dementia, and 294.1 Dementia Due to Head Trauma.

294.8   Dementia Not Otherwise Specified.   Individuals with this disorder fulfill the core criteria for Dementia but there is insufficient evidence to establish a specific etiology.

Amnestic Disorders

294.0   Amnestic Disorder Due to a General Medical Condition.
Individuals with this disorder fulfill the core criteria for Amnestic Disorder and there is evidence (e.g., history, physical examination, laboratory) that the disturbance is caused by the direct physiological consequences of a general medical condition (including physical trauma).

> Sidney is a 36-year-old mailman who lives with his elderly mother. His main passion, besides delivering the mail, is carving and painting wooden bird decoys that are commonly used by duck hunters. Sidney has never hunted himself but proudly displays the decoys in his living room and at local hobby shows. One night Sidney and his friend went to an advanced class on carving bird feathers in wood. As the class progressed Sidney found it difficult to follow the teacher's instructions. Soon he began to feel ill and developed a severe headache. He asked his friend to drive him home early. As they entered the car Sidney suddenly became confused and repeatedly asked his friend, "Where am I?" His confusion increased and he became agitated.
>
> The friend became frightened and took Sidney to the local hospital emergency room where he was examined by the emergency physician and admitted. At admission, Sidney had a temperature of 104°C, was confused, and disoriented. Blood and cerebrospinal fluid were drawn for laboratory tests. Sidney was admitted with a diagnosis of viral encephalitis. The diagnosis was later changed to herpes simplex encephalitis. Sidney was hospitalized for 3 weeks during which his agitation and confusion resolved. However, he developed amnesia and had great difficulty remembering any new information. Six months after his acute illness he still had a significant memory loss and was unable to remember what had happened the day before. The diagnosis is Amnestic Disorder Due to Herpes Encephalitis

29x.xx   Substance-Induced Persisting Amnestic Disorder.   Individuals with this disorder fulfill the core criteria for Amnestic Disorder and there is evidence from the history, physical examination, or laboratory findings that the memory disturbance is etiologically related to the persisting effects of substance use.

The specific codes for substance-induced persisting Amnestic Disorder are determined by the specific substance: 291.1 alcohol; 292.83 sedatives, hypnotics, anxiolytics; other (or unknown) substance).

> Ruth is a 31-year-old woman who was found lying unconscious in her closed garage with the car running. Her friend reported that Ruth had been depressed over breaking up with her boyfriend of 5 years. An ambulance was called and Ruth was given oxygen and rushed to the hospital where she was admitted to the intensive care unit. She regained consciousness but was initially confused and disoriented. When her confusion resolved Ruth was unable to remember what had happened. She continued to be unable to remember some past events and also had difficulty learning new information. The diagnosis is Carbon Monoxide-Induced Persisting Amnestic Disorder

294.8   Amnestic Disorder Not Otherwise Specified.   Individuals with this disorder fulfill the core criteria for Amnestic Disorder but there is insufficient evidence to establish a specific etiology.

294.9   Cognitive Disorder Not Otherwise Specified.   Individuals with this disorder have cognitive dysfunction presumed to be due to the direct physiological effects of a general medical condition that does not meet the core criteria for Delirium, Dementia, or Amnestic Disorder.

Necessary Clinical Information

- Current and past medical illnesses

- Current physical symptoms

- Routine laboratory values (e.g., CBC, differential, electrolytes)

- Memory function

- State of consciousness (e.g., disoriented, confused)

- Current and past alcohol and substance abuse

- Exposure to toxins

- Recent behavioral changes

- Specific cognitive deficits (e.g., aphasia, apraxia, agnosia, etc.)

Making a Diagnosis

The diagnosis of Delirium, Dementia, or Amnestic Disorder depends on the presence of characteristic disturbances of consciousness, memory, and/or other cognitive functions in association with a medical condition or substance (injected, ingested, or inhaled) that is etiologically related to the disturbance. The Cognitive Disorders group is one of only three diagnostic groups in DSM-IV that requires the identification of both specific behavioral symptoms and a causative physiological agent for a diagnosis (the other two groups are Mental Disorders Due to a General Medical Condition and Substance-Related Disorders).

The process of diagnosis for Cognitive Disorders consists of two steps. The initial recognition that the patient's symptoms are consistent with one of the recognized syndromes of cognitive impairment and the search for an underlying physiological cause for the patient's behavioral symptoms. Establishing the link between the behavioral symptoms and the medical condition or substance can be the most difficult part of the diagnosis. Often, this connection is based on a temporal correlation between the psychological change and physiological agent rather than an established cause-and-effect relationship. For example, if a patient who develops cognitive impairment also has a medical illness, that disorder is usually cited as the cause of the cognitive disturbance. These and other problems in the diagnosis of Cognitive Disorders will be discussed in the next section. This section will provide a stepwise series of questions and guidelines that can be used in DSM-IV diagnosis of uncomplicated Cognitive Disorders.

1. Does the patient have a disturbance of consciousness?

A disturbance of consciousness may be severe or mild ranging from unconsciousness to a slightly reduced awareness of the environment. If the patient does not have a disturbance of consciousness, all of the delirium diagnoses are excluded including: Delirium Due to a General Medical Condition, Substance-Induced Delirium, Delirium Due to Multiple Etiologies, and Delirium Not Otherwise Specified. If the patient is unconscious, the diagnosis of delirium is excluded. However, the patient may have an extended period of disturbed consciousness when he or she awakes.

The patient's impaired consciousness may be very mild. For example, he may appear preoccupied because of a reduced ability to focus, sustain, or shift attention. The impairment may be subtle and is often dismissed by the examiner on psychological grounds, with the explanation that the patient is upset about his or her illness or other aspects of life. The examiner should watch for this symptom and note whether the patient is aware of his reduced attention and can offer some explanation for it such as a preoccupation with other worries. If the patient is unaware of the impairment, it may be caused by a general medical condition or substance. If the patient does have an impairment of consciousness, the other components required for the diagnosis of Delirium should be pursued.

2. Does the patient have an impairment in cognition?

Deficits may appear in several different areas including: memory, orientation, perception, language ability, intentional motor activity, object recognition, abstract reasoning, short- and long-term planning, and other executive activities. Delirium and dementia cannot be distinguished solely on the basis of the type of cognitive impairment.

- If the patient's only cognitive impairment is a memory disturbance (either retrograde or anterograde) and the patient is fully conscious, the diagnosis is one of the following Amnestic Disorders: Amnestic Disorder Due to a General Medical Condition, Substance-Induced Persisting Amnestic Disorder, or Amnestic Disorder Not Otherwise Specified.

- If the patient has a disturbance of consciousness and an impairment in cognition that tends to fluctuate during the day, the diagnosis is one of the following deliriums: Delirium Due to a General Medical Condition, Substance-Induced Delirium, Delirium Due to Multiple Etiologies, Delirium Not Otherwise Specified. This does not preclude the possibility that the patient's delirium is superimposed on a preexisting dementia or amnestic disorder.

- If the patient has a memory disturbance and an aphasia, apraxia, agnosia, or disturbance in executive functioning without a disturbance of consciousness, the diagnosis is Dementia. This does not preclude the possibility that the patient's dementia is superimposed on a preexisting amnestic disorder.

3. What is the temporal basis of the patient's disturbance?

Delirium and dementia can sometimes be differentiated by the time course of the appearance of symptoms and their change over time.

- If the patient's cognitive impairments develop slowly (usually weeks or months) and remain stable with little fluctuation during the day, the diagnosis is Dementia.

- If the patient's cognitive impairments develop rapidly (usually hours or days) or worsen rapidly and fluctuate during the course of the day, the diagnosis is Delirium.

- The diagnosis of Dementia of the Alzheimer's Type is based on a course characterized by a gradual onset and continuing cognitive decline. It is the only specific dementia that does not require evidence in the history, physical examination, or laboratory findings of a specific medical condition or substance that is etiologically related to the Cognitive Disorder.

4. Is there an identifiable general medical condition or substance etiologically related to the disturbance?

The diagnosis of a specific Delirium, Dementia, or Amnestic Disorder, with the exception of Dementia of the Alzheimer's Type, requires the identification of one or more general medical conditions or substances (e.g., drugs of abuse, medications, toxic agents) that are judged to be the cause of the disorder. Sometimes the patient may have all of the symptoms of Delirium, Dementia, or Amnestic Disorder without evidence of a specific pathophysiologic etiology. When there is insufficient evidence to establish a specific etiology, the appropriate diagnoses are Delirium Not Otherwise Specified, Dementia Not Otherwise Specified, or Amnestic Disorder Not Otherwise Specified.

If the patient is fully conscious, has multiple cognitive impairments including a disturbance in memory, and has focal neurological signs and symptoms or evidence of cerebral vascular disease, the diagnosis is Vascular Dementia.

Common Problems in Making a Diagnosis

There are four types of problems that occur in the diagnosis of Cognitive Disorders.

1. The patient's cognitive deficits may not meet the criteria for one of the cognitive impairment syndromes.
2. It may be difficult to identify a medical condition or substance that is etiologically related to the cognitive impairment.
3. The patient may fulfill the criteria for more than one cognitive impairment syndrome.
4. The patient may have symptoms of cognitive impairment in association with the symptoms of a mood, anxiety, or psychotic disorder.

Patients Who Almost Fulfill the Diagnostic Criteria

There are four situations in which a patient almost fulfills the criteria for Cognitive Disorder. First, the patient may fit the criteria for one of the three core Cognitive Disorder syndromes but a physical etiology for the disorder cannot be determined with certainty. Either physical signs and symptoms are missing or the relationship between the physical and cognitive symptoms is uncertain. For example, a patient may show clear deficits in memory and no obvious evidence of a physical illness. Alternatively, the patient may have evidence of a disease process such as systemic lupus erythematosus that could, under some circumstances, produce cognitive impairment without clear evidence that it is responsible.

The best verification of the causal relationship between the physical and cognitive symptoms is the presence of repeated episodes and remissions of the medical disorder, each accompanied by the occurrence or exacerbation of the cognitive symptoms. However, the causal connection can also be established if the patient has characteristic medical symptoms, such as neurological deficits or physiological signs of intoxication or withdrawal, that are known to be strongly associated with cognitive symptoms.

Second, a patient with cognitive impairment may have multiple medical conditions, exposure to multiple substances, or a combination of the two that could produce the deficits. It may be difficult to determine the specific causative agent. For example, a patient may have chronic obstructive pulmonary disease, a myocardial infarction, hypertension, renal failure, and be taking several medications.

Third, the patient may not fulfill all the requirements for a specific cognitive syndrome. For example, early in the course of a serious medical illness a patient's cognitive changes may be equivocal and insufficient to fulfill the criteria necessary for the diagnosis of a specific Cognitive Disorder. In some cases the patient's initial symptoms may be change in behaviors rather than cognition. Given time these symptoms may mature into a typical cognitive syndrome.

Fourth, a patient may fulfill the criteria for cognitive impairment syndrome and have an associated medical condition that clinical experience suggests cannot solely explain the changes in the patient's mental status. For example, if a patient develops Delirium and the only observable medical condition is an upper respiratory tract infection, it is unlikely that this is the sole physical cause of the cognitive impairment. The resolution of these diagnostic dilemmas depends on the type of information available and how the clinician interprets the diagnostic criteria. A narrow interpretation of the criteria leads to increased uncertainty and more nonspecific diagnoses.

The Cognitive Disorders group addresses some of these problems by grouping diagnoses according to three levels of diagnostic certainty. The first level includes specific diagnoses (e.g., Substance-Induced Delirium and Dementia Due to Other General Medical Conditions) that are used when the patient's symptoms fit one of the three cognitive impairment syndromes and there is an identifiable general medical condition or substance that is etiologically related to the impairment. The second level includes three diagnoses (Delirium Not Otherwise Specified, Dementia Not Otherwise Specified, and Amnestic Disorder Not Otherwise Specified) that are used when the patient fulfills the requirements for one of the cognitive impairment syndromes but there is insufficient evidence to establish a specific etiology.

The third level contains one diagnosis, Cognitive Disorder Not Otherwise Specified. This diagnosis is used when the patient has a cognitive deficit that does not meet the criteria for any of the three standard cognitive impairment syndromes and there is objective evidence of an accompanying systemic illness or central nervous system dysfunction. The Not Otherwise Specified diagnoses, especially Cognitive Disorder Not Otherwise Specified, are used at some cost. They indicate degrees of clinical suspicion rather than diagnostic certainty.

If the role of a diagnosis is to convey meaningful information about the course of an illness and its appropriate treatment the Not Otherwise Specified diagnoses are not very effective. Therefore, they should only be used as a last resort when no specific diagnosis can be made. Given this caveat, these three levels ensure that the clinician can find a diagnosis for most patients who are suspected of having a cognitive deficit caused by a medical condition or substance even if they do not completely fulfill the criteria for a specific Cognitive Disorder.

Example 1

Milton is a 55-year-old telephone repair man who was perched on the elevated tower of his service truck repairing telephone lines after a hurricane, when he suddenly developed weakness in his left arm and difficulty speaking. His co-workers lowered him to the ground and rushed him to the hospital. The physical examination revealed that Milton had had a stroke. His speech difficulty was characterized by fluent but incoherent speech and difficulty understanding what other people said to him. What diagnosis(es) should the patient receive?

Milton's main cognitive impairment is aphasia. He is fully conscious so all of the delirium diagnoses are excluded. The diagnosis of Cognitive Disorder hinges on whether the patient has memory impairment. If there is evidence of a memory impairment, his diagnosis is Vascular Dementia. If there is no memory impairment, he does not have Cognitive Disorder and the diagnosis is Wernicke's aphasia.

Example 2

Sam is a 43-year-old man who was bowling with his team in a championship league tournament when he suddenly forgot why he was there. He was able to continue bowling but could not remember his score or when it was his turn to bowl. His wife drove him home where he spent the remainder of the day watching television and helping her prepare dinner. The following morning his memory had returned. A subsequent physical examination and laboratory tests revealed no abnormalities. What is the patient's diagnosis?

Sam had a brief impairment of memory (Transient Global Amnesia) that is not associated with any detectable general medical condition or substance. Because he fulfills the criteria for amnestic syndrome without a related physical etiology, the diagnosis is Amnestic Disorder Not Otherwise Specified. The disorder may be related to a temporary physiological alteration in the brain produced by localized ischemia or seizures.

Example 3

Samantha is a 37-year-old mother of three children who has a diagnosis of systemic lupus erythematosus and is presently taking 70 mg of prednisone a day. The dose of prednisone was increased 3 days ago because the patient developed increased evidence of renal involvement of her lupus. Today, as Samantha was making breakfast for her husband and children, she briefly became disoriented, had difficulty speaking clearly, and paying attention to what people were saying to her. The symptoms passed after a few minutes but then reappeared several times over the next 3 hours. In between episodes she seemed to interact normally. Samantha's husband called her physician who admitted her to the hospital. That evening the patient had a brief episode of seeing and talking to her mother who died 2 years previously. What is her diagnosis?

Samantha's case raises two diagnostic questions. First, do her symptoms meet the criteria for cognitive impairment syndrome? Second, what is the physical etiology of her cognitive impairment? Samantha's disorientation, language difficulty, and visual hallucinations represent changes in cognition that are consistent with delirium syndrome. However, the criteria for delirium syndrome also requires that a patient have a disturbance in consciousness. It is left to the clinician's judgment to decide if Samantha's periodic difficulty paying attention to people constitutes a sufficient disturbance of consciousness to fulfill the criteria for delirium syndrome.

The question of etiology arises because both Samantha's medical condition and medication can produce behavior and cognitive changes. In this case it is difficult to sort out which of the two is responsible for the patient's current cognitive changes. Therefore, if Samantha is judged to have fulfilled the criteria for delirium syndrome, the best diagnosis would be Delirium Due to Multiple Etiologies (293.0 Delirium Due to Systemic Lupus Erythematosus and 292.81 Steroid Delirium).

Example 4

Lewis is a 54-year-old man who is the owner and operator of a successful striptease club. Although he is usually jovial and optimistic, his wife reports that there has been a significant change in his personality over the last several weeks and his mood has become increasingly labile. Sometimes he is excessively friendly and happy, at other times he is irritable or sad. The staff of the nightclub report that they don't know how he will react from minute to minute.

Recently, Lewis also began having difficulty planning and organizing the club's business activities and the couple's yearly vacation. He often forgets the little details necessary to run the business on a day-to-day basis. Several of the artists that Lewis employs in the club have called his wife complaining about confusion over their future booking. The patient's wife is convinced that he is going through a midlife crisis and may be depressed. The patient has no obvious physical illnesses or symptoms. What diagnosis(es), if any, should Lewis receive?

Lewis has several equivocal symptoms of cognitive impairment including a mild memory disorder and difficulty planning and organizing his business and leisure activities. In addition, he has a significant change in personality. It is possible that these symptoms are related to depression or some other psychiatric disorder. However, the combination of a significant personality change and mild cognitive impairment, especially in a person over the age of 40, should also raise the question of an underlying organic disorder and stimulate a physical evaluation. If Lewis' memory deficit is persistent and can be objectively documented, he could receive a diagnosis of Dementia Due to Other General Medical Conditions. If a specific medical problem, such as a brain tumor, is subsequently discovered, the diagnosis would be changed to Dementia Due to a Brain Tumor. If the memory deficit is elusive, Lewis should not receive any Cognitive Disorders diagnosis.

Example 5

Carrie is a 29-year-old secretary who works for the chief executive of a frozen yogurt company. One day Carrie was taking notes during a conference in which her boss was discussing several new yogurt flavors. She suddenly became confused, disoriented, unable to focus on her work, and unable to understand what her boss and the other conference participants were saying. Her boss reports that he realized something was wrong when she mixed up marketing information about the different flavors. The episode started abruptly and ended in approximately 5 minutes with little sequela other than some drowsiness.

The patient reported one similar episode 3 weeks before and two previous episodes of fainting. She saw her physician after the first episode of confusion but the examination did not reveal any abnormalities. He suggested that the fainting might have been due to hypoglycemia or heat exhaustion. He made an appointment for her with a neurologist. What diagnosis(es), if any, should Carrie receive?

Carrie's confusion, disorientation, difficulty focusing on her work and language disturbance meet the criteria for delirium syndrome. The history of an identical previous episode with abrupt onset and full remission of symptoms, and the two previous fainting spells suggest that she may have a seizure disorder. This may or may not be verified when she sees the neurologist. Currently, Carrie has no abnormal physical symptoms or laboratory results that might identify an etiologic cause for her symptoms. Because she fulfills the criteria for delirium syndrome, her current diagnosis would be 780.89 Delirium Not Otherwise Specified. If the neurological examination demonstrated that she had a seizure disorder, the diagnosis would change to 293.0 Delirium Due to a General Medical Condition or, more specifically, 293.0 Delirium Due to a Seizure Disorder.

Example 6

Sadie is a 77-year-old woman who has been hospitalized for treatment of a chronic urinary tract infection. The day after her admission she began pressing the nurse call button attached to her bed. When the nurse appeared Sadie couldn't remember why she had called the nurse. Eventually, the nurses disconnected her call button. Sadie responded by yelling for help whenever anyone walked past her room. The patient in the next bed complained and Sadie was moved to a single room where her behavior continued. Two days later the nurses noted in the medical record that she was disoriented, confused, had difficulty communicating with nurses and family members, was unable to concentrate on instructions from the hospital staff, and had become increasingly belligerent. Her awareness of her surroundings fluctuated during the day, becoming worse in the evening. What is Sadie's diagnosis(es)?

The patient fulfills the criteria for delirium syndrome. However, the etiology of her delirium is uncertain. A urinary tract infection is normally not sufficient to produce delirium syndrome unless there is some additional illness or pathological process compromising the patient's cerebral functioning. Therefore, it would be incorrect to only make a diagnosis of 293.0 Delirium due to a urinary tract infection because it would not indicate the probable multiple etiologies for the patient's delirium. One solution might be to give her a second diagnosis of 780.09 Delirium Not Otherwise Specified to indicate that the diagnosis is still uncertain.

Patients Who Fulfill the Criteria for More Than One Cognitive Disorder

The Cognitive Disorders group includes the three core syndromes of Delirium, Dementia, and Amnestic Disorder. It is not uncommon for a patient to fulfill the criteria for more than one of these syndromes. Each of the specific diagnoses in the Cognitive Disorders group contains guidelines that stipulate the diagnosis(es) that should be used when the patient fulfills the criteria for more than one syndrome.

Example 7

Mildred is a 75-year-old woman with a 2-year history of progressive memory loss, disorganization, and difficulty planning and carrying out her daily activities. She has been living in a nursing home for the last 6 months. She has no detectable medical problems that could account for her cognitive decline. For the last several days she has been increasingly confused and has had periods when she was unaware of her surroundings. In addition she appears to be responding to visual hallucinations and is unable to talk coherently. What is the patient's diagnosis(es)?

The patient's memory loss, disorganization, and difficulty planning and carrying out daily activities (impairment in executive functions) fulfill the criteria for dementia syndrome. The recent onset of fluctuating periods of awareness, visual hallucinations, and a language disturbance meet the criteria for delirium syndrome. The most likely diagnosis for the dementia is Dementia of the Alzheimer's Type. The criteria for this diagnosis stipulate that the patient's cognitive deficits do not occur exclusively during the course of delirium. Because the memory deficits, disorganization, and impairment of executive functions occurred before the onset of the delirium syndrome, this requirement is fulfilled. The diagnosis of Dementia of the Alzheimer's Type depends on the predominant features and time of onset. In this case, the presence of delirium superimposed on the dementia after the age of 65 leads to a diagnosis of 290.3 Dementia of the Alzheimer's Type, With Late Onset, With Delirium.

Cognitive Impairment Associated With Other Psychiatric Disorders

Cognitive impairment is a common symptom of many psychiatric disorders. When it occurs the diagnostic challenge is to determine whether the cognitive impairment has a psychogenic or organic etiology. In some circumstances the patient may have multiple psychiatric illnesses with different etiologies. In other cases a disorder with a physical etiology may mimic a nonorganic disorder.

Example 8

Mario is a 63-year-old podiatrist who prides himself on his clinical competence. "I never forget a foot," he once told his wife. Recently, he reduced the number of hours he spends in his practice because of his medical problems that include diabetes and chronic renal disease. His wife states that Mario began complaining about problems with his memory and feeling depressed approximately 4 weeks ago. Mario was concerned most about the difficulty he had remembering the clinical details of his practice. His wife thinks that the depression was precipitated by financial problems in his practice due to his reduced clinical activity.

Mario sleeps poorly, has little energy, seems more indecisive than usual, and seems to take little pleasure in activities that he used to enjoy. His wife reports that he has difficulty concentrating on his clinical practice and seems to be having difficulty making simple decisions. She also reports that he had a previous episode of severe depression 10 years before. He did not complain of memory problems during that episode. During the interview Mario seemed confused and had difficulty remembering what he had done during the day. What is the patient's diagnosis(es)?

The patient displays symptoms of cognitive impairment and depressed mood. He also has two medical illnesses that could be etiologically related to his symptoms of cognitive impairment. The patient meets the criteria for the diagnosis of Major Depressive Disorder, Recurrent. The main diagnostic question is whether his memory complaints and other cognitive symptoms are caused by his depression or a separate Cognitive Disorder.

Indecisiveness and diminished ability to think or concentrate are common symptoms of a major depressive episode and do not necessarily imply Cognitive Disorder. The patient began to complain about his memory problems at the same time that he became depressed. However, patients who have Dementia or Amnestic Disorder generally become depressed after the cognitive impairment has developed and try to deny or minimize the problem rather than highlight it. The patient could be given formal memory testing to determine if he has a true memory deficit. If so, he might fit the criteria for a diagnosis of Dementia Due to Multiple Etiologies, presumably related to his medical problems. An alternative approach would be to treat him for the depression and observe whether his complaints of memory loss and other cognitive symptoms resolve.

Example 9

Brian, a 27-year-old male construction worker, was brought into a hospital emergency room by his brother who reported that he suddenly became upset a few hours before admission after a fight with his foreman. The foreman, who is a woman, became angry with Brian when he began pestering another woman construction worker and making lewd suggestions to her. She told Brian to stop or he would be fired. In the hospital Brian was acutely agitated with loose disorganized thoughts and speech. He was convinced that evil forces were trying to invade his body and had difficulty focusing his attention when he was examined by the physician. He appeared to be having hallucinations but this could not be verified. Throughout the examination Brian kept repeating, "She's a queer bitch. She's a queer bitch." The brother reports that Brian has never had a similar episode.

The physical examination revealed that Brian had a temperature of 100°C and a blood pressure of 170/95. There were no other significant physical findings. Brian's laboratory tests were normal and there was no evidence of alcohol, cocaine, opioids, sedatives, or hypnotics in his urine. He was admitted to the hospital. Three days later his symptoms began to spontaneously remit. He would not talk about the events surrounding the initiation of the episode. Brian was discharged a week later fully functional with no residual symptoms. What is the patient's diagnosis(es)?

This patient presents a mixed clinical picture containing symptoms that are consistent with delirium syndrome or a nonorganic psychotic disorder. The diagnosis of delirium syndrome requires that the patient have a disturbance of consciousness. The clinician must judge whether the patient's difficulty focusing his attention during the examination is sufficient to fulfill the requirement for a disturbance of consciousness. The patient's loose, disorganized thoughts do fulfill the requirement for changes in cognition. However, there is no clear evidence of a substance or medical condition, other than the elevated blood pressure, that could be etiologically related to the cognitive changes.

It is possible that the patient ingested a toxic agent or substance (e.g., hallucinogen, phencyclidine) that was not included in the laboratory tests. His reluctance to talk about the episode makes this difficult to determine. The sudden onset of the disorder and rapid remission without evidence of previous similar episodes suggests the presence of some acute organic process rather than a schizophrenia-like psychosis. The definitive diagnosis may depend on whether he has subsequent episodes. If the patient's reduced attention is considered to be a disturbance of consciousness, the patient fulfills the criteria for a diagnosis of Delirium Not Otherwise Specified. He also fulfills the criteria for a diagnosis of Brief Psychotic Disorder.

Example 10

Sharon is a 31-year-old woman who hit her head on the door frame as she was getting out of her car 2 days ago. She was dizzy for a few moments and then resumed her usual activities complaining of a headache. A few hours later she seemed confused and began having problems with her memory. The deficit was confined to retrograde memory with little or no impairment in her ability to learn new information. Sharon's memory impairment was selective. She had particular difficulty remembering information about her job, the divorce proceedings with her husband, and the death of her mother 3 months before. She was able to remember important events in the news for the past year. A physical and neurological examination revealed no abnormalities. The problems with her memory began to clear spontaneously after several days. What is Sharon's diagnosis(es)?

Sharon fulfills the criteria for amnestic syndrome because she has a memory impairment characterized by the inability to recall previously learned information. There is no requirement in the criteria that this impairment be global versus selective. Sharon also had a physical trauma that could be etiologically related to the memory deficit. She could receive the diagnosis of 294.8 Amnestic Disorder Not Otherwise Specified despite the fact that she did not lose consciousness after bumping her head and had no evidence of a physical abnormality during a subsequent examination. The selective nature of her memory deficit, related to emotionally charged personal issues, also raises the possibility of a diagnosis of 300.12 Dissociative Amnesia.

Precedence of Diagnosis

Many of the cases in preceding sections discuss diagnostic dilemmas that arise when patients have symptoms consistent with more than one diagnosis. The diagnoses may belong to just the Cognitive Disorders group or to other diagnostic groups as well. When these conflicts occur they are often resolved using the rules of diagnostic precedence that are included in the criteria for many diagnoses (Table 3–1). However, these rules are not infallible and in some circumstances we have seen that they are mutually exclusive. Therefore, the rules of diagnostic precedence, rather than taken as hard and firm, should be seen as

Table 3–1 Precedence of diagnosis for cognitive disorders	
Cognitive disorder	**Disorders taking precedence**
Delirium Due to a General Medical Condition Substance Intoxication Delirium Substance Withdrawal Delirium Delirium Due to Multiple Etiologies	Not better accounted for by preexisting, established, or evolving dementia
Delirium NOS	Does not meet criteria for any specific delirium
Dementia of the Alzheimer's Type	Does not meet criteria for another central nervous system disorder or systemic condition that causes dementia Does not occur exclusively during delirium Not better accounted for by another Axis I disorder
Vascular Dementia Dementia Due to Other General Medical Conditions Dementia Due to Multiple Etiologies	Does not occur exclusively during delirium
Substance-Induced Persisting Dementia	Does not occur exclusively during delirium Not better accounted for by substance intoxication or withdrawal
Dementia NOS	Does not meet criteria for any specific dementia
Amnestic Disorder Due to a General Medical Condition	Does not occur exclusively during delirium or dementia
Substance-Induced Persisting Amnestic Disorder	Does not occur exclusively during delirium or dementia Not better accounted for by substance intoxication or withdrawal
Amnestic Disorder NOS	Does not meet criteria for any specific amnestic disorder
Cognitive Disorder NOS	Does not meet criteria for any specific cognitive disorder

Note. NOS = Not Otherwise Specified.

guidelines. They suggest other diagnoses that should be considered before a specific diagnosis is made and they indicate the circumstances under which the diagnosis in question may be excluded if the patient fulfills the criteria for other diagnoses. Table 3–1 presents a list of disorders that may take precedence over specific Cognitive Disorders.

Discussion of Clinical Vignettes

Vignette 1: Grandma Doesn't Know Me Anymore

Mary is a 72-year-old retired widow who has always been independent and functioned at a high level. Approximately 5 years ago her daughter began to notice subtle changes in her behavior. Mary had always been compulsive about keeping her house clean but now began to neglect general housework, ignoring dirty floors and dishes. Instead, she obsessively focused on cleaning the sink and toilet in the bathroom. Next, she began to develop significant problems with her memory and tried to compensate for these problems by posting notes around her apartment to remind her of things she needed to remember. Her memory problems progressed to the point that she couldn't remember her granddaughter's name nor how to drive home in her car. Mary's most striking deficit was her diminished capacity to do basic arithmetic as demonstrated by her inability to balance a checkbook.

Her clinical presentation could be summarized as a progressive impairment of memory and a disturbance in higher cognitive functions associated with abstract reasoning and mathematics. These deficits caused a significant impairment in her daily functioning and represented a significant decline from her previous higher level of functioning. These symptoms fulfill the core criteria for the diagnosis of Dementia. The lack of focal neurological signs excludes the diagnosis of Vascular Dementia. The absence of signs and symptoms of a general medical condition or substance use excludes the diagnoses of Dementia Due to Other Medical Conditions or Substance-Induced Persisting Dementia. This leaves Dementia of the Alzheimer's Type as the most likely diagnosis.

Vignette 2: I'm Fine, Let Me Go

Tom is a 19-year-old man who was struck by a car and briefly knocked unconscious as he was riding his bicycle on the highway. The serious nature of his injury can be underestimated because he keeps proclaiming, "I'm fine," and wants to leave. His ability to communicate with the observers makes them feel uncertain whether they have the right to restrain him and tends to obscure his obvious recent memory deficit and shifting awareness of the environment. However, his repeated questions about the event ("What happened?, Where am I?") demonstrate his recent memory impairment. His agitation is apparent when he insists on leaving the scene of the accident ("I need to go home"). Tom's brief period of unconsciousness means that he probably had a concussion and makes it important that he be observed for at least 24 hours. The presence of a disturbance of consciousness and cognitive changes (i.e., memory deficit, disorientation, unconsciousness) fulfill the criteria for the diagnosis of 293.0 Delirium Due to a General Medical Condition or more specifically, Delirium due to head trauma.

Key Diagnostic Points

- The distinguishing feature of Delirium is a disturbance of consciousness accompanied by some changes is cognition.

- The distinguishing feature of Dementia is a memory impairment accompanied by at least one major cognitive disturbance (i.e., aphasia, apraxia, agnosia, or disturbance in executive functions).

- The distinguishing feature of Amnestic Disorder is a memory impairment without other cognitive deficits.

- Anterograde memory loss (the inability to remember and retrieve new information) rarely has a purely psychological cause.

- Dissociative amnesia is usually retrograde, often selective, and usually related to the inability to recall important personal information.

Common Questions in Making a Diagnosis

1. John, a 58-year-old man, had a cardiac arrest while attending a sales meeting. His colleagues called the paramedics and tried to administer cardiopulmonary resuscitation (CPR). The paramedics arrived 15 minutes later and found the patient unconscious with no heart beat. They resuscitated John with cardiac defibrillation and treated him with intravenous medication to stabilize his heart rhythm. John fluctuated in and out of consciousness as he was transported to the hospital. Two days later he was fully awake but seemed confused, did not remember what had happened, and had difficulty remembering his business transactions and events in his private life for the previous several months. What is John's diagnosis?

   Answer: John has an impairment of retrograde memory. It is too early to tell if his memory impairment is temporary or permanent. The presumed etiology of the impairment is cerebral anoxia subsequent to a cardiac arrest. The appropriate diagnosis would be Amnestic Disorder Due to a General Medical Condition (cerebral anoxia). The memory impairment is transient if it lasts for 1 month or less and chronic if it lasts for more than 1 month.

2. Sarah is a 74-year-old woman who was diagnosed with breast cancer 5 years ago and treated with a simple mastectomy and chemotherapy. Sarah has been doing well with no evidence of recurrence of the cancer since her original treatment. During the last 5 months her husband reports that she has been having increasing difficulty remembering little details of everyday life. She frequently forgets her keys and other objects around the house, repeatedly asks directions to familiar places, and has difficulty planning daily activities. When asked, Sarah denies problems with her memory and says that she has been very busy recently and feels a little depressed. Her husband has observed that Sarah has some difficulty falling asleep at night but attributes that to her afternoon naps. He also states that she seems to nibble at her food, rarely finishes a meal, and has lost 5 pounds in the last month. What is Sarah's diagnosis(es)?

   Answer: Sarah presents a complicated clinical picture. She has some symptoms of depression including a mildly depressed mood, insomnia, and anorexia with weight loss. Despite these symptoms she currently does not meet the criteria for a specific Mood Disorder. She also has evidence of cognitive impairments including progressive memory loss and difficulty planning and organizing her daily activities. Her cognitive impairments fulfill the criteria for dementia syndrome. The etiology of her cognitive deficits is less certain. One possibility is a recurrence of her breast cancer with metastases to the brain. This can be evaluated with a neurological examination and a CAT scan. If a metastatic brain tumor is present, the diagnosis would be Dementia Due to Other General Medical Condition or more specifically Dementia due to a metastatic brain tumor. However, it is unlikely that this problem would develop slowly over a 5-month period or that it would develop without focal neurological signs and symptoms. Another possibility is a progressive dementia. The most likely dementia is 290.00 Dementia of the Alzheimer's Type, uncomplicated with late onset.

3. John, a middle-aged man in his 40s, was brought to the local hospital emergency room by the police. He was well known to the staff of the emergency room. At this admission John was disoriented and drifting in and out of consciousness. When he was conscious he was agitated with a hand tremor and appeared to be seeing people who were not present. Laboratory tests showed no evidence of alcohol, cocaine, amphetamines, sedative-hypnotics, or benzodiazepines in the patient's blood. Physical examination revealed a recent bruise on the patient's head, a heart rate of 110, and a blood pressure of 170/98. What is the patient's diagnosis(es)?

   Answer: John fulfills the criteria for delirium syndrome. He has a disturbance of consciousness, disorientation, and visual hallucinations. The delirium probably has multiple etiologies. His increased heart rate, blood pressure, tremor, and agitation suggest that he is in the early stages of alcohol withdrawal. The bruise on his head suggests that his cognitive changes may also be due to head trauma. The appropriate diagnosis would be Delirium Due to Multiple Etiologies or more specifically, 293.0 Delirium due to head trauma and 291.0 Alcohol Delirium with onset during withdrawal.

4. Mary is a 57-year-old woman who began developing problems with her memory over the last couple of years. Approximately 6 months ago she began to have difficulty walking and complained of some weakness in her right leg. This was followed by difficulty speaking. Her physical examination was normal with the exception of the gait disturbance, leg weakness, and mild hypertension of 160/95. What is the patient's diagnosis(es)?

   Answer: The development of memory impairment and a language distur-bance associated with focal neurological symptoms fulfills the criteria for a diagnosis of 290.47 Vascular Dementia with communication disturbance.

5. Gloria is a 76-year-old retired school teacher who lives alone in a small house. Her husband died 3 years ago. She spends most of her time shopping with friends, visiting her daughter and grandchildren who live in a nearby town, and tending her garden. Gloria's garden is her passion and she has won the first prize in the local garden show several times during the last 10 years. He garden is meticulously arranged with separate plots for flowers and veg-etables. Each day during the summer, she picks a bouquet of flowers and arranges them in a vase on the coffee table in her living room. One Sunday afternoon, a few months ago, Gloria's daughter, son-in-law, and grandchil-dren came to visit and stay for dinner. Her daughter noticed that the flowers on the coffee table appeared wilted and mentioned this to her mother. Gloria responded, "That's strange, I just put them in that vase today, or was it yes-terday?" She seemed briefly confused and then proclaimed, "No matter, I'll get some more." When dinner was served one of the grandchildren began to eat, suddenly gagged and said, "Ugh, the chicken is raw, Grandma." Gloria replied, "My goodness, so it is. I'm sure I cooked it long enough. Well, I'll just cook it a little more."

   These small events troubled Gloria's daughter who knew that her mother was always very careful and precise about her cooking and housekeeping chores. She mentioned them to her husband who replied, "You are reading too much into them, honey." Gloria's friends also seemed unconcerned as one said, "She's the same Gloria I've known for 30 years." Over the next few weeks and months similar events occurred more frequently. Gloria left the oven on, forgot where she parked her car, and seemed to have difficulty organizing the spring planting for her garden. Eventually the garden ap-peared as a hodgepodge with flowers and vegetables mixed together in the same plot. Gloria explained the garden to her daughter, "I was trying out a new arrangement, dear." Her daughter insisted that she see the family doctor who found no evidence of any general medical condition. What diagnosis(es), if any, should Gloria receive?

Answer: Gloria has increasing signs of memory impairment and inattention to the common details of everyday life. The initial changes are subtle and only apparent to her daughter who knows Gloria's usual behavior and daily routines. The persistent and progressive nature of the problems have alarmed the daughter who realizes that something is wrong despite the reassurances of her husband and her mother's friends. Gloria's increasing memory problems and difficulty organizing her garden fulfill the criteria for dementia syndrome. The lack of any general medical conditions or substances that are etiologically related to the these cognitive deficits suggests a tentative diagnosis of Dementia of the Alzheimer's Type, uncomplicated with late onset.

Mental Disorders Due to a General Medical Condition

Clinical Vignette

Why Are You Eating With Your Fingers?

Bert is a 45-year-old man who was hit in the forehead by a baseball one afternoon as he was playing with his friends. He was unconscious briefly and disoriented when he awoke for a few minutes. Bert was taken to the hospital where a skull X ray and examination did not reveal any abnormalities. His wife, Cindy, was told to observe him for 24 hours and to call for a follow-up appointment if he was having problems. Bert seemed to do well for the next few days and the incident was forgotten.

Several weeks later Cindy began to notice some changes in his behavior. Bert had always been quiet, polite, and conservative but now he was increasingly irritable, curt, and inappropriate with her and other people. On one occasion, several weeks after the accident, they were at a party when Bert suddenly began making lewd comments about other women at the party. He put his arm around his wife's shoulder, pointed to a young woman across the room, and commented, "Boy she's got a nice pair on her. I wonder if they're real." Cindy was surprised and distressed by Bert's comments because they were crude and seemed so unlike him. Furthermore, the comments were loud enough for people around him to turn and take notice. She pulled Bert away from the group and said, "What's wrong with you? You've never acted like that before. I'm embarrassed to be with you when you act that way." Bert ignored her comments and walked away to another part of the room.

A few minutes later Cindy heard some angry voices and turned around to see a woman slap Bert across the face. She hurried over to her husband, who was quite angry, and tried to calm him. The woman, who was also angry, was yelling at Bert. Her husband, one of Bert's friends, was trying to intercede. He turned to Cindy and said, "Bert shouldn't drink if he can't handle his liquor." His wife explained that Bert had walked over to her, made a few inane comments, and then placed his hand on her breast. When she slapped him, he was surprised and angry. Cindy gradually calmed Bert and the couple left the party.

The next morning at breakfast Bert continued to act strange. He started to eat his scrambled eggs with his fingers rather than using a fork. Cindy watched and then quietly asked, "Why are you eating with your fingers?" Bert exploded, threw the eggs across the kitchen and began yelling at her. Cindy became frightened and went into another room to call the family physician. She explained that Bert's behavior had changed over the last few weeks. "He acts like a different person," she said. The physician asked if Bert was under stress at work and suggested that Cindy bring Bert to see him. In the doctor's office Bert remained irritable and moody. At first he was angry, then he became quiet and withdrawn. The physician suggested that Bert might be depressed and decided to admit him to the hospital for further evaluation.

The hospital staff took a detailed medical history including information about Bert's recent head trauma. A psychiatric consultation was requested to evaluate Bert's behavior changes. The psychiatrist discovered that Bert was irritable, had difficulty making plans for the future, and had a labile affect. The psychiatrist suggested that the symptoms were consistent with an organic process rather than depression. Several tests were performed during the next two days including a nuclear magnetic resonance (NMR) scan. The scan showed damage to the frontal cortex of Bert's brain, presumably due to the blow from the baseball.

Core Concept of the Diagnostic Group

The core concept of the Mental Disorders Due to a General Medical Condition diagnostic group is the occurrence of a mental disorder in association with a general medical condition that is judged to be its cause. The symptoms of the mental disorder in this group must not fulfill the criteria for a Mental Disorder Due to a General Medical Condition found in another DSM-IV diagnostic group.

Definitions

correlation   The degree to which two separate phenomenon vary together. For example, a patient becomes more irritable when he has a cold.

cause   Two phenomenon are correlated and one produces the other. For example, a patient's increased irritability and lability are caused by a tumor in his frontal lobe.

Synopses and Diagnostic Prototypes
of the Individual Disorders

Several other diagnostic groups contain specific diagnoses for disorders that are judged to be caused by a general medical condition. The specific disorders and their diagnostic groups are shown in Table 4–1. The Mental Disorder Due to a General Medical Condition group includes three diagnoses: Catatonic Disorder Due to a General Medical Condition, Personality Change Due to a General Medical Condition, and Mental Disorder Not Otherwise Specified Due to a General Medical Condition.

293.89   Catatonic Disorder Due to a General Medical Condition.

Individuals with this disorder have catatonia as manifested by motoric immobility, excessive purposeless motor activity, extreme negativism, peculiarities of voluntary movement, echolalia, or echopraxia. There is evidence from the history, physical examination, or laboratory findings that the disturbance is caused by the direct physiological consequences of a general medical condition.

> Ross is a 29-year-old man who was brought to a local hospital by ambulance. His mother reported that she found him lying in bed unresponsive that morning. She explained that her son had been under treatment for personality problems for the last year but that he had never been like this before. The physical examination revealed a young man who was mute with rigid muscles and some posturing of his limbs. His blood pressure, heart rate, and temperature were abnormally elevated and he was sweating profusely. The physician drew blood for laboratory tests and then spoke with Ross' mother again to gather more information about his medical his-

Table 4–1	Mental Disorders Due to a General Medical Condition in other diagnostic groups	
Diagnosis	**Diagnostic group**
Delirium Due to a General Medical Condition Amnestic Disorder Due to a General Medical Condition Dementia Due to a General Medical Condition	Delirium, Dementia, Amnestic Disorder, and Other Cognitive Disorders
Psychotic Disorder Due to a General Medical Condition	Schizophrenia and Other Psychotic Disorders
Mood Disorder Due to a General Medical Condition	Mood Disorders
Anxiety Disorder Due to a General Medical Condition	Anxiety Disorders
Sexual Dysfunction Due to a General Medical Condition	Sexual Disorders
Sleep Disorder Due to a General Medical Condition	Sleep Disorders

tory. She explained that Ross had been taking tranquilizers for his nerves for several months and showed the doctor a bottle of chlorpromazine (Thorazine) tablets. A few minutes later the results from the laboratory tests were returned and revealed that Ross' white blood count and serum creatinine kinase enzyme levels were abnormally high. The physician made a diagnosis of neuroleptic malignant syndrome and began supportive treatment.

310.1   Personality Change Due to a General Medical Condition.

Individuals with this disorder have a persistent personality disturbance that represents a change from the individual's previous characteristic personality pattern. There is evidence from the history, physical examination, or laboratory findings that the disturbance is caused by the direct physiological consequences of a general medical condition.

Labile type: if the predominant feature is affective lability

Disinhibited type: if the predominant feature is poor impulse control (e.g., sexual indiscretions)

Aggressive type: if the predominant feature is aggressive behavior

Apathetic type: if the predominant feature is marked apathy and indifference

Paranoid type: if the predominant feature is suspiciousness or paranoid ideation

Other type: for example, personality change associated with a seizure disorder

Combined type: if more than one feature predominates in the clinical picture

Unspecified type.

Vernon is a 37-year-old man who was diagnosed with temporal lobe epilepsy 17 years ago. The disorder was discovered after Vernon experienced several episodes of déjà vu followed by repeated automatic movements of his fingers and hand. He was unaware of the hand movements until they were reported to him by observers. At the time his seizures were diagnosed Vernon was a junior in college. He led an active social life, dated several women, was reasonably easy going, and had a good sense of humor.

   In the last 15 years Vernon's epilepsy has been moderately well controlled by anticonvulsant agents, although he still has an occasional seizure. During that time his parents and sister have noticed a slow but persistent change in his behavior. The change was subtle at first but gradually became more pronounced. Vernon became more emotional about things he was involved in or read in the newspapers. He began to talk about a "greater spiritual meaning" that infiltrated everything and became excessively concerned about moral issues of right and wrong.

Discussions with Vernon were no longer casual. His parents and friends noticed that he displayed an unusual intensity and sticky quality in conversations that made it difficult for them to end the discussion. At the same time Vernon became increasingly wordy and circumstantial when he spoke and often launched into vague philosophical monologues that no one could understand. Gradually, he became less and less interested in women and concentrated his energies on writing philosophical tracts and the story of his life. He began to carry a large briefcase containing many pages of outlines and notes for his projects. Each sheet of paper was filled with long verbose paragraphs and detailed notes in the margins.

Fifteen years after the initial diagnosis of temporal lobe epilepsy there was little left of the old Vernon. His sense of humor and easy going manner had disappeared to be replaced by an overly serious and suspicious man whom his family barely recognized. The diagnosis is Personality Change Due to a General Medical Condition, Other Type

293.9 Mental Disorder Not Otherwise Specified Due to a General Medical Condition. Individuals with this disorder have a mental disturbance that is due to a general medical condition but the criteria have not been met for a specific Mental Disorder Due to a General Medical Condition.

Necessary Clinical Information

*   Evidence of a general medical disorder that could cause the mental disorder (e.g., neurosyphilis, tumor, infection, cerebrovascular accident).

*   Recent changes in personality that are not characteristic for the individual (e.g., irritable, labile, disinhibited, impulsive, apathetic, aggressive, paranoid, or grandiose behavior).

*   Catatonic behavior.

Making a Diagnosis

Almost all of the diagnostic groups in DSM-IV contain a specific diagnosis for a mental disorder caused by a general medical condition. The reason for creation of a specific diagnostic group called Mental Disorder Due to a General Medical Condition is unclear because the diagnosis of Personality Change Due to a General Medical Condition could have been placed in the Personality Disorders section. Presumably the category was created because there was no other diagnostic group that could reasonably contain the diagnoses of Catatonic Disorder Due to a General Medical Condition and Mental Disorder Not Otherwise Specified Due to a General Medical Condition. Notwithstanding the specific disorder of catatonia, this diagnostic category includes all disorders of behavior or personality that are caused by a general medical condition yet do not fit into another specific diagnostic category such as the Mood Disorders or Cognitive Disorders.

An individual's personality consists of a pervasive and enduring set of behaviors, reactions, and attitudes. As such, it is not normally modified to any substantial degree by day-to-day interactions with other people or the environment. Therefore, any significant personality change, especially if it occurs over a short period of time, requires investigation. If a general medical disorder has been previously identified in a patient, the potential behavioral changes commonly associated with that disorder may already be anticipated.

For example a frontal lobe cerebral hemorrhage might be expected to produce a frontal lobe behavioral syndrome. Under these circumstances the diagnosis is relatively straightforward. However, if a behavior change is the first indication of illness, the differentiation between a general medical etiology and a purely psychological etiology may be difficult. In these cases the diagnosis of Mental Disorder Due to a General Medical Condition usually relies on the identification of certain typical behavioral signs and symptoms that are characteristic of organic-induced disorders, or the subsequent identification of an underlying general medical condition that is etiologically related to the mental disorder.

If the changes are subtle or gradual they are often initially recognized only by family members or intimate friends who have known the patient for many years. In that case, the individual is rarely brought for evaluation until the changes become more persistent and intense. If the initial change is sudden and catastrophic, such as a catatonic reaction or substance intoxication, the patient is more likely to be brought for immediate evaluation. In either situation the first step in the evaluation of any significant change in behavior is to search for an underlying general medical condition. The following questions outline one approach to the diagnosis.

1. Is the patient catatonic?

Every patient who is catatonic requires a medical evaluation to exclude a possible metabolic or substance-related etiology for the disorder. This should include a detailed history from family or friends, a physical examination including a detailed neurological exam, urine and blood drug screens, and routine blood tests. If all of these are negative, the diagnosis of Catatonic Disorder Due to a General Medical Condition can be tentatively excluded.

2. Does the patient have a classic organic behavior syndrome (frontal lobe syndrome or epileptic personality)?

- Damage to the frontal lobe of the brain can produce two types of personality changes called *frontal lobe syndromes*. If the damage is localized to the orbital areas of the frontal lobe, the patient may have a sociopathic type of behavior characterized by disinhibition of aggression and sexuality, impulsivity, lability of affect, paranoia, grandiosity, and little appreciation of the social consequences of the abnormal behavior. If the damage is localized to the convexity of the frontal lobe, the patient may have a more retarded or depressed type of behavior, characterized by the inability to initiate activity independently, lack of engagement, apathy, indifference, and withdrawal. Some patients show a combination of these two patterns. The appearance of frontal lobe behavior should lead to a complete neurological evaluation.

- Epileptic personality is generally associated with long-term temporal lobe seizures and is characterized by intensified emotional responses, excessive seriousness, stickiness in social interactions, excessive religiosity, self-righteousness, hyposexuality, and periodic rage and paranoia. The presence of temporal lobe seizures can be confirmed by specialized electroencephalogram (EEG) recordings.

3. Does the patient have changes in specific personality traits that do not meet the criteria for any other diagnostic group?

If the patient's predominant symptoms are cognitive impairment, depression, anxiety, mania, or psychosis, the diagnosis of Mental Disorder Due to a General Medical Condition is excluded. The diagnosis for patients with these symptoms, when they are caused by a general medical condition, can be found in other DSM-IV diagnostic categories based on the phenomenology of the symptom (e.g., Mood Disorders; Anxiety Disorders; Delirium, Dementia, Amnestic Disorder, and Other Cognitive Disorders).

The diagnosis of Personality Change Due to a General Medical Condition is reserved for patients whose predominant symptoms include exaggerated personality traits that do not fit into one of the other main diagnostic groups and do not generally present in the context of a characteristic syndrome. These symptoms include disinhibited behavior with poor control over sexual or aggressive impulses, affective lability, aggressive behavior, apathetic behavior, and paranoid behavior. The behaviors may occur in isolation, in combination with each other, or combined with other psychiatric symptoms. They rarely meet the criteria for a specific personality disorder.

Although there are no syndromes that are characteristic of Personality Change Due to a General Medical Condition, some symptom presentations are more suggestive of a general medical etiology than others. For example, the sudden appearance of personality changes at any age or the gradual appearance of personality changes in a middle-aged patient is likely to be caused by a general medical condition. When these symptoms are observed the patient should receive a full medical and neurological examination to search for any underlying general medical condition that could cause the symptoms.

Common Problems in Making a Diagnosis

There are two main problems that occur in the diagnosis of Mental Disorders Due to a General Medical Condition.

1. It is often difficult to identify a general medical condition that is responsible for the mental disorder. The mere presence of such a condition does not necessarily mean that it is the etiology of the patient's mental disorder. Correlation does not always imply causality.
2. It is often difficult to distinguish changes in personality from changes in mood, anxiety, or cognition. Often, the patient has symptoms that fit into several different diagnostic categories.

Patients Who Almost Fulfill the Diagnostic Criteria

The two main criteria for the diagnosis of Mental Disorders Due to a General Medical Condition are the presence of a constellation of unusual behaviors that represent a change from an individual's previous characteristic behavior and the presence of a general medical condition that is etiologically related to these changes.

Example 1

Tracy is a 39-year-old woman who has always been even-tempered. However, she has become increasingly irritable and moody during the last few weeks since she lost her job. Two days after she lost her job Tracy was in an automobile accident. In the accident she hit her head and was knocked unconscious for a few minutes. Tracy was dizzy for 2 or 3 days after the accident. A follow-up neurological examination 1 week after the accident revealed no lasting sequela. What diagnosis(es), if any, should Tracy receive?

Tracy's irritable and labile affect follows two traumatic events, the loss of her job and significant head trauma. Conceivably, either trauma or something else could be responsible for the change in her behavior. It would be prudent to reevaluate her neurological status if her irritability and lability continue. However, at the present time it would be difficult to make a diagnosis of Personality Change Due to a General Medical Condition because there is no evidence that the head trauma is responsible for her behavioral changes. An additional question is whether her behavioral changes are substantial enough to consider them a significant personality disturbance.

Example 2

Patrick is a 48-year-old man who has become increasingly paranoid and suspicious during the last several weeks. He has always been a reasonable man and the paranoid behavior is a distinct change from his previous personality. A medical and neurological examination revealed no abnormalities. What diagnosis(es), if any, should Patrick receive?

Significant changes in personality, especially in a middle-aged patient, suggest that an underlying general medical condition is the cause. In Patrick's case no medical condition was discovered. Therefore, the diagnosis of Personality Change Due to a General Medical Condition cannot be made. It is possible that Patrick is developing late-onset Schizophrenia, Paranoid Type or a Delusional Disorder. Nevertheless, the possibility of a general medical cause for his disorder should not be dismissed and he should have periodic medical evaluations if his behavior continues to deteriorate. The inability to discover a general medical condition responsible for the patient's altered behavior is a common problem in the diagnosis of Mental Disorders Due to a General Medical Condition.

Personality Changes Associated With Other Psychiatric Disorders

Although some patients with Mental Disorder Due to a General Medical Condition have typical symptoms of a personality change such as lability, disinhibition, aggression, apathy, or paranoia, many others have a mixed clinical presentation that includes symptoms from the other large diagnostic categories in DSM-IV. To complicate matters further, the typical personality change behaviors listed above are frequently misinterpreted as mood, anxiety, psychotic, or dissociative symptoms. For example, a disinhibited type of personality change could be mistaken for a hypomanic or manic episode with associated hypersexuality.

Example 3

Audrey is a 36-year-old woman with multiple sclerosis. Two months ago her husband noticed that she was becoming increasingly withdrawn and apathetic. She took little interest in her usual daily activities and seemed to move through the day in slow motion. Audrey also had difficulty concentrating, organizing her work, and making plans for future activities. Her husband wondered if she was depressed. What diagnosis(es), if any, should Audrey receive?

Audrey has had a recent personality change characterized by apathy, indifference, psychomotor retardation, withdrawal, anhedonia, and difficulty concentrating. Because she also has multiple sclerosis, a central nervous system disorder that can affect various areas of the brain, she meets the criteria for a diagnosis of Personality Change Due to a General Medical Condition Apathetic Type. However, Audrey also has several symptoms of depression including a diminished interest in daily activities. Therefore, the differential diagnosis includes Mood Disorder Due to a General Medical Condition. The decision of which diagnosis to use depends on the clinician's judgment about which symptoms predominate. In Audrey's case, the lack of a prominent depressed mood, despite the other symptoms of depression, suggests that a diagnosis of Personality Change Due to a General Medical Condition would be appropriate.

Precedence of Diagnosis

Several of the cases in preceding sections discuss diagnostic dilemmas that arise when patients have symptoms consistent with more than one diagnosis. The competing diagnoses are always in different diagnostic categories (e.g., Mental Disorder Due to a General Medical Condition or Mood Disorders). When these conflicts occur they are often resolved using the rules of diagnostic precedence included in the criteria for each diagnosis in this diagnostic group. These rules are summarized in Table 4–2. Each of the diagnoses in the column titled *Disorders taking precedence* should be considered and excluded before a specific Mental Disorder Due to a General Medical Condition diagnosis is made.

Table 4–2   Precedence of diagnosis for a mental disorder due to a general medical condition

Mental disorder	Disorders taking precedence
Catatonic Disorder Due to a General Medical Condition	Does not occur exclusively during Delirium Not better accounted for by another mental disorder
Personality Change Due to a General Medical Condition	Does not meet criteria for dementia Does not occur exclusively during delirium Not better accounted for by another mental disorder
Mental Disorder NOS Due to a General Medical Condition	Does not meet criteria for any specific Mental Disorder Due to a General Medical Condition

Note.   NOS = Not Otherwise Specified.

Discussion of Clinical Vignette

Why Are You Eating With Your Fingers?

Bert is a 45-year-old man who was struck in the forehead by a baseball. He was dizzy and disoriented for several minutes but did not lose consciousness. Several weeks later he began to behave erratically. Bert became more irritable, aggressive and explosive. He also became sexually inappropriate, making lewd comments and physically touching one woman's breasts. Despite the negative reactions of other people, he seemed unaware of the inappropriate nature of his behavior.

These symptoms of general disinhibition fit the characteristic picture of a frontal lobe syndrome caused by a lesion to the orbital areas of the frontal lobe. The NMR scan verified damage to the frontal lobe area. Personality changes of this type that alter social interactions and intrude on the rights of other people are often misdiagnosed. This is especially true in the early stages of the disorder when the behavioral changes are subtle and there are still no significant cognitive deficits.

Key Diagnostic Points

- The symptoms of a Personality Change Due to a General Medical Condition are usually exaggerated character or personality traits that do not meet the criteria for any other diagnostic category.

Common Questions in Making a Diagnosis

1. Gary is a 20-year-old student who is in the first semester of his senior year in college. During the last 4 weeks he has been increasingly irritable and argumentative with his girlfriend. He is also doing poorly academically and spends much of the day playing pool or watching television. Gary's girlfriend and parents are worried about him and have encouraged him to see a physician at the student health service. The examination did not reveal any physical abnormalities. Gary's medical history included a viral respiratory illness 2 months before and an incident 4 months previously when he was knocked unconscious while working for a construction firm. Subsequent evaluations did not demonstrate any neurological deficits resulting from the accident. During the examination Gary was mainly concerned about finding a good job after he graduated. What diagnosis(es), if any, should Gary receive?

   Answer: Gary's behavior has changed significantly over a period of 4 weeks. It is not clear whether this is a unique change or whether he has had previous periods when he is irritable, argumentative, and not concentrating on his studies. There are several possible etiologies for his behavior. The head trauma or the viral illness could have produced some brain damage leading to his personality changes. The changes could also be due to his worries about finding a job after graduation, changes in the relationship with his girlfriend, or other undetermined factors. Neuropsychiatric testing and brain imaging studies should help determine whether his behavior changes are due to brain damage. His symptoms have some of the qualities of a frontal lobe syndrome. If this is confirmed by tests, the diagnosis would be Personality Change Due to a General Medical Condition.

2. Jane is a 27-year-old woman who experiences two or three brief periods of a minute or two each day when she feels detached from her surroundings and her own body. Sometimes she cannot remember what happens during these periods. Friends have observed these episodes and describe her as acting distant, as if she is in a dreamlike state. A neurological evaluation has demonstrated some abnormal EEG patterns, although the physician was unable to provoke one of her dissociative states during the examination. What diagnosis(es), if any, should Jane receive?

Answer: Jane's dissociative episodes are consistent with temporal lobe seizures even though no seizure activity was noted on her EEG. Because they are brief episodes that do not represent a persistent personality change, she cannot receive the diagnosis of Personality Change Due to a General Medical Condition. The appropriate diagnosis is Mental Disorder Not Otherwise Specified Due to a General Medical Condition.

Substance-Related Disorders

Clinical Vignettes

Vignette 1: Money Is No Object

Stephen is a 35-year-old surgeon who is the member of a prominent local group practice. He joined the practice 4 years ago after finishing his surgical residency at a prestigious university training program. Stephen worked hard to achieve his current position. He grew up in a lower middle-class family with five brothers and sisters. His father was a skilled laborer who worked hard to support the family but never made much money. Stephen put himself through college and medical school on scholarships and loans. By the time he had finished medical school he owed $125,000.

Stephen met his wife Joan during his last year of school and they were married when he graduated. Joan continued to work as a secretary for the next 3 years. Their combined salary was enough to pay living expenses and the interest on his loans. Stephen's son was born during his third year of training and his daughter 2 years later. With the birth of his second child Stephen became increasingly concerned about making money to pay off his loans and support his family. Because the training program did not allow him to moonlight as a physician when he wasn't on duty at the hospital, he decided to invest in a risky, but potentially lucrative, financial enterprise with one of his friends. He had no difficulty borrowing several thousand dollars from a company that specialized in making loans to physicians. The initial investments provided a good return and he made $10,000 in the first year, which he used for a down payment on a new house. A few months later he finished training and joined the group practice.

Stephen did well in his first year of practice. He loved surgery and was liked and respected by his patients and colleagues. He began to pay off his loans, bought two new cars, furniture for the house, and invested more money with his friend. Suddenly he had money for everything he wanted. For the first time in his life he felt free and financially secure. He and his wife began to socialize with a group of wealthy young professionals who lived fast and seemed to have unlimited amounts of money to spend for new cars, houses, food, and drugs. Stephen began to feel pressured to be accepted by his new friends and keep up with them financially. He worked hard over the next 3 years, his practice grew, and he invested more money in risky investments that provided the high return he needed to support his new, expensive life style. Soon he had acquired all the personal possessions and trappings of a successful physician.

In his fourth year of practice Stephen's luck changed. An economic recession produced a reversal in his financial affairs and he lost a substantial amount of money in his investments. He responded by working harder in his practice but his wife and co-workers noted subtle changes in his behavior. He became moody and irritable. Sometimes he was alert, full of energy, and almost euphoric. At other times he was angry and sensitive to the slightest actual or imagined criticism, or he was depressed. He seemed to be losing weight and his wife sometimes heard him vomiting in the bathroom early in the morning. The operating room staff complained that he behaved erratically during operations, often exploding and yelling at the staff. His wife became concerned about his behavior and depression. He responded to her questions with irritation and curt, superficial comments. Finally, Stephen's colleagues became concerned enough about his behavior to insist that he see someone for a professional evaluation.

Reluctantly, Stephen made an appointment to see a psychiatrist. In the first interview he reported feeling alternately elated and depressed over the last few months. When depressed his sleep was poor with vivid, unpleasant dreams and his appetite was poor. He lost approximately 9 pounds during that time. The psychiatrist inquired about other details of Stephen's life including: medical illnesses, suicidal thoughts, stresses at work, drug and alcohol use, and his relationship with his wife. Stephen answered some questions directly and dismissed others as irrelevant. He seemed irritated with the interview and became impatient to leave. When the psychiatrist asked him about drug use Stephen seemed insulted and laughed. The psychiatrist pressed further and Stephen became angry stating, "I didn't want to come here. My partners forced me to. You shrinks always think the worst of someone. How much longer are you going to interrogate me?" The psychiatrist listened quietly and then asked again whether Stephen was using drugs. Stephen was silent, looked down, and slowly nodded.

Vignette 2: Doctor, I'm Still Anxious

Christie is a 32-year-old married woman who works as a sales clerk in a local department store. She has been mildly to moderately depressed and anxious most of her life. Several years ago she began having stomach discomfort and pain and went to see her family physician. He made a diagnosis of "nervous stomach," told her she had to learn how to manage stress, and prescribed diazepam, a minor tranquilizer. The doctor cautioned her to use the tranquilizers as he prescribed them. Christie found the medication helpful in reducing her anxiety, although it made her drowsy and she had some difficulty concentrating on her work and driving. After a few weeks she tried to decrease the amount of medication she was taking. Each time her anxiety returned. She continued to follow the doctor's instructions, seeing him every few months for a check-up and prescription refill.

As time went on the effects of the medication seemed to wear off and she found herself taking more than he prescribed. She asked her physician for more medication but he was reluctant to prescribe a larger dose. After she had pestered him with several telephone calls and unscheduled appointments, he increased her dose. The additional medication helped and her anxiety diminished, although the drowsiness increased. A few months later she started feeling more anxious and found herself increasing the dose on her own without talking to the physician. Her drowsiness increased and she began to experience a slight impairment of coordination. Christie was now using the medication faster than the physician prescribed it. She called him and asked for more. Her physician was even more reluctant than before to prescribe additional medication but finally wrote her another prescription for the same dose of diazepam and told her that he would not increase the dose.

Feeling ignored by her own doctor, Christie again tried to decrease the medication on her own. As in the previous attempt, her anxiety soon returned and seemed worse than before she started the medication. In response, she made an appointment to see a physician in a nearby community and convinced him to give her a prescription for diazepam. This was the first in a series of visits to new physicians and local hospital emergency rooms where she asked for diazepam. Soon she was spending a significant amount of time driving around the community trying to obtain tranquilizers from various sources. She also continued to pester her own doctor for more medication. After several months, her family physician told her that he felt uncomfortable continuing to prescribe diazepam for her and suggested that she would benefit from seeing a psychiatrist. Christie was angry, protested that she didn't need psychiatric care, and accused her physician of trying to abandon her. The doctor insisted, and referred Christie to a local psychiatrist along with a note asking the physician to prescribe her diazepam.

Christie reluctantly made an appointment with the psychiatrist. When they met she gave him the note and began to explain that she was only seeing him for medication. The psychiatrist was noncommittal and asked about the personal problems that led to her referral. They spoke for about an hour. At the end of the session he concluded that Christie was depressed as well as anxious and offered to prescribe antidepressant medication. Christie asked about the diazepam and the psychiatrist replied that he would not prescribe the tranquilizer. Christie pleaded saying, "What do I do when I'm anxious? I can't even sleep." The psychiatrist was adamant stating, "In my opinion you don't need a tranquilizer." Christie was furious, took the prescription for the antidepressant medication, and left. She continued to seek tranquilizers from various sources, including her family doctor, for the next several months. She also began to see the psychiatrist and take antidepressant medication. Her use of tranquilizers remained a major topic of discussion in her sessions with the psychiatrist.

Core Concept of the Diagnostic Group

The core concept of the Substance-Related Disorders group is the occurrence of adverse social, behavioral, psychological, and physiological effects caused by seeking or using (i.e., ingesting, injecting, or inhaling) one or more substances from the 12 classes of abused substances below.

- Alcohol
- Inhalants
- Amphetamines
- Nicotine
- Caffeine
- Opioids

- Cannabis
- Phencyclidine
- Cocaine
- Sedatives, Hypnotics, or Anxiolytics
- Hallucinogens
- Other or Unknown Substances

Criteria Applicable to Multiple Disorders

There are four sets of general criteria that apply to multiple disorders in the Substance-Related Disorders group: substance dependence, substance abuse, substance intoxication, and substance withdrawal.

Criteria for Substance Dependence

The criteria used in the diagnosis of Substance Dependence fall into two groups. The first group includes the physiological signs and symptoms of tolerance and withdrawal. The second group includes repeated behavior problems associated with the continued use of the substance. Tolerance is defined as the need for a gradually increasing amount of a drug to produce a desired physiological or psychological effect previously produced by a smaller amount of drug. It is usually caused by the enhanced metabolism of the substance in the user's body. As tolerance develops, the user is able to endure doses of the substance that would significantly impair a naive user.

Concomitant with tolerance, users often experience a group of symptoms associated with the cessation of the substance use. The symptoms associated with the withdrawal syndrome for a specific substance are often specific to each general category of substance. Some withdrawal syndromes appear within a few hours after the user stops the substance, whereas others appear in subsequent days or weeks. However, not all substances have a clearly defined withdrawal syndrome. The prototypic substances that have associated tolerance and withdrawal syndromes are opioids, alcohol, and cocaine.

The second group of criteria associated with the diagnosis of Substance Dependence includes repeated behavior problems associated with the continued use of the substance. These problems include behavior related to obtaining the substance, frequently called "drug-seeking behavior," and behavior associated with the actual ingestion or use of the substance. It also includes behavioral problems that appear to be a result of the pharmacologic effects of the substance.

Substance dependence is usually manifest by compulsive use of a substance. Patients may spend a large amount of time trying to get the substance from physicians or other sources. Those who are dependent on a substance are frequently unable to control the amount of substance they use or the length of time it is used. This lack of control may be manifest by unsuccessful efforts to reduce or stop using the substance despite a persistent wish to do so. They may continue to use the substance, often in situations in which it is physically hazardous to do so, despite the awareness of persistent serious problems it causes.

A second group of problems may relate to the pharmacologic effects of the substance as well as the time and activities spent in obtaining the substance. It includes the reduction or cessation of occupational, domestic, educational, and social activities or the inability to fulfill obligations associated with these activities. Recurrent legal or interpersonal problems may also develop with continued substance use. The specific criteria for Substance Dependence include:

A maladaptive pattern of substance use, leading to clinically significant impairment or distress, as manifested by three (or more) of the following, occurring at any time in the same 12-month period:

(1) tolerance, as defined by either of the following:

    (a) a need for markedly increased amounts of the substance to achieve intoxication or desired effect

    (b) markedly diminished effect with continued use of the same amount of the substance

(2) withdrawal, as manifested by either of the following:

    (a) the characteristic withdrawal syndrome for the substance (refer to Criteria A and B of the criteria sets for Withdrawal from the specific substances)

    (b) the same (or a closely related) substance taken to relieve or avoid withdrawal symptoms

(3) the substance is often taken in larger amounts or over a longer period than was intended

(4)   there is a persistent desire or unsuccessful efforts to cut down or control substance use
(5)   a great deal of time is spent in activities necessary to obtain the substance (e.g., visiting multiple doctors or driving long distances), use the substance (e.g., chain-smoking), or recover from its effects
(6)   important social, occupational, or recreational activities are given up or reduced because of substance use
(7)   the substance use is continued despite knowledge of having a persistent or recurrent physical or psychological problem that is likely to have been caused or exacerbated by the substance (e.g., current cocaine use despite recognition of cocaine-induced depression, or continued drinking despite recognition that an ulcer was made worse by alcohol consumption)

Specify if:
    With Physiological Dependence: evidence of tolerance or withdrawal (i.e., either Item 1 or 2 is present)
    Without Physiological Dependence: no evidence of tolerance or withdrawal (i.e., neither Item 1 nor 2 is present)

The course modifiers below can be applied to Substance Dependence but not Substance Abuse. However, the diagnoses of Substance Abuse and Substance Dependence are hierarchical in the sense that once an individual meets the criteria for dependence, the person can no longer qualify for a diagnosis of abuse for that substance. Therefore, although they have different criteria, DSM-IV stipulates that the determination of whether an individual is in partial or full remission from dependence must consider substance use behavior found in the criteria sets for both Substance Dependence and Substance Abuse.

Early Full Remission: For at least 1 month but for less than 12 months; no criteria for Dependence or Abuse have been met.

Early Partial Remission: For at least 1 month, but less than 12 months; one or more criteria (but not the full criteria) for Dependence or Abuse have been met.

Sustained Full Remission: No criteria for Dependence or abuse have been met at any time for the last 12 months or longer.

Sustained Partial Remission: At least one of the criteria for Dependence or Abuse has been met for 12 months or longer but the full criteria have not been met.

On Agonist Therapy: The patient is on a prescribed agonist medication and no criteria for Dependence or Abuse have been met for that class of medication for at least the past month (other than tolerance to, or withdrawal from, the agonist).

In a Controlled Environment: The individual is in an environment where access to alcohol and controlled substances is restricted and no criteria for Dependence or Abuse have been met for at least the past month.

Criteria for Substance Abuse

The criteria for the diagnosis of Substance Abuse relate to the potential or actual consequences associated with the use of a substance. The criteria are identical for all 12 classes of substances. The specific criteria for Substance Abuse include the following:

A. A maladaptive pattern of substance use leading to clinically significant impairment or distress, as manifested by one (or more) of the following, occurring within a 12-month period:

   (1) recurrent substance use resulting in a failure to fulfill major role obligations at work, school, or home (e.g., repeated absences or poor work performance related to substance use; substance-related absences, suspensions, or expulsions from school; neglect of children or household)
   (2) recurrent substance use in situations in which it is physically hazardous (e.g., driving an automobile or operating a machine when impaired by substance use)
   (3) recurrent substance-related legal problems (e.g., arrests for substance-related disorderly conduct)
   (4) continued substance use despite having persistent or recurrent social or interpersonal problems caused or exacerbated by the effects of the substance (e.g., arguments with spouse about consequences of intoxication, physical fights)

B. The symptoms have never met the criteria for Substance Dependence for this class of substance.

Criteria for Substance Intoxication

Most classes of substances have unique and characteristic intoxication syndromes consisting of specific behavioral, psychological, and physiological signs and symptoms. These signs and symptoms are presented in detail in the section containing the synopses of the individual Substance-Related Disorders. The generic criteria below apply to all substance intoxication diagnoses.

A. The development of a reversible substance-specific syndrome due to recent ingestion of (or exposure to) a substance. **Note:** Different substances may produce similar or identical syndromes.

B. Clinically significant maladaptive behavioral or psychological changes that are due to the effect of the substance on the central nervous system (e.g., belligerence, mood lability, cognitive impairment, impaired judgment, impaired social or occupational functioning) and develop during or shortly after use of the substance.

C. The symptoms are not due to a general medical condition and are not better accounted for by another mental disorder.

Criteria for Substance Withdrawal

Most classes of substances have unique and characteristic withdrawal syndromes consisting of specific behavioral, psychological, and physiological signs and symptoms. These signs and symptoms are presented in detail in the section containing the synopses of the individual Substance-Related Disorders. The generic criteria below apply to all substance withdrawal diagnoses.

A. The development of a substance-specific syndrome due to the cessation of, or reduction in, substance use that has been heavy and prolonged.

B. The substance-specific syndrome causes clinically significant distress or impairment in social, occupational, or other important areas of functioning.

C. The symptoms are not due to a general medical condition and are not better accounted for by another mental disorder.

Definitions

anxiolytic   Another name for medications that relieve anxiety such as benzodiazepines.

macropsia   A perceptual state in which objects seem larger than they actually are.

micropsia   A perceptual state in which objects seem smaller than they actually are.

nodding off   Sedation or a sense of drowsiness that occurs after the initial experience of a high with an injection of an opioid such as heroin.

polydrug abuse   The use of more than one drug at the same time (e.g., heroin and cocaine; hallucinogens and anxiolytics).

psychomotor agitation An abnormal increase in physical and emotional activity.

rush An immediate high that occurs shortly after an intravenous injection of an opioid such as heroin.

Synopses and Diagnostic Prototypes of the Individual Disorders

The specific diagnoses in the Substance-Related Disorders group can be arranged into three large categories: 1) dependence and abuse; 2) intoxication, withdrawal, and not otherwise specified diagnoses; and 3) substance-induced psychiatric syndromes. DSM-IV lists all of the diagnoses for a specific class of substances together under one heading. However, it is simpler, more efficient, and less redundant to first separate them into the three larger categories above.

The criteria for dependence and abuse will be discussed in the first subsection below. The second category, including criteria for intoxication, withdrawal, and not otherwise specified diagnoses, will be discussed in the second subsection. These criteria are generally specific to each class of substances. However, Alcohol Use Disorders and Sedative, Hypnotic, or Anxiolytics Use Disorders have identical criteria as do Amphetamine and Cocaine Use Disorders.

The intoxication and withdrawal criteria for each class of substance will be synopsized. Most of the synopses are followed by a vignette that provides a clinical example of the diagnosis. Each vignette is a prototype in the sense that it represents a typical patient from that specific diagnostic category. The prototypes provide a more lifelike portrayal of the diagnosis than the criteria alone. They also provide a clinical baseline that can be used in the discussion of problems associated with the diagnosis of these disorders and as a standard for comparison even if they do not exhaust all the possibilities for the clinical presentation of a specific diagnosis. The last category includes substance-induced syndromes that mimic other psychiatric disorders (e.g., anxiety, psychosis, mood disorder). These will be discussed in the third subsection.

Substance Dependence and Abuse

Table 5–1 provides a summary of DSM-IV codes for Substance Dependence and Abuse for each of the 12 categories. The criteria for these three diagnoses are exactly the same for all 12 classes of substances and have been discussed above (see section on Criteria Applicable to Multiple Disorders). The DSM-IV codes are listed in Table 5–1 for convenience and comparison. The names of specific Substance Dependence and Abuse diagnoses are constructed as follows: Alcohol Dependence or Alcohol Abuse, Opioid Dependence or Opioid Abuse, Cannabis Dependence or Cannabis Abuse. The diagnosis of Polysubst-

Table 5–1 DSM-IV codes for specific substance dependence and abuse diagnoses		
Substance	Dependence	Abuse
Alcohol	303.90	305.00
Amphetamine	304.40	305.70
Caffeine	---	---
Cannabis	304.30	305.20
Cocaine	304.20	305.60
Hallucinogen	304.50	305.30
Inhalant	304.60	305.90
Nicotine	305.10	---
Opioid	304.00	305.50
Phencyclidine	304.90	305.90
Sedative, Hypnotic, Anxiolytic	304.10	305.40
Other or unspecified	304.90	305.90
Polysubstance	304.80	---

ance Dependence has slightly different criteria than the other dependence syndromes. A synopsis of this diagnosis is presented below.

Polysubstance-Related Disorder

304.80   Polysubstance Dependence.   Individuals with this disorder have a pattern of maladaptive use of at least three classes of substances (not including nicotine and caffeine) and meet the full criteria for Substance Dependence for the substances considered as a group but not for any single substance.

Substance Intoxication, Withdrawal, and Not Otherwise Specified Diagnoses

Most classes of substances have unique intoxication and withdrawal syndromes with specific behavioral, psychological, and physiological signs and symptoms. There are two exceptions. The Alcohol Use Disorders and the Sedative, Hypnotic, or Anxiolytics Use Disorders have identical criteria, as do Amphetamine and Cocaine Use Disorders. Hallucinogens are associated with a specific intoxication syndrome but not withdrawal. Instead, patients who use these substances sometimes experience flashbacks (292.89 Hallucinogen Persisting Perception Disorder) that may be analogous to a withdrawal syndrome.

   A synopsis of the intoxication and withdrawal criteria for each class of substance will be presented in this section. Most synopses are followed by a prototypic vignette. Summaries of the behavioral, psychological, and physiological signs and symptoms of intoxication are listed in Table 5–2 and withdrawal in Table 5–3 for each class of abused substances.

Table 5–2 Behavioral, psychological, and physiological symptoms of intoxication

Substance	Behavioral and psychological changes of intoxication	Clinical signs and symptoms of intoxication
Alcohol (303.00) or Sedative, Hypnotic, *or* Anxiolytic (292.89)	Inappropriate sexual/ aggressive behavior Mood lability Impaired judgment Impaired social/occupational functioning	One of the following: 1. Slurred speech 2. Incoordination 3. Unsteady gait 4. Nystagmus 5. Impairment of attention and memory 6. Stupor or coma
Amphetamine (or related substance) (292.89) *or* Cocaine (292.89)	Euphoria or affective blunting Changes in sociability Hypervigilance Interpersonal sensitivity Anxiety, tension, or anger Stereotyped behaviors Impaired judgment Impaired social/occupational functioning	Two of the following: 1. Tachycardia or brady-cardia 2. Pupillary dilation 3. Elevated or lowered blood pressure 4. Perspiration or chills 5. Nausea or vomiting 6. Evidence of weight loss 7. Psychomotor agitation or retardation 8. Muscular weakness, respiratory depression, chest pain, or cardiac arrhythmias 9. Confusion, seizures, dyskinesias, dystonias, or coma
Caffeine (305.90)	No specific behavioral or psychological changes normally occur with caffeine intoxication other than those listed as clinical signs and symptoms to the right.	Five of the following: 1. Restlessness 2. Nervousness 3. Excitement 4. Insomnia 5. Flushed face 6. Diuresis 7. Gastrointestinal distur-bance 8. Muscle twitching 9. Rambling flow of thought and speech 10. Tachycardia or cardiac arrhythmia 11. Periods of inexhausti-bility 12. Psychomotor agitation

(continued)

Table 5–2   Behavioral, psychological, and physiological symptoms of intoxication
(continued)

Substance	Behavioral and psychological changes of intoxication	Clinical signs and symptoms of intoxication
Cannabis (292.89)	Impaired motor coordination Euphoria Anxiety Sensation of slowed time Impaired judgment Social withdrawal	Two of the following: 1. Conjunctival injection 2. Increased appetite 3. Dry mouth 4. Tachycardia
Hallucinogen (292.89)	Marked anxiety or depression Ideas of reference Fear of losing one's mind Paranoid ideation Impaired judgment Impaired social/occupational functioning	Two of the following: 1. Pupillary dilation 2. Tachycardia 3. Sweating 4. Palpitations 5. Blurring of vision 6. Tremors 7. Incoordination
Inhalant (292.89)	Belligerence Assaultiveness Apathy Impaired judgment Impaired social/occupational functioning	Two of the following: 1. Dizziness 2. Nystagmus 3. Incoordination 4. Slurred speech 5. Unsteady gait 6. Lethargy 7. Depressed reflexes 8. Psychomotor retardation 9. Tremor 10. Generalized muscle weakness 11. Blurred vision or diplopia 12. Stupor or coma 13. Euphoria

Opioid (292.89)	Initial euphoria followed by
	   apathy
	Dysphoria
	Psychomotor agitation or retardation
	Impaired judgment
	Impaired social/occupational
	   functioning
		Pupillary constriction and
		One of the following:
		1. Drowsiness or coma
		2. Slurred speech
		3. Impairment in attention or memory

Table 5–2   Behavioral, psychological, and physiological symptoms of intoxication *(continued)*

Substance	Behavioral and psychological changes of intoxication	Clinical signs and symptoms of intoxication
Phencyclidine (292.89)	Belligerence Assaultiveness Impulsiveness Unpredictability Psychomotor agitation Impaired judgment Impaired social/occupational functioning	Two of the following: 1. Vertical or horizontal nystagmus 2. Hypertension or tachycardia 3. Numbness or diminished responsiveness to pain 4. Ataxia 5. Dysarthria 6. Muscle rigidity 7. Seizure or coma 8. Hyperacusis

Alcohol Use Disorders

303.00   Alcohol Intoxication.   Patients with this disorder have recently used alcohol and have clinically significant maladaptive behavioral or psychological changes developing during, or shortly after the alcohol ingestion (e.g., inappropriate sexual or aggressive behavior, mood lability, impaired judgment, and impaired social or occupational functioning). The patient also has at least one of the following signs.

1. Slurred speech
2. Incoordination
3. Unsteady gait
4. Nystagmus
5. Impairment of attention and memory
6. Stupor or coma

Ted is a newly enlisted 19-year-old sailor who went drinking with his shipmates when their destroyer put into port for resupply. Soon after they entered a local bar one of Ted's friends challenged him to a beer-drinking contest. When Ted tried to decline one of the other sailors said, "What's the matter, can't you hold your liquor?" The others laughed and Ted reluctantly agreed to the contest.

An hour later, after five beers, Ted noticed a young woman sitting next to the bar. He staggered over to her table and sat down. She seemed annoyed and said, "My boyfriend went to the bathroom. He'll be right back." Ted paid no attention, put his arm around the girl, and pulled her close to him. As she struggled to get away her boyfriend appeared. He grabbed Ted and dragged him off the chair. Ted got angry and swung at the boyfriend but missed. After a brief fight Ted ended up on the floor with a bloody nose and one tooth knocked out. His shipmates hauled him back to the ship.

291.8   Alcohol Withdrawal.   Patients with this disorder have stopped (or reduced) the consumption of alcohol after prolonged and heavy use. At least two of the following have developed within several hours to days after stopping. (Specify if there are perceptual disturbances.)

1. Autonomic hyperactivity (e.g., sweating or pulse greater than 100)
2. Increased hand tremor
3. Insomnia
4. Nausea or vomiting
5. Transient visual, tactile, or auditory hallucinations or illusions
6. Psychomotor agitation
7. Anxiety
8. Grand mal seizures

Allison is the 38-year-old wife of a wealthy and successful business executive who is devoted to his work. The couple decided early in their marriage that they would not have children. Allison was trained as a social worker and worked full time for 3 or 4 years before meeting her husband. She continued to work part time for a couple of years after her marriage but eventually became frustrated, feeling that, despite the endless work, she had little effect on the problems around her.

Allison finally quit her job when the couple moved to an expensive suburb several miles outside the city. The couple joined a country club and Allison spent her time doing volunteer work in a local children's hospital and playing tennis with her friends. Her husband was too busy to spend much time at the club. Allison had always confined her drinking to social occasions but now began drinking more as she felt increasingly lonely and empty. Lunch at the club, after tennis, usually included one or two cocktails. Later in the day, after her volunteer work or shopping, she frequently stopped at a local restaurant with friends and had a few cocktails before going home. Allison's husband often worked late so she had one or two more drinks while preparing dinner for herself. Finally, before bed she had a nightcap. Her husband's job required periodic business trips lasting several days. Allison sometimes accompanied him but found the trips lonely and boring. On the days he was away her drinking increased substantially in the evenings.

One morning, after her husband had been gone for several days, Allison awoke late in the morning sweating, feeling nauseous and anxious as her heart raced. Her hands shook as she got out of bed and went into the bathroom where she vomited in the toilet. She felt like she couldn't sit still and began pacing around her room and down the hall to the living room. She poured some liquor into a glass and tried to drink

Table 5–3 Clinical signs and symptoms of Withdrawal	
Substance	**Clinical signs and symptoms of withdrawal**
Alcohol (291.8) *or* sedative, hypnotic, *or* anxiolytic (292.0)	Two of the following: 1. Autonomic hyperactivity (e.g., sweating or pulse greater than 100) 2. Increased hand tremor 3. Insomnia 4. Nausea or vomiting 5. Transient visual, tactile, or auditory hallucinations or illusions 6. Psychomotor agitation 7. Anxiety 8. Grand mal seizures
Amphetamine (or related substance) (292.0) *or* cocaine (292.0)	Dysphoric mood and two of the following: 1. Fatigue 2. Vivid, unpleasant dreams 3. Insomnia or hypersomnia 4. Increased appetite 5. Psychomotor retardation or agitation
Nicotine (292.0)	Four of the following: 1. Dysphoric or depressed mood 2. Insomnia 3. Irritability, frustration, or anger 4. Anxiety 5. Difficulty concentrating 6. Restlessness 7. Decreased heart rate 8. Increased appetite or weight gain
Opioid (292.0)	Three of the following: 1. Dysphoric mood 2. Nausea or vomiting 3. Muscle aches 4. Lacrimation or rhinorrhea 5. Pupillary dilation, piloerection, or sweating 6. Diarrhea 7. Yawning 8. Fever 9. Insomnia

without spilling it. Within a half hour she began to calm down, her hands stopped shaking, and she felt better. Allison got dressed and went to the club for tennis.

291.9 Alcohol-Related Disorder Not Otherwise Specified. Patients with this disorder have symptoms associated with the use of alcohol that cannot be classified as any specific Alcohol Use Disorder.

Amphetamine-Related Disorders

292.89   Amphetamine Intoxication.   Patients with this disorder have recently used amphetamine or a related substance (e.g., methylphenidate) and have clinically significant maladaptive behavioral or psychological changes developing during, or shortly after use of the amphetamine or related substance (e.g., euphoria or affective blunting; changes in sociability; hypervigilance; interpersonal sensitivity; anxiety, tension, or anger; stereotyped behaviors; impaired judgment; or impaired social or occupational functioning). The patient also has at least two of the following signs. (Specify if the patient has perceptual disturbances.)

1. Tachycardia or bradycardia
2. Pupillary dilation
3. Elevated or lowered blood pressure
4. Perspiration or chills
5. Nausea or vomiting
6. Evidence of weight loss
7. Psychomotor agitation or retardation
8. Muscular weakness, respiratory depression, chest pain, or cardiac arrhythmias
9. Confusion, seizures, dyskinesias, dystonias, or coma

> Tim is a 19-year-old college student who was studying for his final examinations. He paid little attention to his school work during the semester and had to learn all of the material for several courses in a few days. As in the past, he took amphetamines to stay awake and study. Tim stayed awake for 3 days, with minimal sleep. Whenever he became sleepy he took more pills. Initially, he felt wide awake, confident, and had an increased sense of well being.
>
> By the third day Tim's roommate noticed some changes in his personality. Tim was increasingly irritable and tense. Casual comments or interruptions angered him. He seemed easily startled by the smallest sound and watched his roommate and other people closely when they entered his room. On the fifth day his roommate returned to find Tim vomiting and sweating profusely, his pupils widely dilated. He seemed confused. An empty pill bottle lay on the desk. Tim's roommate and friends stayed with him for the next 2 days until his confusion cleared and he fell asleep.

292.0   Amphetamine Withdrawal.   Patients with this disorder have stopped (or reduced) the consumption of amphetamine (or related substance) after prolonged and heavy use. Dysphoric mood and at least two of the following have developed within a few hours to several days after stopping.

1. Fatigue
2. Vivid, unpleasant dreams
3. Insomnia or hypersomnia

4. Increased appetite
5. Psychomotor retardation or agitation

> Adam is an 18-year-old adolescent who is known as a "speed freak" by his acquaintances. He spends most of his time hustling at the local pool hall and video game arcade. Adam routinely mainlines (i.e., injects intravenously) heavy doses of amphetamine in runs of several days at a time. For the first 2 or 3 days his performance at pool and video games improves substantially. Regulars at the pool hall know from experience not to bet money when they play against him during these periods. As the run continues he becomes less sociable and soon stops playing.
>
> Adam abruptly quits taking amphetamine when he becomes weak from not eating and has no remaining money or drugs. A few hours after the last dose of amphetamine he crashes and becomes depressed. The intensity of the depression varies and can be severe. It usually peaks in 2 to 3 days but can last for several days or a few weeks. Adam is exhausted after a run and usually sleeps for hours. His sleep is punctuated by frequent, vivid nightmares of being chased, assaulted, or caught in serious accidents. When he finally wakes he has an insatiable appetite that lasts several days. After he accumulates enough money for more amphetamine he begins another run that follows the same pattern.

292.9 Amphetamine-Related Disorder Not Otherwise Specified. Patients with this disorder have symptoms associated with the use of amphetamine (or a related substance) that cannot be classified as any specific Amphetamine Use Disorder.

Caffeine-Related Disorders

305.90 Caffeine Intoxication. Patients with this disorder have recently consumed caffeine in excess of 250 mg (e.g., more than 2–3 cups of brewed coffee) and have five of the following signs developing during or shortly after use.

1. Restlessness
2. Nervousness
3. Excitement
4. Insomnia
5. Flushed face
6. Diuresis
7. Gastrointestinal disturbance
8. Muscle twitching
9. Rambling flow of thought and speech
10. Tachycardia or cardiac arrhythmia
11. Periods of inexhaustibility
12. Psychomotor agitation

Derick is a 29-year-old certified public accountant who is starting a small accounting firm with two of his colleagues. This year they received several last-minute tax
returns to complete for individuals who did not want to file extensions for their
returns. All three partners were forced to work late hours. Three days before the
deadline for filing taxes there were still several returns to finish. Derick realized that
they would have to work all night on the returns to finish them in time for their
clients. The partners met for a brief working dinner. Derick was already beginning
to get sleepy. He had a couple of cups of coffee, finished the discussion with his
colleagues, and went back to his office to work.

Three hours later Joe, one of the partners, walked into Derick's office. He was
sitting at his desk with his eyes barely open. Joe said, "You look a little sleepy,
partner." Derick's eyes jerked open, "I guess so, I was never good at this late night
stuff. I'm a morning person." Joe looked at him for a minute. "No problem," he said,
"You need some more coffee." Derick looked up, "I don't know how much more
coffee I can drink." Joe left for a minute and returned with two cups. After they
finished the coffee Joe gave him a little bottle of pills. "Secret weapon for accoun-
tants," he joked. Derick looked at them, "I don't take drugs," he said. Joe laughed,
"Hey, this is just instant coffee. You know, caffeine pills, over the counter stuff.
Each pill is like a cup of coffee. It's easier than making coffee." Derick shrugged
and took the bottle.

A couple of hours later he began to get sleepy again and took two pills. During
the next 7 hours he took seven more pills. Derick continued working but felt increasingly restless and nervous. He went to the bathroom to urinate every half hour.
He could feel his heart racing. At one point, as Joe passed his office, Derick was
pacing the floor in front of his desk holding one of the returns. He turned to look at
Joe and said, "I can't sit still." Joe laughed and replied, "Hey, lay off those caffeine
pills, you're going to overdose on them."

292.9   Caffeine-Related Disorder Not Otherwise Specified.   Patients with
this disorder have symptoms associated with the use of caffeine that cannot be
classified as any specific Caffeine Use Disorder.

Cannabis-Related Disorder

292.89   Cannabis Intoxication.   Patients with this disorder have recently used
cannabis and have clinically significant maladaptive behavioral or psychological
changes developing during, or shortly after use of the cannabis (e.g., impaired
motor coordination, euphoria, anxiety, sensation of slowed time, impaired judgment, social withdrawal). The patient also has at least two of the following signs.
(Specify if the patient has perceptual disturbances.)

1. Conjunctival injection
2. Increased appetite

3. Dry mouth
4. Tachycardia

Doug is a single 25-year-old repairman for a large home appliance company. On weekends he often goes to parties with his girlfriend. Drugs are often available at the parties but he and his girlfriend rarely use them. However, at a recent party one of his friends offered him some marijuana to smoke. His girlfriend, who rarely used drugs, was initially reluctant to participate but finally agreed to join him. The couple lay on a bed and Doug rolled a joint. As they smoked his girlfriend became withdrawn, anxious, and frightened. She stood up but found it difficult to walk and lay back down on the bed feeling even more anxious. Doug stopped smoking and began trying to calm her. Gradually, over the next hour she relaxed and her anxiety changed to a mild sense of euphoria. As the effects of the drug wore off she complained that her mouth was dry and asked Doug to get her something to drink. When he returned she said, "I'm starved. Let's get out of here and get something to eat."

292.9   Cannabis-Related Disorder Not Otherwise Specified.   Patients with this disorder have symptoms associated with the use of cannabis that cannot be classified as any specific Cannabis Use Disorder.

Cocaine-Related Disorders

292.89   Cocaine Intoxication.   Patients with this disorder have recently used cocaine and have clinically significant maladaptive behavioral or psychological changes developing during, or shortly after use of the cocaine (e.g., euphoria or affective blunting; changes in sociability; hypervigilance; interpersonal sensitivity; anxiety, tension, or anger; stereotyped behaviors; impaired judgment; or impaired social or occupational functioning). The patient also has at least two of the following signs. (Specify if the patient has perceptual disturbances.)

1. Tachycardia or bradycardia
2. Pupillary dilation
3. Elevated or lowered blood pressure
4. Perspiration or chills
5. Nausea or vomiting
6. Evidence of weight loss
7. Psychomotor agitation or retardation
8. Muscular weakness, respiratory depression, chest pain, or cardiac arrhythmias
9. Confusion, seizures, dyskinesias, dystonias, or coma

Stan is a 28-year-old undercover police officer in the narcotics squad. His job is to buy drugs from local dealers. When he makes a purchase he alerts the other officers in the squad who make the arrest. Stan spent several months cultivating a relationship with Slim, a small dealer known to be well connected to local cocaine suppliers. One time, while Stan waited in Slim's apartment for drugs, a woman began smoking crack. She packed a small glass pipe with a chunk of a white crystal-like substance, lit it, and began inhaling. Within a few seconds she settled back in the chair with a contented look on her face. Her eyes were wide open and her pupils were dilated. Suddenly she began to sweat profusely and vomited. Slim asked how she was doing. The woman seemed slightly confused, turned slowly toward him, and said, "Hey baby, I'm cool." A few seconds later she became agitated, angry, and began looking around the room. Slim and another woman tried to calm her. After several minutes her agitation subsided and she sat down on the couch.

292.0   Cocaine Withdrawal.   Patients with this disorder have stopped (or reduced) the consumption of cocaine after prolonged and heavy use. Dysphoric mood and at least two of the following have developed within a few hours to several days after stopping.

1. Fatigue
2. Vivid, unpleasant dreams
3. Insomnia or hypersomnia
4. Increased appetite
5. Psychomotor retardation or agitation

Greg is a 31-year-old man who owned a small contracting business that employed four other construction workers and a secretary. He worked hard and the business seemed to be growing. Approximately 1 year ago his employees began noticing changes in his behavior. He became irritable and touchy. Little things in the office that he had always ignored began to bother him. He had difficulty sitting still and frequently got up to go to the bathroom. When he returned he seemed calmer. His secretary began to suspect that he was using drugs. She confronted Greg but he denied using drugs and was angry that she asked.

Greg's behavior began to have an effect on the business. He missed appointments and gradually the company's work declined. His secretary kept track of the company bank accounts and noticed that Greg was continually withdrawing money. When she asked him about the money he was evasive and told her to mind her own business. Finally, as the money continued to disappear he laid off three of his workers. Greg was on the verge of bankruptcy. He tried to borrow money but he was unsuccessful. One morning he came into the office looking tired and withdrawn. His secretary was alarmed and asked him if he was sick. Greg shook his head and said, "I haven't been sleeping too well." Then he slumped into a chair and began crying. "I'm useless. I might as well be dead, for all it's worth. I feel like killing myself." His secretary tried to talk with him but he didn't respond. Finally, she called the other worker and drove him to the hospital emergency room. Greg was seen by a physician and admitted to the psychiatric unit with a diagnosis of Cocaine Withdrawal.

292.9   Cocaine-Related Disorder Not Otherwise Specified.   Patients with this disorder have symptoms associated with the use of cocaine that cannot be classified as any specific Cocaine-Related Disorder.

Hallucinogen-Related Disorders

292.89   Hallucinogen Intoxication.   Patients with this disorder have recently used a hallucinogen and have clinically significant maladaptive behavioral or psychological changes developing during, or shortly after use of the hallucinogen (e.g., marked anxiety or depression, ideas of reference, fear of losing one's mind, paranoid ideation, impaired judgment, or impaired social or occupational functioning) and perceptual changes that occur in a state of full wakefulness and alertness (e.g., intensification of perceptions, depersonalization, derealization, illusions, hallucination, synesthesias). The patient also has at least two of the following signs.

1. Pupillary dilation
2. Tachycardia
3. Sweating
4. Palpitations
5. Blurring of vision
6. Tremors
7. Incoordination

> Hal is a 16-year-old adolescent who recently began experimenting with drugs. Recently, he and three friends decided to take some lysergic acid diethylamide (LSD). Hal describes the experience as follows. "When I took the acid nothing happened for about a half hour. Then I began sweating and my vision changed and everything became blurry. Colors started to seem brighter and more intense. The music we were listening to seemed more meaningful than it ever had before. I was suddenly aware of smells I had never noticed. I could feel my heart beating much faster than usual and my kidneys making urine. At first I began to worry that I was losing my mind. When I became anxious one of my friends said, 'Hey man, it's OK, just let it happen. Nothing's wrong.' After a couple of hours other things began to change. I started hearing colors. I know it sounds crazy. I can't explain it but that's what happened. Gradually I began feeling like I was one with the universe. Nothing separated me from the rest of the world. It was profound. like a religious experience."

292.89   Hallucinogen Persisting Perception Disorder (Flashbacks).
Patients with this disorder have previously used a hallucinogen and reexperience one or more of the perceptual symptoms that were experienced while intoxicated with the hallucinogen (e.g., geometric hallucinations, false perceptions of move-

ment in the peripheral visual fields, flashes of color, intensified colors, trails of images of moving objects, positive afterimages, halos around objects, macropsia, and micropsia).

> Margaret is a 22-year-old woman who used LSD twice, 2 months ago. Her LSD trips were pleasant and consisted mainly of perceptual alterations that made colors and objects seem far more brilliant and intense than usual, and distorted objects so they appeared to be melting. Three days ago Margaret was walking down the street near her home when she suddenly noticed something moving out of the corner of her eye. She turned, but didn't see anything. Following this she noticed that a garbage truck appeared to leave a visible trail or afterimage, as if it were dropping rubbish, when it passed by her in the street. The perceptual distortions lasted for several seconds and then disappeared. Margaret was startled by the experience and didn't initially connect it with her LSD trips. She had another flashback on the next day. Margaret told one of her friends who reassured her and admitted that she had also had flashbacks after taking LSD and they had eventually disappeared.

292.9   Hallucinogen-Related Disorder Not Otherwise Specified.   Patients with this disorder have symptoms associated with the use of a hallucinogen that cannot be classified as any specific Hallucinogen-Related Disorder.

Inhalant-Related Disorders

292.89   Inhalant Intoxication.   Patients with this disorder have intentionally used or briefly been exposed to volatile inhalants and have clinically significant maladaptive behavioral or psychological changes developing during, or shortly after exposure to the volatile inhalants (e.g., belligerence, assaultiveness, apathy, impaired judgment, impaired social or occupational functioning). The patient also has at least two of the following signs.

1. Dizziness
2. Nystagmus
3. Incoordination
4. Slurred speech
5. Unsteady gait
6. Lethargy
7. Depressed reflexes
8. Psychomotor retardation
9. Tremor
10. Generalized muscle weakness
11. Blurred vision or diplopia
12. Stupor or coma
13. Euphoria

Larry, a 17-year-old high school senior, was enrolled in an advanced placement chemistry course. He was intelligent and did well academically. However, he often played around in the chemistry laboratory in a manner that was dangerous to himself and others. In one incident he poured acid on a student. The student's shirt was ruined and he narrowly avoided injury. The teacher threatened to expel Larry from the class if he ever did anything similar again.

A few weeks later, during chemistry lab, Larry began inhaling an organic solvent to get high. Several seconds later he became belligerent and began stumbling around the room. His speech became slurred, as if he were drunk. Soon he became dizzy and sat down in the corner of the room. The episode passed after 5 or 10 minutes but he still seemed unsteady as he walked. Larry's father, who was a physician, was very concerned when he heard about the episode that evening and had Larry examined by one of his colleagues to make sure he had no liver or lung damage. Larry killed himself 3 years later.

292.9 Inhalant-Related Disorder Not Otherwise Specified. Patients with this disorder have symptoms associated with the use of an inhalant that cannot be classified as any specific Inhalant-Related Disorder.

Nicotine-Related Disorders

292.0 Nicotine Withdrawal. Patients with this disorder have stopped (or reduced) the consumption of nicotine after prolonged and heavy use for at least several weeks. At least four of the following have developed within 24 hours after stopping.

1. Dysphoric or depressed mood
2. Insomnia
3. Irritability, frustration, or anger
4. Anxiety
5. Difficulty concentrating
6. Restlessness
7. Decreased heart rate
8. Increased appetite or weight gain

Brenda is a 44-year-old woman who works as a senior editor for an advertising agency. She smokes heavily. Brenda began smoking in college and gradually increased her cigarette consumption until she was smoking two to three packs a day. She finds it difficult to work without smoking. Recently, her agency established a no-smoking policy throughout the office. Brenda and her colleagues were forced to smoke outside the building. They soon began to feel like outcasts who were escaping from the office to indulge in some immoral vice. She and most of the other smokers crossed the street and hid behind the corner of another building to smoke so they could not be seen from the office. Because it took too much time to leave the building, her smoking was significantly reduced.

Within a day or two Brenda began to have trouble working. She felt depressed and had difficulty concentrating on her work. She was irritable with the people who worked for her and impatient when they asked for help with their projects. She was restless and couldn't wait until her next smoking break. In between breaks she began to eat junk food and gained 5 pounds in the first week. She tried several methods to stop smoking, including nicotine patches and group therapy, but none were successful. Finally, she began thinking about changing her job.

292.9   Nicotine-Related Disorder Not Otherwise Specified.   Patients with this disorder have symptoms associated with the use of nicotine that cannot be classified as any specific Nicotine Use Disorder.

Opioid-Related Disorders

292.89 Opioid Intoxication.   Patients with this disorder have recently used an opioid and have clinically significant maladaptive behavioral or psychological changes developing during, or shortly after use of the opioid (e.g., initial euphoria followed by apathy, dysphoria, psychomotor agitation, or retardation, impaired judgment, or impaired social or occupational functioning). The patient also has pupillary constriction (or pupillary dilation due to anoxia from severe overdose) and at least one of the following signs. (Specify if the patient has perceptual disturbances.)

1. Drowsiness or coma
2. Slurred speech
3. Impairment in attention or memory

Jamie is a 17-year-old high school dropout whose boyfriend Matt has recently joined a local motorcycle gang. The gang members used drugs extensively and Matt's initiation to the gang required that he receive a "fix" or injection of intravenous heroin. It was his first experience with heroin and he enjoyed it. He tried to convince Jamie to try heroin. She was fearful and initially resisted.

One night Matt and Jamie were riding with the gang and they stopped at a local gang hangout. Several of the female gang members gathered around Jamie and started teasing her about not trying heroin. She finally agreed to try a "fix." One of the women dissolved some heroin in a spoon, drew it into a syringe, put a tourniquet on Jamie's arm, and injected the heroin into her vein. Jamie felt a sudden "rush" or "high" that she later described as akin to an orgasm. This was followed by a sense of euphoria. Matt glanced at her face and noticed that she had a slightly dazed look with tiny pupils. After a few minutes Jamie became lethargic and began to nod off. The effects peaked in about 20 to 30 minutes and gradually began to wear off.

292.0   Opioid Withdrawal.   Patients with this disorder have stopped (or reduced) using an opioid after prolonged and heavy use or have been given an opioid antagonist. At least three of the following have developed within minutes to several days later.

1. Dysphoric mood
2. Nausea or vomiting
3. Muscle aches
4. Lacrimation or rhinorrhea
5. Pupillary dilation, piloerection, or sweating
6. Diarrhea
7. Yawning
8. Fever
9. Insomnia

> Sean is a 27-year-old man who arrived at a local hospital emergency room late one night complaining of feeling depressed and suicidal. He was admitted to the psychiatric ward for observation. A few hours later, in the middle of the night, he began vomiting and complaining of muscle aches, stomach cramps, diarrhea, and difficulty sleeping. The nurse initially thought that he was developing a viral syndrome. However, when she examined his arms she discovered several needle "tracks." Sean admitted that he began injecting heroin a few weeks ago. He injected his last heroin approximately 6 hours before his admission to the hospital. The nurse called the ward psychiatrist who examined Sean and prescribed medication to treat the symptoms of his withdrawal syndrome.

292.9   Opioid-Related Disorder Not Otherwise Specified.   Patients with this disorder have symptoms associated with the use of an opioid that cannot be classified as any specific Opioid-Related Disorder.

Phencyclidine-Related Disorders

292.89   Phencyclidine Intoxication.   Patients with this disorder have recently used phencyclidine (or a related substance) and have clinically significant maladaptive behavioral changes developing during, or shortly after use of the substance (e.g., belligerence, assaultiveness, impulsiveness, unpredictability, psychomotor agitation, impaired judgment, or impaired social or occupational functioning). The patient also has at least two of the following signs within an hour of using the substance. (Specify if the patient has perceptual disturbances.)

1. Vertical or horizontal nystagmus
2. Hypertension or tachycardia
3. Numbness or diminished responsiveness to pain
4. Ataxia

5. Dysarthria
6. Muscle rigidity
7. Seizure or coma
8. Hyperacusis

> Alex is a 17-year-old male who was brought to the emergency department of a large
> hospital by the police. His leg was bleeding from a laceration he got after getting
> into a fight with another man. However, he apparently was unaware of his injury or
> did not feel it. The police reported that the patient was belligerent and assaultive
> when they took him into custody. It took three officers to control him. Alex was
> calmer and noncommunicative by the time the physician saw him. A friend, who
> accompanied the patient, reported that Alex had smoked some "special grass" that
> he bought from a drug dealer who said it would give him a nice "buzz." A few
> minutes after smoking the drug Alex became belligerent and picked a fight with a
> man sitting nearby who made an offhand comment to him. The physical examina-
> tion revealed that the patient had horizontal nystagmus and moderate hypertension
> (170/105). He stumbled when he tried to walk and his muscles seemed rigid and
> stiff.

292.9   Phencyclidine-Related Disorder Not Otherwise Specified.   Patients
with this disorder have symptoms associated with the use of phencyclidine (or
related substances) that cannot be classified as any specific Phencyclidine-Related
Disorder.

Sedative-, Hypnotic-, or Anxiolytic-Related Disorder

292.89   Sedative, Hypnotic, or Anxiolytic Intoxication.   Patients with this
disorder have recently used a sedative, hypnotic, or anxiolytic and have clinically
significant maladaptive behavioral or psychological changes developing during, or
shortly after the ingestion (e.g., inappropriate sexual or aggressive behavior, mood
lability, impaired judgment, and impaired social or occupational functioning). The
patient also has at least one of the following signs.

1. Slurred speech
2. Incoordination
3. Unsteady gait
4. Nystagmus
5. Impairment of attention and memory
6. Stupor or coma

> Stephanie is a 28-year-old woman who has been going out with a man who is ver-
> bally abusive to her. Two nights ago she got into an argument with him that esca-
> lated to the point that he abruptly left her apartment yelling that he never wanted to
> see her again. Stephanie began crying and called a friend for consolation. The friend

told her, "I never could understand what you saw in that man. You're better off getting rid of him. If he left me, I'd celebrate." Her friend's support didn't make Stephanie feel much better.

As the evening wore on she became more and more depressed and began to feel suicidal. Finally, she took a handful of sleeping pills that her roommate kept in the medicine cabinct. Twenty minutes after she took the pills she became frightened and called her boyfriend to tell him. He rushed over to the apartment, arriving approximately 15 minutes later. Stephanie was lying asleep on her bed. He shook her until she woke and tried to get her to stand and walk. Stephanie awoke and tried to stand. She had poor coordination and was unable to walk straight. Her speech was slurred when she replied to his questions. Her boyfriend took her to the emergency room of the local hospital and stayed with her through the night.

292.0   Sedative, Hypnotic, or Anxiolytic Withdrawal.   Patients with this disorder have stopped (or reduced) use of a sedative, hypnotic, or anxiolytic after prolonged and heavy use. At least two of the following have developed within several hours to days after stopping. (Specify if there are perceptual disturbances.)

1. Autonomic hyperactivity (e.g., sweating or pulse greater than 100)
2. Increased hand tremor
3. Insomnia
4. Nausea or vomiting
5. Transient visual, tactile, or auditory hallucinations or illusions
6. Psychomotor agitation
7. Anxiety
8. Grand mal seizures

Caroline is a 46-year-old woman who has had chronic difficulty sleeping. Several months ago she visited a physician who prescribed short-acting barbiturates to help her sleep. Caroline initially took the medication before bed as prescribed. After 2 or 3 months she found that the prescribed dose was no longer sufficient for sleep. She asked her physician for additional medication but he refused to increase the prescription and instead suggested that she decrease the medication and eventually stop it. Caroline responded by seeing another physician for a prescription.

The amount of barbiturates she took for sleep gradually increased over the next few months. She began to experience difficulty concentrating on her work in the afternoons. Eventually she ran low on medication and had difficulty getting another prescription. One night she was forced to take less than half of her usual dose. The medication had little effect and she was unable to sleep. Late the next morning she felt anxious, nauseated, and began experiencing a moderate hand tremor. She went to the local emergency room for treatment where she was given a diagnosis of barbiturate withdrawal.

292.9   Sedative-, Hypnotic-, or Anxiolytic-Related Disorder Not Otherwise Specified.   Patients with this disorder have symptoms associated with the use of a sedative, hypnotic, or anxiolytic that cannot be classified as any specific Sedative-, Hypnotic-, or Anxiolytic-Related Disorder.

Other (or Unknown) Substance Use Disorder

292.89   Other (or Unknown) Substance Intoxication.   Patients with this disorder have an intoxication syndrome that is caused by a recently used substance that is not one of the 11 commonly abused classes of substances listed above or that is unknown. The signs and symptoms of this intoxication syndrome vary depending on the substance.

> Brad is a 17-year-old male who was rushed to the hospital by his friends when he became disoriented and confused after smoking something he bought from an acquaintance on the street corner. A physical examination revealed mild hypertension of 160/95 and a tachycardia of 105. Urine and blood tests for common abused substances were negative for cocaine, phencyclidine, opioids, alcohol, sedatives, and amphetamines. Brad's friends did not know what he had smoked but described it as a brown, sticky substance with some crystals. Brad's symptoms cleared after 3 or 4 hours and he was released from the hospital. The final diagnosis was Unknown Substance Intoxication.

292.0   Other (or Unknown) Substance Withdrawal.   Patients with this disorder have a withdrawal syndrome that is caused by cessation or reduction of use of a substance that is not one of the 11 commonly abused classes of substances listed above or that is unknown. The signs and symptoms of this withdrawal syndrome vary depending on the substance.

292.9   Other (or Unknown) Substance-Related Disorder Not Otherwise Specified.   Patients with this disorder have symptoms associated with the use of other (or unknown) substances that cannot be classified as any specific Substance Use Disorder.

Substance-Induced Psychiatric Syndromes

Every class of abused substance, except nicotine, has the capacity to produce or mimic symptoms of other psychiatric disorders (e.g., Delirium; Dementia; and Amnestic, Psychotic, Mood, Anxiety, Sex, and Sleep Disorders) during intoxication or withdrawal. Several substances (e.g., alcohol, inhalants, sedatives, other substances) have the capacity to produce Dementia or Amnestic Disorder that persists after the acute effects of the intoxication or withdrawal have disappeared.

The primary organization of DSM-IV is phenomenological. Therefore, these syndromes are listed in this section for convenience but the full criteria for their diagnosis and clinical vignettes are presented in the diagnostic group to which they are phenomenologically similar. For example, the criteria and clinical vignette for a Substance-Induced Psychotic Disorder would appear in the chapter on Schizophrenia and Other Psychotic Disorders. In each case the diagnosis should specify whether the syndrome occurs during intoxication or withdrawal. The names of specific Substance-Induced Psychiatric Syndromes are constructed as follows:

Code	Substance	Psychiatric Syndrome	Onset Condition
291.8	Alcohol-Induced	Anxiety Disorder	with onset during withdrawal
	(291.8 Alcohol-Induced Anxiety Disorder with onset during withdrawal)		
292.81	Inhalant-Induced	Delirium	with onset during intoxication
	(292.81 Inhalant-Induced Delirium with onset during intoxication)		

Table 5–4 presents a list of nine psychiatric syndromes, the clinical criteria for their diagnosis, the substances that may induce the syndrome, and the appropriate DSM-IV codes. Eight psychiatric syndromes have one DSM-IV code if they are alcohol-induced and a second code for all of the remaining substances that may induce the syndrome. Sleep Disorder has a single DSM-IV code that is used for all sleep-inducing substances. The clinical criteria included in the table are a synopsis of the complete criteria set for each Substance-Induced Disorder and represent the salient components of the criteria set. The following two criteria are common to all of the diagnoses in Table 5–4.

1. There is evidence from the history, physical examination, or laboratory findings of substance intoxication or withdrawal, and the symptoms fulfilling the clinical criteria developed during or within a month of significant substance intoxication or withdrawal.
2. The disturbance is not better accounted for by a psychiatric disorder that is not substance-induced.

Necessary Clinical Information

* Identity of substance(s) used

* History of substance(s) used

* History of substance use emergencies and treatment

* Cognitive impairment (confusion, disorientation, impaired attention, rambling thought, drowsiness, etc.)

Table 5–4   Substance-induced psychiatric syndromes

Psychiatric syndrome	Clinical criteria	Inducing substances	DSM-IV codes
Delirium	A disturbance of consciousness and cognition that develops over a short period of time (hours to days), fluctuates during the day, and is not better explained by a preexisting, established or evolving dementia	Alcohol Amphetamine; cannabis; cocaine; hallucinogen; inhalant; opioid; phencyclidine; sedative, hypnotic, anxiolytic; other	291.0 292.81
Persisting dementia	Memory impairment and one of the following: aphasia, apraxia, agnosia, or disturbance in executive functioning. Does not only occur during delirium.	Alcohol Inhalant; sedative, hypnotic, anxiolytic; other	291.2 292.82
Persisting amnestic disorder	Memory impairment manifested by inability to learn new or recall old information. Does not only occur during delirium or dementia.	Alcohol Sedative, hypnotic, anxiolytic; other	291.1 292.83
Psychotic disorder with delusions	Prominent delusions. Does not only occur during delirium or dementia.	Alcohol Amphetamine; cannabis; cocaine; hallucinogens; inhalant; opioid; phencyclidine; sedative, hypnotic, anxiolytic; other	291.5 292.11
Psychotic disorder with hallucinations	Prominent hallucinations. Does not only occur during delirium or dementia.	Alcohol Amphetamine; cocaine; hallucinogen; inhalant; opioid; phencyclidine; sedative, hypnotic, anxiolytic; other	291.3 292.12

Table 5–4 Substance-induced psychiatric syndromes *(continued)*			
Psychiatric syndrome	Clinical criteria	**Inducing substances**	**DSM-IV codes**
Mood disorder	A disturbance in mood characterized by either (or both) of the follow-ing: 1) depressed mood or diminished interest and pleasure in activities; or 2) elevated, expansive or irritable mood. Does not only occur during delirium.	Alcohol Amphetamine; cocaine; hallucinogen; inhalant; opioid; phencyclidine; sedative, hypnotic, anxiolytic; other	291.8 292.84
Anxiety disorder	Prominent anxiety, panic attacks, obsessions, or compulsions. Does not only occur during deliri-um or dementia.	Alcohol Amphetamine; caffeine; cannabis; cocaine; hallucino-gen; inhalant; phencyclidine; sedative, hypnotic, anxiolytic; other	291.8 292.89
Sexual dysfunction	Clinically significant sexual dysfunction	Alcohol Amphetamine; cocaine; opioid; sedative, hyp-notic, anxiolytic; other	291.8 292.89
Sleep disorder	A prominent disturbance in sleep	Alcohol Amphetamine; caffeine; cocaine; opioid; seda-tive, hypnotic, anxio-lytic; other	291.8 292.89

- Physiological signs (tachycardia, hypertension, hypotension, hyperpyrexia, pupillary dilatation or constriction, etc.)

- Neurological signs (slurred speech, incoordination, ataxia, dystonia, tremor, seizure, etc.)

- Psychomotor agitation or retardation

- Changes in mood, perception, and thought

- Changes in personality, mood, anxiety

- Urine drug screening, blood alcohol level

- Changes in social or family life
- Current and past legal problems

Making a Diagnosis

The diagnosis of Substance-Related Disorder requires the identification of the abused substance(s) and the description of its current pattern of use. There are three ways to identify the abused substance: 1) the patient specifies the substance(s); 2) the substance(s) is detected in the patient's urine or blood; 3) the patient has characteristic physiological, behavioral, or psychological signs and symptoms of intoxication or withdrawal from the substance(s).

1. Does the patient admit to using a substance?

If the patient admits to using a substance, the clinician's job is simplified. Generally, it is best to assume that the patient is telling the truth and also knows what drugs he or she has been using, unless there is a compelling reason not to believe him. The next step is to determine which of the following three diagnostic categories best describes the patient's current substance use: 1) dependence or abuse, 2) intoxication or withdrawal, or 3) a substance-induced psychiatric syndrome. If the patient denies using drugs the task of diagnosis is more difficult but not impossible.

2. Does the patient have abnormal physiological signs or symptoms?

Almost all intoxication and withdrawal syndromes are accompanied by abnormal physiological signs or symptoms. These abnormalities include increases or decreases in normal autonomic physiological functions such as heart rate, temperature, respiration, production of mucous, frequency of urination and bowel movements, eye movement, pupillary reactivity and size, sweating, coordination, and blood pressure. The presence of these physiological changes suggests that the patient may be in a state of active intoxication or withdrawal. The absence of at least one or two abnormal autonomic physiological signs or symptoms usually, but not always, excludes the diagnosis of current substance intoxication or withdrawal.

3. Does the patient have a history of substance abuse?

If the patient admits to a history of substance abuse the likelihood that the patient's current symptoms can be explained by substance intoxication or withdrawal is much higher.

4. Has the patient experienced recent related legal problems?

Legal difficulties related to the patient's behavior while intoxicated are a frequent consequence of substance abuse. These may include arrests for disorderly conduct or driving while intoxicated. Patient's who are reluctant to admit significant substance use may acknowledge recent legal difficulties. Further questioning may uncover the associated substance abuse.

5. Does the patient have maladaptive behavioral or psychological changes?

There are two types of behavior associated with substance use: 1) behavior changes that are caused by the physiological effects of the substance, and 2) behavior that is associated with obtaining and using substances. Recent maladaptive behavioral or psychological changes such as those listed in Tables 5–2 and 5–4 are often an early clue to substance intoxication. Several of these changes such as agitation, belligerence, and impaired judgment tend to overlap from one substance class to another. Therefore, the change in personality or behavior is often as important or more important than the type of behavior.

The behavioral and psychological changes in substance withdrawal are usually restricted to anxiety or dysphoric mood, accompanied by physiological or neurological changes. The behavior associated with obtaining and using substances may also help in the diagnosis. Individuals who abuse substances often fail to fulfill their educational, family, and occupational obligations. They may spend a considerable amount of time trying to obtain drugs (i.e., drug-seeking behavior). Continued substance use may also exacerbate previous interpersonal problems or stimulate new arguments about drug use.

Common Problems in Making a Diagnosis

The problems that arise in the diagnosis of Substance-Related Disorders are similar to those of other diagnostic categories. There are three main problems.

1. The patient may come close to fulfilling the criteria for the diagnosis yet not actually fulfill it. The clinician must weigh the clinical information and decide whether the evidence is sufficient to make a working diagnosis despite the uncertainty.
2. The patient may exhibit signs and symptoms from several diagnoses.
3. The patient may have unusual signs and symptoms that do not normally occur in typical intoxication or withdrawal syndromes.

Patients Who Almost Fulfill the Diagnostic Criteria

The diagnosis of Substance-Related Disorder generally depends on the identification of a specific substance that is being abused, as well as a characteristic pattern of behavioral, psychological, and physiological signs and symptoms. The most obvious problems in diagnosis occur when some of the information necessary to fulfill the criteria for a specific diagnosis is missing. Either the abused drug cannot be identified or some of the necessary signs and symptoms are not present.

Example 1

Marshall, an agitated 17-year-old male, is brought to a hospital emergency room having visual hallucinations. The patient has some pupillary dilation and a mild tremor. He is awake, alert, and fearful that he is going crazy. His friends report that the symptoms occurred suddenly during the afternoon. They think he swallowed something 2 or 3 hours before the symptoms started but do not know what the substance was. Urine and blood toxicology did not show evidence of any abused substance. The patient has no previous history of psychotic behavior. What is Marshall's diagnosis(es)?

This is a common patient presentation in an urban hospital emergency room. The patient has a psychotic disorder. The important diagnostic question is whether the psychosis was caused by an abused substance. The patient's friends report that they think he took some type of substance a few hours before the psychosis developed. It is easy to assume that they are correct and that the patient's psychosis is due to the substance. However, there are other possibilities. The patient's friends may be wrong and he may not have ingested anything. On the other hand, he may have taken an aspirin. Because there were no traces of drugs in the urine or blood there is no objective evidence that he took a drug.

There is other evidence suggesting that the patient's psychosis is substance-induced. Visual hallucinations are more likely to occur in an organic-induced psychosis than a nonorganic psychosis. In addition, the patient has abnormal physiological signs and no previous history of psychotic behavior. Therefore, it is reasonable to make a working diagnosis of Hallucinogen Intoxication. If the patient has substance-induced psychosis, the symptoms should resolve over a day or two as the substance is metabolized and eliminated from the patient's body.

In this case, the physician is making a judgment that Hallucinogen Intoxication is the most likely diagnosis based on the patient's clinical signs and symptoms despite the absence of an identified substance. If this is unacceptable, an alternative diagnosis would be Brief Psychotic Disorder.

Example 2

Stacy is a 33-year-old woman who is applying for a job at a fast-food restaurant. She is mildly hypervigilant, tense, irritable, and easily offended. Her physical examination is normal with the exception of a blood pressure of 165/95. A routine urine screen for drugs indicates the presence of trace amounts of cocaine. What is Stacy's diagnosis(es)?

In this case the patient has maladaptive behavior and psychological symptoms consistent with Cocaine Intoxication. She also has objective evidence of cocaine in her urine. Despite this, she does not completely fulfill the criteria for Cocaine Intoxication because she has only one abnormal physiological sign (i.e., hypertension).

The clinician could probe further for another general physiological sign such as nausea, perspiration, or muscle weakness to fulfill the criteria. These signs are usually subjective and can often be elicited in patients who have no Substance-Related Disorder. However, the presence of cocaine in the patient's urine in addition to the other physiological and behavioral signs and symptoms should be sufficient to justify a diagnosis of Cocaine Intoxication even though the complete criteria are not fulfilled.

Patients Who Fulfill the Criteria for More Than One Substance-Related Disorder

Unfortunately, the signs and symptoms of the various intoxication and withdrawal syndromes are not pathognomonic. There is considerable overlap between the various disorders. For example, hypertension, incoordination, and insomnia may be seen in several of the syndromes. This may produce a problem if a patient displays a confusing set of signs and symptoms that fulfill the criteria for more than one substance intoxication or withdrawal syndrome. Under these circumstances it is almost impossible to make a complete substance-related diagnosis without the identification of specific drugs in the patient's urine or blood.

Example 3

Kevin is a 23-year-old man who is a known drug abuser. One night, while visiting a friend, he was given a sample of a new batch of drugs and injected it intravenously. He rapidly became confused, drowsy, and his breathing slowed markedly. After a few minutes he became unresponsive. His friend called the paramedics who arrived to find Kevin with dilated pupils, no heartbeat, and turning blue from anoxia. He died a few minutes later despite their attempts at resuscitation. At autopsy his blood was found to contain heroin and cocaine. What is Kevin's diagnosis(es)?

Addicts frequently take more than one drug at the same time to experience the combined effects of the drugs. An intravenous injection of a mixture of heroin and cocaine (or an amphetamine) is a frequent, potentially lethal combination called a "speedball." Intoxication with both heroin and cocaine may produce respiratory depression and coma. Cocaine produces a pupillary dilation and opioids normally produce pupillary constriction. However, in large doses opioids can produce pupillary dilation due to the anoxia from the overdose. This patient's diagnosis is Cocaine Intoxication and Opioid Intoxication.

Example 4

Ann is a 27-year-old woman who is in an outpatient drug treatment program for her polydrug abuse. The program requires weekly urine screening for drugs. One day she arrived for a group therapy session and seemed depressed. She complained of feeling tired and sleeping poorly. Her mood was labile and she seemed to have mildly impaired coordination. The group members immediately accused her of using drugs. She denied taking drugs and explained that she was tired from working all night. A toxicology screen detected diazepam and traces of cocaine in her urine. What is Ann's diagnosis(es)?

Benzodiazepines such as diazepam are commonly used by addicts to treat the effects of cocaine withdrawal. In this case, Ann has a dysphoric mood, fatigue, and insomnia that fulfill the criteria for Cocaine Withdrawal. She has taken diazepam to counteract these feelings. Her labile mood and impaired coordination fulfill the criteria for a diagnosis of Sedative, Hypnotic, and Anxiolytic Intoxication.

Substance-Related Disorders That Mimic Other Disorders

Each class of abused substances in the Substance-Related Disorders group contains diagnoses for substance-induced syndromes that mimic other psychiatric disorders (e.g., anxiety, mood, psychotic). The diagnosis of these syndromes can be a challenge because their symptoms are phenomenologically identical to those of similar non-substance-induced disorders. The clinician must decide whether the syndrome is etiologically related to an abused substance, independent of a substance, or comorbid with a substance intoxication.

Example 5

Derek is a 21-year-old man who was admitted in acutely psychotic condition to a psychiatric hospital. He has auditory hallucinations and is extremely paranoid with delusions that the devil is after him. He has no previous psychiatric history. His parents report that Derek's friends told them that he smoked some type of cigarette several days before he became psychotic. The parents thought that the friend said the cigarettes were musty or dusted. Derek's urine and blood contained no detectable drugs. What diagnosis(es), if any, should Derek receive?

Derek's differential diagnosis includes a substance-induced psychosis and a Brief Psychotic Disorder. Hallucinogens, amphetamine, cocaine, and phencyclidine can produce psychosis. Hallucinogen psychosis generally abates within 1–2 days after the drug has been metabolized. Amphetamine or cocaine can also produce a psychosis during intoxication. However, traces of these drugs should be found in the patient's blood or urine while the patient is psychotic. Phencyclidine can produce an immediate psychosis during intoxication and a late-occurring psychosis several days after the initial intoxication. There may or may not be phencyclidine in the patient's blood or urine at that time.

The term "angel dust" is a common name for phencyclidine. It is often sprinkled on marijuana or parsley flakes. The resulting dusted leaf is smoked to inhale the phencyclidine. Because there was no phencyclidine found in the patient's blood or urine, the diagnosis is uncertain. One approach is to make a working diagnosis of Phencyclidine Psychotic Disorder, with delusions and Brief Psychotic Disorder. A definitive diagnosis may depend on the patient's report of drug use after the psychotic episode resolves. Subsequent episodes without evidence of drug use would reinforce the diagnosis of Brief Psychotic Disorder.

Precedence of Diagnosis

The precedence of diagnosis for all Substance-Related Disorders is the same. First, if the patient's signs and symptoms can be accounted for by a general medical condition or another mental disorder, these take precedence over the diagnosis of Substance-Related Disorder. Presumably this could only occur if a patient was known to have used a specific substance and now has symptoms produced by a general medical condition or mental illness that mimic the substance symptoms. For example, a patient that has used cocaine might present with agitation and nausea secondary to a panic attack. Second, any specific Substance-Related Disorder takes precedence over the Substance Use Disorder Not Otherwise Specified for that class of substance. For example, if the patient meets the criteria for Cocaine Intoxication, this diagnosis will always take precedence over Cocaine Use Disorder Not Otherwise Specified.

Discussion of Clinical Vignettes

Vignette 1: Money Is No Object

Stephen is a young physician who worked hard and sacrificed to become a surgeon. The financial stress he felt from his loans and family obligations led him to make several risky financial investments, which initially proved lucrative and helped stabilize his financial situation. His first years of practice were also profitable and provided him with a sense of financial security. However, this success was also accompanied by entry into a new life style that required more and more money and exposed him to drugs.

The first signs of Stephen's drug abuse were changes in his personality including irritability, euphoria, increased interpersonal sensitivity, anger, and erratic behavior in the operating room. The behavior changes were accompanied by physiological signs including weight loss and vomiting. These symptoms fulfill part of the criteria for Cocaine Intoxication. Stephen's other symptoms, including depression accompanied by insomnia and vivid, unpleasant dreams fulfill part of the criteria for Cocaine Withdrawal.

The likely clinical scenario is a combination of cocaine abuse, punctuated with periods of abstinence, leading to depression and withdrawal. However, the definitive diagnosis of Substance-Related Disorder requires confirmation of the abused substance in addition to the fulfillment of the behavioral and physiological criteria. Stephen must directly acknowledge that he uses cocaine or the drug must be detected in a chemical test of his urine.

Vignette 2: Doctor, I'm Still Anxious

Christie is a 32-year-old woman who is anxious and depressed. She originally saw her physician with complaints of stomach discomfort and pain. He diagnosed a nervous stomach and prescribed diazepam. The tranquilizer decreased her anxiety but it returned when she tried to stop the medication. After a few months her anxiety began to increase again as she became tolerant to the prescribed dose. She responded by taking more medication and asking the physician to prescribe a higher dose. He increased the dose once and refused to do so again when she became tolerant to the new dose. Christie responded by going from doctor to doctor in an attempt to obtain diazepam.

There is no indication that she experienced any of the symptoms of intoxication or withdrawal during this period other than some breakthrough anxiety when she tried to stop the medication, persistent drowsiness, and mild impairment in coordination. These do not fulfill the criteria for the diagnoses of Sedative, Hypnotic, or Anxiolytic Intoxication or Abuse.

Her continued driving while she was experiencing drowsiness and impaired coordination does fulfill the criteria for Substance Abuse. However, her increasing tolerance for the diazepam, the amount of time she spent in trying to obtain the drug, and her unsuccessful efforts to cut down on the use of the medication, fulfill the criteria for the diagnosis of Substance Dependence. This diagnosis takes precedence over the diagnosis of Substance Abuse.

Key Diagnostic Points

- Substance-induced (i.e., organic) psychiatric syndromes meeting the criteria for other diagnostic categories, such as major depression, are included in those categories rather than in the Substance-Related Disorders category.

- The diagnosis of a specific substance dependence requires evidence of either substance tolerance or withdrawal.

- The two main categories of criteria used in the diagnosis of substance dependence relate to the physiological effects of the substance and the behavioral problems associated with the use of the substance.

- The signs and symptoms of Alcohol Intoxication and Alcohol Withdrawal are identical to those of Sedative, Hypnotic, or Anxiolytic Intoxication and Sedative, Hypnotic, or Anxiolytic Withdrawal.

- The perceptual changes in Hallucinogen Intoxication occur while the patient is in a state of full wakefulness and alertness.

- Nystagmus, hypertension, and numbness or diminished responsiveness to pain are the hallmarks of Phencyclidine Intoxication.

- Pupillary dilation is a sign of intoxication with some central nervous system stimulants (amphetamine, cocaine, hallucinogens) and a sign of withdrawal with some central nervous system depressants (opioids).

- Psychopathology occurring within 1 month after substance use may be etiologically related to the substance use.

Common Questions in Making a Diagnosis

1. Oscar is a 27-year-old successful businessman who complains of having mood swings, on and off, for the last several weeks. Sometimes he feels alert and full of energy. He currently feels depressed and reports problems with sleeping. When he does sleep, he often has unpleasant dreams. He also reports a weight loss of approximately 7 pounds over the last 3 months and denies dieting. The patient's physical examination is normal except for some mild hypertension. When he is asked if he takes drugs he is evasive and reluctant to talk further. What is Oscar's diagnosis(es)?

   Answer: Oscar's symptoms include a dysphoric mood, unpleasant dreams, insomnia, weight loss, and mild hypertension. He fulfills the psychological and physiological criteria for Cocaine Withdrawal. His clinical presentation is consistent with periods of Cocaine Intoxication followed by Cocaine Withdrawal. Neither diagnosis can be made definitively unless he acknowledges that he has been using cocaine or there is evidence of cocaine in a toxicology screen of his urine.

2. Vincent is a 33-year-old man who has been arrested three times in the last year for driving while intoxicated. His wife tells him that he drinks too much but he says he can stop any time. What is Vincent's diagnosis(es)?

   Answer: Recurrent substance-related legal problems fulfills the criteria for the diagnosis of Alcohol Abuse.

Schizophrenia and Other Psychotic Disorders

Clinical Vignettes

Vignette 1: It's a Conspiracy

Johannes is a 38-year-old machinist who escaped from East Germany at the age of 26, leaving a wife and small daughter behind. He planned to smuggle them out to freedom after he immigrated to the United States and made enough money to pay for their escape. During his flight Johannes was shot in the leg by communist border guards and subsequently taken to a hospital in West Germany. After several months of treatment, he was discharged with a permanent limp.

He immediately tried to get in touch with his wife and daughter through the anti-Communist underground but discovered that his wife had been arrested and his daughter had been given to another family to raise. Feeling helpless, he proceeded with his plan to immigrate to the United States and moved to Chicago. When he arrived he began looking for work as a skilled machinist with the hope of making enough money to return to Europe and bribe Communist officials to free his wife and child.

Johannes was not successful in finding work as a machinist in the United States. Instead, he could only find work as a laborer at unskilled, menial jobs. He was alone and despaired of ever seeing his wife or child again. He blamed the Communists for his problems and began joining anti-Communist groups and attending their meetings. Gradually, his suspicion and anxiety grew that there were other forces involved in his inability to achieve his wife and child's freedom. He began reading right-wing, anti-Catholic, and anti-Semitic literature sold by various hate groups. Soon he became convinced that there was a conspiracy of communists, rabbis, and priests who controlled the government and kept him from reuniting with his family.

Once Johannes made this discovery, his anxiety diminished. He began to feel that he had an obligation or mission to warn people about the conspiracy. To fulfill this mission he constructed a set of sandwich-board signs proclaiming "Communism is treason, priests are traitors, and Communism is rabbinish." Johannes wore these signs as he peddled hate literature to people on the streets of Chicago. Passersby stopped to argue with him but he remained steadfast in his convictions, eventually becoming agitated if they continued to argue and accusing them of being members of the conspiracy. His small apartment was gradually filled from floor to ceiling with hate literature, leaving only a narrow path from the living room to the kitchen and his tiny bedroom. He made enough money selling his literature to lead a meager, isolated existence and feed himself.

Johannes was arrested once for loitering and interviewed by a court psychiatrist. He denied any history of hallucinations or hospitalizations for psychiatric problems. There was no evidence of negative symptoms, disorganized speech, or disorganized or catatonic behavior. A physical examination revealed no underlying medical disorder or evidence of substance abuse. The psychiatrist reported that Johannes' affect was restricted but not flat. When the psychiatrist tried to ask Johannes why he sold hate literature, he first tried to explain his conspiracy theories. When the psychiatrist seemed unconvinced, Johannes became more guarded and refused to talk further. The psychiatrist concluded that there was no indication that he was a danger to himself or others and therefore could not be involuntarily hospitalized.

Vignette 2: He Killed My Friend

The police are summoned to an apartment by an agitated young woman named Alice. When they enter they see Tom, a 28-year-old man, lying unconscious on the floor with a bloody knife next to him. He has a deep laceration in his abdomen and is bleeding profusely. Lying near him is a dead 23-year-old woman who has multiple stab wounds in her chest and abdomen and is subsequently found to be 3 months pregnant. The floor and walls are covered with blood. Several empty beer bottles are scattered around the room. Alice tells the following story to the police.

She and her dead friend Pam visited Tom to buy some drugs earlier in the day. Although the two women used drugs casually, Tom had a history of heavy drug use and had been on a drug binge for the last couple of days. When they arrived, Tom was acting strange. He seemed nervous and repeatedly glanced around the hall and room before asking them to come in. He asked if they had been followed. Alice replied, "no," but the question made her feel uncomfortable.

Tom continued to talk about his concerns that someone or something was after him. After a few minutes he became calmer and the women asked to buy some drugs. Tom told them to sit down and wait for him as he disappeared into a back room. In a few minutes he reappeared with a container of a ground-up leafy substance that looked like marijuana. He asked the two women if they wanted to try some of the drug before they bought it. They answered yes and Tom rolled two cigarettes, handed one to the women, and lit one for himself.

The three of them sat quietly smoking the drug for several minutes. Alice reported that she and her friend began to feel "spaced-out." Tom became more agitated. His eyes seemed to jump back and forth as he glanced around the room. He tried to talk but his words were slurred. When he got up he had difficulty walking, staggering as if he was drunk. He walked past them and stumbled and hitting his leg hard on the edge of the coffee table. A knife on the table clattered off onto the floor. Alice looked down and saw that Tom had a deep cut on his leg that was bleeding. She was surprised that he didn't seem to feel any pain.

Tom looked wildly around the room and began yelling about trying to stop the devil from talking to him. The women became frightened and got up to leave. Suddenly Tom picked up the knife that had fallen on the floor and began to yell at Pam. "You're the devil. Stop looking at me. Stop talking." He ran toward her and stabbed her repeatedly with the knife. Pam's blood splattered on Alice's blouse as she ran out of the room screaming. She ran to a nearby apartment and called the police.

The paramedics arrived shortly after the police and took Tom to the hospital where the abdominal laceration was sutured. His physical examination revealed horizontal nystagmus and a blood pressure of 170/90. Tom remained semistuporous for the next 2 days. When he regained consciousness a psychiatrist interviewed him. During the session with the psychiatrist Tom was calm and cooperative. He denied any memory of the events surrounding his injury and Pam's murder and stated that he could not have killed her. He also denied any history of previous psychiatric problems or hospitalizations.

Core Concept of the Diagnostic Group

The core concept of the Schizophrenia and Other Psychotic Disorders group is the presence of one or more of the following symptoms: a significant distortion in the perception of reality; an impairment in the capacity to reason, speak, and behave rationally or spontaneously; and an impairment in the capacity to respond spontaneously with appropriate affect and motivation. These distortions occur in the absence of an impairment of consciousness or memory.

Criteria Applicable to Multiple Disorders

The Schizophrenia and Other Psychotic Disorders group, similar to most diagnostic categories in the DSM-IV, contains basic criteria sets that apply to some or all of the diagnoses in the group. There are three sets of basic criteria. The first set applies to all of the disorders in the group and essentially defines the requirements for the core concept of psychosis. The second set of criteria defines the attributes that are common to all of the schizophrenic disorders. A third set of basic criteria contains requirements about the etiology, social impairment, and diagnostic precedence, that apply to many, but not all, of the disorders in the diagnostic group. The criteria in these three sets commonly overlap. For example, the common criteria set for Schizophrenia includes the main criterion for psychosis and general criteria.

Main Criterion for Psychosis

All of the illnesses in the Schizophrenia and Other Psychotic Disorders group include in their diagnostic criteria set the requirement for one or more of the following psychotic symptoms: delusions, hallucinations, or disorganized speech and thought. These criteria define the psychological concept of psychosis in DSM-IV, but imply nothing about the etiology of the disorder nor its consequences. The remaining criteria for each diagnosis differentiate the disorders according to the phenomenology of the psychotic symptoms and their duration, etiology, and associated symptoms.

Common Criteria Set for Schizophrenia

Schizophrenia is a group of Psychotic Disorders that are phenomenologically distinct, yet share certain common features. The common criteria set for the diagnosis of Schizophrenia is listed in DSM-IV separately from the criteria for the individual schizophrenia subtypes. The diagnosis of a specific schizophrenic subtype requires that the patient meet the common criteria and additional criteria that distinguish the specific subtype from each other. The common criteria set for Schizophrenia contains six parts.

A. *Characteristic symptoms:*   Two (or more) of the following, each present for a significant portion of time during a 1-month period (or less if successfully treated):

    (1)   delusions
    (2)   hallucinations
    (3)   disorganized speech (e.g., frequent derailment or incoherence)
    (4)   grossly disorganized or catatonic behavior
    (5)   negative symptoms, i.e., affective flattening, alogia, or avolition

    Note: Only one Criterion A symptom is required if delusions are bizarre or hallucinations consist of a voice keeping up a running commentary on the person's behavior or thoughts, or two or more voices conversing with each other.

B. *Social/occupational dysfunction:*   For a significant portion of the time since the onset of the disturbance, one or more major areas of functioning such as work, interpersonal relations, or self-care are markedly below the level achieved prior to the onset (or when the onset is in childhood or adolescence, failure to achieve expected level of interpersonal, academic, or occupational achievement).

C. *Duration:* Continuous signs of the disturbance persist for at least 6 months. This 6-month period must include at least 1 month of symptoms (or less if successfully treated) that meet Criterion A (i.e., active-phase symptoms) and may include periods of prodromal or residual symptoms. During these prodromal or residual periods, the signs of the disturbance may be manifested by only negative symptoms or two or more symptoms listed in Criterion A present in an attenuated form (e.g., odd beliefs, unusual perceptual experiences).

D. *Schizoaffective and Mood Disorder exclusion:* Schizoaffective Disorder and Mood Disorder With Psychotic Features have been ruled out because either: (1) no Major Depressive, Manic, or Mixed Episodes have occurred concurrently with the active-phase symptoms; or (2) if mood episodes have occurred during active-phase symptoms, their total duration has been brief relative to the duration of the active and residual periods.

E. *Substance/general medical condition exclusion:* The disturbance is not due to the direct physiological effects of a substance (e.g., a drug of abuse, a medication) or a general medical condition.

F. *Relationship to a Pervasive Developmental Disorder:* If there is a history of Autistic Disorder or another Pervasive Developmental Disorder, the additional diagnosis of Schizophrenia is made only if prominent delusions or hallucinations are also present for at least a month (or less if successfully treated).

The cardinal features of Schizophrenia can be succinctly described as the presence of persistent core psychotic, prodromal, or residual symptoms associated with significant deterioration of previous social and occupational functioning without evidence of a Mood Disorder or organic etiology. The course of the illness should be described according to the following classification scheme.

Episodic With Interepisode Residual Symptoms. The course is characterized by episodes in which Criterion A for Schizophrenia is met and there are clinically significant residual symptoms between episodes (specify if prominent negative symptoms are present).

Episodic With no Interepisode Residual Symptoms. The course is characterized by episodes in which Criterion A for Schizophrenia is met and there are no clinically significant residual symptoms between episodes.

Continuous. The characteristic symptoms of Criterion A for Schizophrenia are met throughout all (or most) of the course (specify if prominent negative symptoms).

Single Episode, in Partial Remission. There is a single episode in which Criterion A for Schizophrenia is met and clinically significant residual symptoms remain (specify if prominent negative symptoms are present)

Single Episode, in Full Remission. There is a single episode in which Criterion A for Schizophrenia is met and no clinically significant residual symptoms remain.

Other or Unspecified Pattern

General Criteria

The general criteria for the Schizophrenia and Other Psychotic Disorders group are similar in content to those for many other diagnostic groups. Like other general criteria in DSM-IV, they apply to many but not all of the diagnoses in the group. There are two general criteria.

1. The disorder is not due to an abused substance or a known nonpsychiatric medical disorder. This criterion applies to all diagnoses in the Schizophrenia and Other Psychotic Disorders group except Substance-Induced Psychotic Disorders and Psychotic Disorder Due to a General Medical Condition, which by definition have an identified organic etiology.
2. The symptoms associated with the disorder are not better accounted for by another psychiatric disorder. This criterion applies to many of the diagnoses in the group. For example, a patient who has nonbizarre delusions cannot receive a diagnosis of a Delusional Disorder if he has ever met Criterion A for Schizophrenia described below. Similarly, the diagnosis of Schizophrenia, Schizophreniform Disorder, Delusional Disorder, or Brief Psychotic Disorder cannot be made if the patient meets the criteria for a specific Mood Disorder or has mood episodes of significant duration with respect to the psychotic symptoms.
   There are two reasons for these exclusion criterion. First, they serve as a reminder to the clinician that although the patient's clinical presentation at any specific point in time may fulfill the criteria for the diagnosis of a disturbance, such as Brief Psychotic Disorder, this may mask the existence of a more pervasive disorder such as Schizophrenia or another type of disorder such as a Mood Disorder. Second, there is an established hierarchy or precedence of diagnosis in the Schizophrenia and Other Psychotic Disorders group that guides the clinician in making a diagnosis in those cases in which the patient displays symptoms that fulfill the criteria for more than one diagnosis. This hierarchy is presented in more detail in the section on the Precedence of Diagnosis below.

Definitions

catalepsy   A condition of diminished responsiveness and continually maintained immobile position

catatonia   A psychotic syndrome that is characterized by muscular rigidity and a lack of response to outside stimuli. Catatonic patients may also have periods of acute agitation.

delusion   A falsely held belief that cannot be influenced or corrected by reason or contradictory evidence. Delusions are often characterized as nonbizarre or bizarre. Nonbizarre delusions involve situations that could occur in everyday life, such as the belief that the patient is being followed, loved by an important person, or ill with a serious disease. Bizarre delusions involve fantastic situations that could never occur in reality. They include the patient's belief that he is possessed by Satan, influenced at a distance by alien creatures, or has the power to directly influence the minds of other people by mental telepathy.

echolalia   A repetition of a recently heard sound or phrase. Often the patient repeats the last words spoken by the interviewer.

disorganized behavior   Behavior that is not goal-directed or guided by any rational, preconceived plan, and may appear random, disconnected, or odd.

disorganized speech   Speech in which the patient's statements are not logically connected to each other and the content of the speech usually makes no sense. Loose associations, derailments, and incoherence are examples of disorganized speech and, presumably, disorganized thought.

hallucination   An organized sensory experience that is a product of the patient's mind and does not exist in the outside world. Hallucinations commonly exit in auditory and visual modalities and less commonly as tactile or gustatory experiences. Typically, patients with Schizophrenia experience auditory hallucinations consisting of a voice that command them to perform some act or comments on their thoughts and actions.

psychosis   A syndrome that includes one or more of the following symptoms: delusions; hallucinations; or disorganized speech, thought, or behavior. The thought disorders commonly include deficits in higher intellectual or executive functions such as the capacity to make and carry out detailed plans.

Synopses and Diagnostic Prototypes
of the Individual Disorders

The brief synopses in this section summarize the specific requirements or criteria that must be fulfilled for each of the diagnostic categories. Each synopsis includes a brief vignette that provides a clinical example of the diagnoses. Each vignette is a prototype in the sense that it represents a typical patient from a specific diagnostic category. The prototypes provide a more lifelike portrayal of the diagnosis than the criteria alone. They also provide a clinical baseline that can be used in the discussion of problems associated with the diagnosis of these disorders and as a standard for comparison even if they do not exhaust all the possibilities for the clinical presentation of a specific diagnosis. All of the Schizophrenia subtypes, with the exception of Residual Type, require that the patient fulfill the common criteria set for Schizophrenia, discussed above, in addition to other specific criteria that uniquely characterize each subtype.

295.30 Schizophrenia, Paranoid Type. A type of Schizophrenia in which the patient is preoccupied with delusions or auditory hallucinations and does not have flat or inappropriate affect, catatonic behavior, disorganized speech, or disorganized behavior.

> A 37-year-old woman works on the evening shift in the post office sorting mail. She began hearing voices making critical comments about her behavior approximately 6 years before and became concerned that someone was trying to influence her mind. At that time she worked as a secretary in a large company. Her work was considered good and she was respected, although people commented that she seemed aloof and somewhat isolated. She was successfully treated with neuroleptic medication that prevented the voices and decreased her concern about external influence of her mind. However, she never regained her former level of competency at work and eventually left her job as a secretary and sought employment at the post office.

295.10 Schizophrenia, Disorganized Type. A type of Schizophrenia in which disorganized speech, disorganized behavior, and flat or inappropriate affect are prominent, and there is no evidence of catatonia.

> A 31-year-old man has been unemployed for 10 years and lives on the streets. He is periodically hospitalized in a state hospital, moves into a halfway house, and eventually left to wander the streets. His speech is generally incoherent and his behavior is odd and disorganized. He displays little affect, except some agitation and periodic outbursts of angry yelling that seems inappropriate and bizarre. The patient spends most of his time picking through the garbage and adorning himself with various bits and pieces of clothes he finds. He responds to antipsychotic medication with a decrease in agitation, but his disorganized speech and loose associations persist and he continues to wander aimlessly.

295.20 Schizophrenia, Catatonic Type. A type of Schizophrenia in which the patient demonstrates two of the following:

1. Motoric immobility as evidenced by catalepsy (including waxy flexibility) or stupor
2. Excessive motor activity (that is apparently purposeless and not influenced by external stimuli)
3. Extreme negativism (an apparently motiveless resistance to all instructions or maintenance of a rigid posture against attempts to be moved) or mutism
4. Peculiarities of voluntary movements as evidenced by posturing (voluntary assumption of inappropriate or bizarre postures) stereotyped movements, prominent mannerisms, or prominent grimacing
5. Echolalia or echopraxia

A 26-year-old man was brought to a hospital emergency room for evaluation. He was mute, immobile, and lying on his back with his arms extended in a bizarre posture. His arms could be moved with some force and stayed in the position in which they were placed. The patient would not follow any instructions from the staff. Two hours after he was given antipsychotic medication, the patient began repeating the words the staff spoke to him and other words he heard spoken nearby (i.e., echolalia). He still refused to follow instructions or answer questions.

295.90 Schizophrenia, Undifferentiated Type. A type of Schizophrenia in which symptoms meeting Criterion A for Schizophrenia are present but criteria for Paranoid, Catatonic, or Disorganized types are not met.

A 42-year-old woman lives in a halfway house in a large eastern city. During the day she sits in the park near her house and talks to the birds while feeding them scraps of bread. She appears preoccupied most of the time and admits to her social worker that she hears the voices of several people talking to her. Her affect is generally flat and she interacts minimally with other people.

295.60 Schizophrenia, Residual Type. A type of Schizophrenia in which either negative symptoms are still present or at least two symptoms listed in Criterion A for Schizophrenia (i.e., delusions, hallucinations, disorganized speech, or grossly disorganized or catatonic behavior) are present in an attenuated form (e.g., odd beliefs, unusual perceptual experiences).

A 38-year-old man has had three hospitalizations in the past during which he was agitated and believed that demons were pursuing him to make him perform indecent acts. He also heard continuous voices telling him that he was a bad person and should kill himself. He was last hospitalized 5 years ago. Currently he lives alone, has no job, and survives on disability payments. He periodically thinks that he hears someone talking but he cannot understand what they are saying. In addition, he has become very concerned about crime in his neighborhood and is convinced that some unidentified group is behind the increase in violence in the city. He talks vehemently about his concerns with neighbors and his social worker.

295.40   Schizophreniform Disorder.   Patients with this disorder meet Criteria A, D, and E of the common criteria set for Schizophrenia discussed above and have symptoms that last at least 1 month and less than 6 months.

> A 25-year-old woman lives alone and works as a maid in a large hotel. She was brought to her local community mental health center by a concerned neighbor who stated that the patient had recently started behaving in an unusual manner. She had apparently missed work several days in a row and had received a letter from the hotel indicating that she had been placed on probation and might lose her job because of her absences. The neighbor reported that the patient had been friendly and talkative until about 2 months ago when she began staying in her apartment and avoiding other people in the neighborhood. Her apartment, which was usually neat, was littered with dirty clothes and garbage. The patient admitted to hearing voices that continually comment on her behavior starting 1–2 months before. She denied depression and drug abuse.

295.70   Schizoaffective Disorder.   Patients with this disorder continuously meet Criterion A for Schizophrenia and experience a Major Depressive Episode, Manic Episode, or Mixed Episode for a substantial period of the illness. The patient has delusions or hallucinations for at least 2 weeks in absence of the mood symptoms. (Specify: *Bipolar Type* if a Manic or Mixed Episode; *Depressive Type* if Major Depressive Episode only.)

> A 21-year-old man is brought to the local mental health clinic by his parents for an evaluation. The patient lives with his parents and attends a local community college. The parents report that there has been a significant change in his personality and behavior in the last few weeks. He has stopped going to classes and spends much of the day in his room reading the Bible. He has little interest in hobbies or other activities he used to enjoy.
>
> His mother relates that she often hears him talking to himself when she passes his room during the day. She also reports that he eats little, seems to have lost weight, and is up all hours of the night walking around the house. The patient indicates that he began hearing voices a couple of months ago. He is convinced that voices are a message from God trying to prevent him from sinning. He reads the Bible to interpret the messages he receives from the voices, but is having difficulty concentrating. About 1 month ago he began feeling depressed and worthless because he could not understand what God wanted from him.

297.1   Delusional Disorder.   Patients with this disorder experience nonbizarre delusions (i.e., involving situations that occur in everyday life) for at least 1 month, have never met Criterion A for Schizophrenia, and function reasonably well aside from the impact or ramifications of their delusions. If mood episodes occur concurrently with the delusions, their total duration is brief.

A 32-year-old married man becomes infuriated whenever his wife glances at other men or talks to them. He frequently accuses her of having affairs with men in the neighborhood despite her repeated denials. On a few occasions he has become so enraged that he hit his wife and refused to allow her to leave the house. The patient's wife reports that he listens to her phone calls and is suspicious whenever a man calls. When she goes out in the evening he insists that she tell him where she is going and with whom. He periodically calls her at work during the day to check on her. The couple has seen a marriage counselor who tried to help the patient understand that his wife was faithful to him. He refused to believe her and left the session enraged. The diagnosis is Delusional Disorder (Jealous Type)

298.8   Brief Psychotic Disorder.   Patients with this disorder experience either delusions, hallucinations, disorganized speech, or grossly disorganized or catatonic behavior for at least 1 day and less than 1 month, with eventual complete recovery.

A 47-year-old woman who is a high school teacher went on a tour to another city with a group of her fellow teachers. To save money, they shared hotel rooms. Two or three days after the trip began, her friends began to notice a change in the patient. She became increasingly anxious and began to talk about people watching her. On the third night she became more delusional, refused to get ready for bed, and began pacing the hotel room looking in the closet and under the bed for people hiding there watching her. Her friends became increasingly alarmed and took her to a nearby hospital where she was examined, given some medication to calm her nerves, and sent back to the hotel with her friends.

The patient continued to be agitated and her husband arrived to take her home on the following day. She was admitted to a local psychiatric hospital near her home. Within 2 days of her admission her delusions and agitation disappeared without medication. The patient was discharged in 5 days with no evidence of psychiatric symptoms. She returned to work and was soon functioning at her previous high level.

297.3   Shared Psychotic Disorder (Folie à Deux).   Patients with this disorder develop a delusion that is similar in content to the already established delusion of another person with whom they have a close relationship.

A 35-year-old man was arrested when he became angry and combative over the purity of the food in a supermarket where he and his wife were shopping. The judge dismissed the charges against the man with the condition that he and his wife consult a psychiatrist about his concerns. In the psychiatric interview the man described his concerns about food purity. "All the food you buy these days is contaminated with pesticides or disease. You have to make sure its been carefully wrapped and then you have to purify it. If you don't it can poison you. The food at that supermarket was filthy, I could see the disease," he said. The patient described a set of elaborate steps he and his wife take to purify food before they eat it. He reports that if he omits any of the purification steps he becomes nervous and ill within a day or two.

The psychiatrist interviewed the man's wife separately. She indicated that they had been married for 8 years. When they were first married she was skeptical about his food concerns. However, she has become increasingly concerned about food purity and now is able to see the food contamination her husband talks about.

293.8x   Psychotic Disorder Due to . . . *[Indicate the General Medical Condition].*   Patients with this disorder develop prominent delusions (293.81) or hallucinations (293.82) that are judged to be caused by a general medical condition and do not occur exclusively during the course of Delirium or Dementia.

A 62-year-old woman is admitted to the hospital upset and mildly confused. Her daughter states that the woman has not been herself for the last few days. The patient reports that she has had some unusual experiences over the last few days that she cannot explain. Two days previously she was cleaning her basement with her 15-year-old granddaughter. Suddenly she heard a noise behind her and turned to look. "I saw a large linoleum dog," she said. "It was dragging a box along the floor. I never saw anything like that before." The patient continued, "When I got into my hospital room I saw a parade of goldfish. They came out of the bowel, up the wall, and swam across the ceiling. Now, that can't be real. Something's wrong."

The patient's only significant medical history was a thyroidectomy performed 25 years before. Laboratory tests demonstrated that the patient was significantly hypocalcemic. When she was treated, the hallucinations disappeared.

29x.xx Substance-Induced Psychotic Disorder.   The disorder includes prominent hallucinations or delusions associated with evidence that the symptoms developed within 1 month of significant substance intoxication or withdrawal, or is etiologically related to medication use or toxin exposure.

The specific codes for Substance-Induced Psychotic Disorder are determined by the specific substance: 291.5 alcohol; 292.11 amphetamines; cannabis; cocaine; hallucinogens; inhalants; opioids; phencyclidine; sedatives, hypnotics, anxiolytics; other (or unknown) substances.

Sam is a 45-year-old unmarried man who lives alone in a single room in a rundown section of the city. He is unemployed and spends most of his time roaming the streets trying to beg money to buy alcohol. Sam has been ill in bed for the last 2 days and unable to buy any wine. Last night he had difficulty sleeping and awoke several times shaking and hearing a man talking to him telling him that he was no good.

Sam has had three previous experiences hearing voices when he has suddenly stopped drinking in the past.

298.9   Psychotic Disorder Not Otherwise Specified.   This disorder includes syndromes with prominent psychotic symptomatology that do not meet the criteria for any specific Psychotic Disorder.

A 29-year-old man complains that he hears someone call his name and talk to him. The voice belongs to a woman and reminds him of his mother who died 15 years ago. He finds the voice comforting and supportive at times when he is under stress. The patient has no other psychotic symptoms. He is married and has worked at the same job for 10 years.

Necessary Clinical Information

The accurate differential diagnosis of a Psychotic Disorder requires the following clinical information.

- History of documented psychiatric illness

- History of socially unusual, odd, or isolative behavior

- History of substance abuse

- History of medical illnesses

- Current experience of hallucinations or odd perceptual experiences

- Disorganized thought or speech

- Delusions

- Negative symptoms (e.g., flat affect, alogia, avolition)

- Depression or mania

- Duration of symptoms

Making a Diagnosis

Unlike anxiety, psychotic symptoms are not ubiquitous in health and disease. They rarely appear in healthy individuals and they are not a common part of many other psychiatric disorders. Almost everyone has experienced anxiety and is aware of the common behavior manifestations of anxiety in themselves and others. Therefore, they do not consider it unusual to see someone with these symptoms.

Individuals who have a Psychotic Disorder usually display behaviors that seem distinctly abnormal or at least odd. Unusual behavior is typically the reason for the patient's clinical evaluation. However, these outward signs of internal disarray are usually not sufficient, in themselves, to make a diagnosis. Not all odd behaviors or beliefs are caused by a Psychotic Disorder. Furthermore, the presence of psychotic symptoms is compatible with several different diagnoses.

Additional information must be collected to fulfill the necessary criteria for a specific diagnosis. Frequently it is difficult to gather the clinical information necessary for the criteria because the patient cannot communicate or is a poor historian. Once the available information is gathered, a few questions can rapidly help exclude inappropriate diagnoses and thereby narrow down the list of possible correct diagnoses. The following questions should help the clinician make a diagnosis in most typical clinical presentations. Specific problems in the diagnosis of Psychotic Disorders will be discussed in the next section.

1. Could the patient's symptoms be produced by drugs or a nonpsychiatric medical illness?

Determine whether the patient has any current nonpsychiatric medical illnesses or substance-related problems. If so, deciding the relationship between these problems and the patient's psychiatric symptoms should be the first step in the diagnostic process. The presence of a nonpsychiatric medical illnesses or substance-related problem in conjunction with psychiatric symptoms does not imply that the former caused the latter.

The occurrence of psychiatric symptoms before the onset of a medical illness or use of a substance suggests that they have an independent etiology. Similarly, the persistence of psychiatric symptoms after adequate treatment of the medical illness or cessation of substance use implies that the two are unrelated. The diagnoses of Psychotic Disorder Due to a General Medical Condition and Substance-Induced Psychotic Disorder can be excluded if there is no evidence that a nonpsychiatric medical disorder or drugs have produced the patient's symptoms.

Note: Assume that an organic etiology for the patient's symptoms has been ruled out for the remaining questions in this section.

2. Does the patient currently meet Criterion A (characteristic symptoms) of the common criteria set for Schizophrenia?

If Criterion A is met, Schizophrenia, Residual Type; Delusional Disorder; and Psychotic Disorder Not Otherwise Specified can be excluded as diagnoses. The first two diagnoses require that Criterion A not be met. The compliance with Criterion A means that the criteria set for one of the specific Psychotic Disorder diagnoses will be fulfilled and the diagnosis of Psychotic Disorder Not Otherwise Specified will not be needed as a "wastebasket" diagnosis.

3. Have the patient's symptoms lasted less than 6 months?

If the patient's symptoms have lasted for less than 6 months, none of the Schizophrenia diagnoses (e.g., Schizophrenia, Paranoid Type, etc.) can be made. The diagnosis of Schizophreniform Disorder requires the same psychotic symptoms as Schizophrenia for at least 1 month and no more than 6 months. The diagnosis of Brief Psychotic Disorder requires fewer psychotic symptoms for at least 1 day and no more than 1 month.

It is frequently difficult to establish the true duration of the patient's psychotic symptoms. The patient may not be able to give an accurate report if he is psychotic. A relative, friend, or neighbor may be a more reliable historian of subtle changes in the patient's behavior that appeared during the prodromal stage of the illness.

4. Does the patient have a major depressive episode (including depressed mood) or manic episode concurrent with symptoms that meet Criterion A of the common criteria set for Schizophrenia?

If the patient does not fulfill the criteria for a Mood Disorder concurrent with symptoms that fulfill Criterion A for Schizophrenia, the diagnosis of Schizoaffective Disorder can be excluded. Symptoms of depression or hypomania are not sufficient to fulfill the criteria for Schizoaffective Disorder if they do not fulfill the criteria for the Mood Disorder.

5. Does the patient have significant disorganized speech and behavior?

- If the patient has disorganized speech or disorganized behavior, Schizophrenia, Paranoid Type, can be excluded.

- If the patient has a flat or inappropriate affect in addition to disorganized speech and behavior, the likely diagnosis is Schizophrenia, Disorganized Type, assuming the duration criteria for Schizophrenia is fulfilled.

- If the patient has disorganized speech or disorganized behavior without flat affect, or bizarre motoric activity, the likely diagnosis is Schizophrenia, Undifferentiated Type, assuming the duration criteria for Schizophrenia is met.

6. Does the patient have unusual or peculiar motor activity?

If the patient's main symptoms include excessive purposeless motor activity, immobility, rigidity, bizarre posture, prominent grimacing, or stereotyped movements, the likely diagnosis is Schizophrenia, Catatonic Type.

7. Does the patient have prominent hallucinations that he or she realizes are not real?

Patients who have hallucinations in the presence of intact reality testing (i.e., they realize the hallucinations are not real), generally have Psychotic Disorder Due to a General Medical Condition or Substance-Induced Psychotic Disorder.

8. Does the patient have bizarre delusions?

If the patient has bizarre delusions, the diagnosis of Delusional Disorder is excluded. Bizarre delusions in the absence of any other significant symptoms is usually associated with a diagnosis of Schizophrenia, Paranoid Type.

Common Problems in Making a Diagnosis

There are three areas of uncertainty in the diagnosis of Schizophrenia and Other Psychotic Disorders.

1. Some patients initially come close but don't actually fulfill the criteria for a specific diagnosis. A further consideration of the diagnostic criteria may or may not resolve the problem.
2. Some patients fulfill the diagnostic criteria for more than one psychiatric disorder during the course of their illness. In these cases, a decision must be made based on the precedence of diagnosis or comorbidity considerations.
3. Finally, some patients have isolated symptoms of psychosis associated with other psychiatric disorders but do not fulfill the criteria for a specific Psychotic Disorder.

Patients Who Almost Fulfill the Diagnostic Criteria

Most patients with symptoms of psychosis clearly either fit or do not fit the criteria for a specific diagnosis. However, there are a number of patients whose symptoms appear to come close to fulfilling the diagnostic criteria for a Psychotic Disorder without actually fulfilling them. Usually this problem relates to only one criterion in the criteria set for a diagnosis. It occurs for three reasons.

First, the clinician may be interpreting the criteria for a specific diagnosis so rigidly that a specific patient cannot be fit into the criteria. For example, the diagnosis of Schizophrenia Disorganized Type requires that the patient have disorganized speech, disorganized behavior, and flat or inappropriate affect. It would be an overly rigid interpretation of the criteria to exclude the diagnosis because the patient has occasional periods of appropriate behavior and lucid speech.

Second, the patient may appear psychotic yet still not fulfill the criteria for a specific diagnosis. Frequently, further inquiry, sometimes after initial treatment, will elicit sufficient information to determine whether or not the patient's symptoms fulfill the criteria for the diagnosis of a specific Psychotic Disorder. For example, a patient who is acutely psychotic may only be able to provide necessary information about his symptoms after the acute psychosis has been controlled by medication.

Third, some patient's symptoms do not fulfill the required criteria because the necessary information cannot be obtained. For example, a patient with obvious psychotic symptoms may not be able to provide an accurate account of when his symptoms began.

Example 1

A disheveled man is seen walking down the street yelling unintelligible comments; making bizarre, seemingly meaningless, gestures to passersby; and periodically stopping to search through trash barrels. When the psychiatric social worker assigned to his case tries to speak with him, his speech is loose and incoherent and his behavior is grossly disorganized. What diagnosis(es), if any, should the man receive?

This man appears seriously ill. His main symptoms are disorganized speech and thinking and bizarre or disorganized behavior. These symptoms fulfill Criterion A of the common criteria set for Schizophrenia. The man's disheveled appearance suggests that he is socially dysfunctional. However, there is no indication of duration of the disturbance, or the presence or absence of an underlying Schizoaffective Disorder, Mood Disorder, or Substance-Related Disorder. Therefore, the patient's symptoms do not meet the remaining common criteria set for Schizophrenia.

Because the possibility of an underlying Mood Disorder cannot be ruled out, the patient cannot be given a diagnosis of a Schizophreniform Disorder, Schizoaffective Disorder, or Brief Psychotic Disorder. The absence of clear evidence of delusions rules out the diagnosis of Delusional Disorder. Finally, the absence of information about substance use or concomitant general medical illnesses makes it impossible to diagnose either Psychotic Disorder Due to a General Medical Condition or Substance-Induced Psychotic Disorder.

This leaves the diagnosis of Psychotic Disorder Not Otherwise Specified. The patient's symptoms meet the criteria for this diagnosis because it basically has no criteria other than gross psychotic symptomatology such as disorganized speech. Most clinicians are unhappy making this "wastebasket" diagnosis. However, the casual observation of abnormal behavior displayed by an individual in public rarely offers enough information to make a definitive diagnosis.

A more detailed evaluation of the patient, perhaps after treatment of his psychotic symptoms, would probably provide enough additional information to make a specific diagnosis. Specifically, an evaluation of the patient's mood and the exclusion of a substance as the etiologic agent for the patient's disorder, would lead to a diagnosis of Schizophrenia.

Example 2

John is a 28-year-old man who is being seen for the first time in a hospital emergency room where he admits to hearing voices that continually make critical comments about his behavior and work, and interfere with his ability to work at his job as a salesclerk. There is no evidence of an underlying medical illness or substance-related problem that might be the cause of his symptoms. He denies feeling depressed or euphoric. When the patient is asked how long he has been hearing the voices, he says he cannot remember. When he is pressed further, he replies, "a few weeks." What diagnosis(es), if any, should John receive?

John's symptoms explicitly meet all of the requirements in the common criteria set for Schizophrenia, with the exception of the requirement that he have continuous signs of the disturbance for at least 6 months. He is either unwilling or unable to be more specific. In lieu of this information, the most reasonable diagnosis is Brief Psychotic Disorder.

This is a common problem in the diagnosis of Psychotic Disorders. The final diagnosis is dependent on a follow-up of the patient to determine whether the symptoms resolve in less than 6 months. If they resolve within 1 month with a full return to the premorbid level of functioning, the diagnosis would remain Brief Psychotic Disorder. If the symptoms fully resolve within 6 months, the diagnosis would be Schizophreniform Disorder. If the disturbance lasts more than 6 months, John's will meet the criteria for the diagnosis of Schizophrenia, Paranoid Type.

Example 3

Sal is a 33-year-old man with flat affect who responds minimally to questions. He is compliant, amotivational, and has difficulty following complicated instructions or making plans. He denies hallucinations or delusions. What diagnosis(es), if any, should Sal receive?

Sal's most striking features are his negative symptoms. His symptoms will meet the criteria for Schizophrenia, Residual Type if they have previously met Criterion A for Schizophrenia.

Example 4

Tom is a 25-year-old man who is grimacing and mute, so it is impossible to obtain any information from him. What diagnosis(es), if any, should Tom receive?

The symptoms of grimacing and mutism fulfill the specific criteria for the diagnosis of Schizophrenia, Catatonic Type. In order to make the diagnosis, the patient's symptoms must also fulfill the common criteria set for Schizophrenia discussed above. However, when a patient is mute, it is always important to make certain that there are no possible underlying organic causes. In this case, a specific Substance-Induced Psychotic Disorder would be a significant diagnosis to exclude.

Example 5

Nicholas is a 33-year-old man who is concerned that members of a satanic cult are after him to try and destroy him. He suspects that there are higher forces, beyond the cult, behind his persecution, but he cannot be more specific about these forces. His concerns have interfered with his work and social life for the past year. What diagnosis(es), if any, should Nicholas receive?

This patient's symptoms could fulfill the criteria for a diagnosis of a Delusional Disorder or Schizophrenia, Paranoid Type, depending on the interpretation of the patient's delusions. A Delusional Disorder requires nonbizarre delusions. The diagnosis of Schizophrenia, Paranoid Type, requires bizarre delusions if the delusions are the only psychotic symptom.

This patient's delusions border on the bizarre because of his references to a higher force. Further, gentle questioning may provide more information about these forces and the details of the delusions. If they go beyond situations that could occur in everyday life, the diagnosis would be Schizophrenia, Paranoid Type.

Example 6

Mario is a 27-year-old man who periodically hears a voice telling him what to do. What diagnosis(es), if any, should Mario receive?

If the symptom lasts for more than 1 day and less than 1 month, the patient can be given a diagnosis of Brief Psychotic Disorder. If the symptom lasts for more than 1 month, the patient must be given a diagnosis of Psychotic Disorder Not Otherwise Specified because the diagnoses of Schizophreniform Disorder and Schizophrenia both require two characteristic symptoms from Part A of the common criteria for Schizophrenia.

Example 7

Reed is a 30-year-old man who reports having bizarre delusions and auditory hallucinations that have lasted for 4 months. He does not have symptoms of a Mood Disorder and there is no evidence for an organic basis to his disorder. He has had two previous similar episodes over the last 2 years. Each episode lasted approximately 3–4 months. He has had no psychotic symptoms between episodes. What diagnosis(es), if any, should Reed receive?

The diagnosis of Schizophrenia requires that a patient have continuous signs of the disturbance for at least 6 months. This period must include at least 1 month of symptoms that fulfill Criterion A of the common criteria set for Schizophrenia. It may also include prodromal or residual periods during which the patient has only negative symptoms or attenuated symptoms from Criterion A, such as odd beliefs or strange perceptual experiences.

Reed does not meet the 6-month requirement for the diagnosis of Schizophrenia based on his active symptoms of delusions and hallucinations. However, further inquiry may determine that he had prodromal or residual symptoms in the periods between the active symptoms. These symptoms may not be evident to most observers. Furthermore, Reed may not spontaneously mention odd beliefs or strange perceptions because they represent a baseline or normal state for the patient. If they are present, he can be given a diagnosis of Schizophrenia.

Patients Who Fulfill the Diagnostic Criteria for More Than One Psychotic Disorder

A patient's symptoms may fulfill the criteria for more than one psychotic diagnosis at the same time. Usually when this occurs, the rules for the precedence of diagnosis (see section on Precedence of Diagnosis) or the general criteria will determine which diagnosis to use. For example, a patient may fulfill the criteria for Brief Psychotic Disorder at a given time. However, if his symptoms have ever met the criteria for Schizophrenia, that diagnosis will take precedence over the diagnosis of Brief Psychotic Disorder.

Sometimes the patient may actually have two comorbid Psychotic Disorders superimposed on each other or overlapping in time. If the patient's symptoms fulfill the criteria for both disorders, he should be given both diagnoses.

Example 8

Paul is a 25-year-old man who began acting strange and talking to himself 2 weeks ago. Last night he was brought to the emergency room of the local hospital, acutely psychotic and paranoid with auditory hallucinations and bizarre delusions. A toxicology screening showed moderate amounts of amphetamine in the patient's urine. What diagnosis(es), if any, should Paul receive?

Amphetamine is a commonly abused psychotomimetic drug that can produce a severe agitated psychosis. The presence of amphetamine in Paul's urine suggests that he has Amphetamine Psychotic Disorder. However, one of the criteria for this diagnosis requires that the symptoms are not better accounted for by a Psychotic Disorder that is not substance-induced.

One indication that he may not have a Substance-Induced Psychotic Disorder is the presence of unusual symptoms that preceded his appearance in the emergency room. In this case he was noted to have been acting strange and talking to himself 2 weeks before he developed an active psychosis. It is possible that Paul was also using amphetamine at that time. However, it is equally possible that he has another, non-substance-induced psychotic disorder such as Schizophrenia.

Unfortunately, the sparse information about his previous behavior is insufficient to make a diagnosis. This diagnostic problem can only be resolved by eliciting further information about his past psychiatric symptoms and by following him closely for several weeks after the acute amphetamine psychosis has resolved. Paul's history suggests that he had an underlying psychosis, such as Schizophrenia, that was exacerbated by the amphetamine. If his symptoms fulfill the criteria for Schizophrenia and Amphetamine Psychotic Disorder, he should receive both diagnoses and the two problems should be treated as comorbid disorders.

Psychotic Symptoms Associated With Other Psychiatric Disorders

Psychotic symptoms may also occur in nonpsychotic psychiatric illnesses such as Mood Disorders, Anxiety Disorders, or Personality Disorders. They may be transient or occur throughout the course of the illness.

Example 9

Irma is a 37-year-old woman whose symptoms meet all of the criteria for a Major Depressive Disorder, Single Episode, that has lasted for approximately 2 months. She also has a delusion that other people can read her mind. The delusion has been present for much of the time that she has been depressed. She had a similar episode 10 years previously that resolved completely after treatment with antidepressant medication. What diagnosis(es), if any, should Irma receive?

Psychotic symptoms associated with a Major Depressive Disorder are usually mood-congruent in the sense that their content is consistent with themes of the depression including: guilt, disease, death, or personal inadequacy. Irma's delusions are mood-incongruent because they do not relate to typical depressive themes and are more consistent with the types of delusions seen in Schizophrenia or a Schizoaffective Disorder.

Their occurrence raises the possibility that she may have the latter disorder. In order to meet the criteria for Schizoaffective Disorder, Irma must have experienced the delusion for at least 2 weeks in the absence of the mood symptoms. In this case the opposite appears to be true. The psychotic symptoms do not occur independent of the mood symptoms that last throughout the illness.

Example 10

Luis is a 47-year-old man who witnessed a serious accident on the highway in which a husband and wife in the front seat of the car were killed and their three children were trapped in the back with minor injuries. He stopped to see if he could help and heard the children screaming and crying for help. Several weeks later he began hearing the voices of children screaming and crying similar to the children in the car. The voices occurred several times a day. What diagnosis(es), if any, should Luis receive?

Luis reports symptoms that are consistent with a diagnosis of a Posttraumatic Stress Disorder related to the serious accident he witnessed. One of the criteria for the diagnosis of this disorder is that the patient persistently relives the traumatic event through illusions, hallucinations, flashbacks, or other symptoms.

Luis' hallucinations are not consistent with the auditory hallucinations found in Schizophrenia and most other Psychotic Disorders. They are not bizarre, do not keep up a running commentary on the patient's thoughts and behavior, are not associated with a significant deterioration of function and do not have a medical or substance-related basis. Technically he could be given a diagnosis of Brief Psychotic Disorder because hallucinations lasting more than 1 day with eventual full return to premorbid levels of functioning fulfill the requirements for that disorder. This diagnosis should be considered if Luis' hallucinations change their character and no longer seem related to the traumatic event.

Precedence of Diagnosis

As in other diagnostic groups, patients may display symptoms that are consistent with more than one psychotic diagnosis. Usually the criteria for the diagnosis of a specific disorder includes rules that indicate how the conflict should be resolved. Table 6–1 lists the disorders that take diagnostic precedence over Schizophrenia and Other Psychotic Disorders.

The most common example of this problem in the Schizophrenia and Other Psychotic Disorders group is the occurrence of symptoms of a Mood Disorder in conjunction with psychotic symptoms. Other potential conflicts occur about the precedence of organic diagnoses over nonorganic diagnoses and vice versa. This reciprocal relationship appears contradictory. However, it serves the purpose of emphasizing that the occurrence of psychotic symptoms and organic factors is not necessarily a cause-and-effect relationship. Table 6–1 should be used as a reminder of those diagnoses that usually must be excluded before a specific diagnosis can be made.

Table 6–1 Precedence of diagnosis for Schizophrenia and Other Psychotic Disorders

Psychotic disorder	Disorders taking precedence

Schizophrenia
  Paranoid Type
  Disorganized Type
  Catatonic Type
  Undifferentiated Type
  Residual Type
	Does not meet criteria for Schizoaffective Disorder, Mood Disorder with psychotic features, other Schizophrenia disorders
	Not due to effects of a substance or general medical condition

Schizophreniform Disorder	Does not meet the criteria for Schizoaffective Disorder, Mood Disorder with psychotic features Not due to effects of a substance or general medical condition
Schizoaffective Disorder	Not due to effects of a substance or general medical condition
Delusional Disorder	Has never met criteria for Schizophrenia Not due to effects of a substance or general medical condition
Brief Psychotic Disorder	Not better accounted for by Mood Disorder or Schizophrenia Not due to effects of a substance or general medical condition
Shared Psychotic Disorder (Folie à Deux)	Not better accounted for by another Psychotic Disorder Not due to effects of a substance or general medical condition
Psychotic Disorder Due to a General Medical Condition	Does not occur exclusively during Delirium or Dementia Not better accounted for by another mental disorder
Substance-Induced Psychotic Disorder	Does not occur exclusively during Delirium or Dementia Not better accounted for by non-substance-induced psychotic disorder
Psychotic Disorder NOS	Does not meet criteria for any other psychotic disorder Not due to effects of a substance or general medical condition

Note. NOS = Not Otherwise Specified.

Discussion of Clinical Vignettes

Vignette 1: It's a Conspiracy

Johannes' main symptom is his fixed delusion, of several years duration, that there is a conspiracy of communists, rabbis, and priests who control the government and keep him from reuniting with his family. He has no history of previous hallucinations or psychiatric hospitalizations. There is no current evidence of disorganized speech, disorganized behavior, or negative symptoms such as flat affect.

The lack of an underlying medical disorder or substance-related problem means that Johannes does not fit the criteria for either Psychotic Disorder Due to a General Medical Condition or Substance-Induced Psychotic Disorder. Similarly, he cannot be given a diagnosis of Schizoaffective Disorder because there is no indication that he has had depression or mania associated with the delusions. The duration of his disorder excludes the possibility of Schizophreniform Disorder or Brief Psychotic Disorder. This leaves two possible diagnoses, Schizophrenia, Paranoid Type, or Delusional Disorder. The decision between these two diagnoses depends on judgments about his social and occupational function and the nature of his delusions.

The diagnosis of Schizophrenia requires that the patient's social and occupational functioning is significantly below the level achieved before the onset of the disturbance. In addition, the patient must have bizarre delusions in the absence of other symptoms of psychosis such as hallucinations, disorganized speech, or disorganized behavior. The criteria for Delusional Disorder requires that the patient have nonbizarre delusions, no significant deterioration of function, and no evidence of odd or bizarre behavior. Nonbizarre delusions involve situations that conceivably could occur in everyday life such as being followed, loved by an individual of a higher status, or being convinced that one has special knowledge or is being malevolently treated by others.

The judgment about Johannes' social and occupational functioning is complicated by his physical injury and immigrant status. He no longer works as a skilled machinist; however it is not uncommon for immigrants to have difficulty finding employment in their previous occupation. Some clinicians might think that Johannes' delusions of a large conspiracy go beyond everyday experiences. This is a matter of clinical judgment. Given the uncertainty in the nature of his delusions and the long-term stability of his illness, the most prudent diagnosis is Delusional Disorder.

Vignette 2: He Killed My Friend

The most striking aspect of this case is the sudden escalation of Tom's psychotic symptoms and violent behavior associated with his subsequent amnesia of the event. The occurrence of these symptoms so soon after he smoked a drug suggests that the behavior is a Substance-Induced Psychotic Disorder. Paranoid psychotic ideation and behavior can be associated with cocaine, amphetamine, hallucinogen, and phencyclidine intoxication. Violence is more commonly associated with phencyclidine intoxication. Furthermore, the patient also demonstrates other signs and symptoms of phencyclidine intoxication including hypertension, horizontal nystagmus, diminished responsiveness to pain, and dysarthria.

Patients who take heavy doses of phencyclidine may also experience amnesia about their activities while they are intoxicated. Therefore, the presumptive diagnosis is Phencyclidine Psychotic Disorder with Delusions, with onset during intoxication. The definitive diagnosis of phencyclidine intoxication would depend on evidence of the drug in the patient's blood or urine or an analysis of residual drug that he smoked. Although there is a possibility that he has another, non-substance-induced disorder, this cannot be determined unless his symptoms reappear more than 1 month after his last use of drugs.

Key Diagnostic Points

- The diagnosis of any psychosis requires that the patient have delusions, hallucinations, or disorganized speech and thought.

- The diagnosis of a Delusional Disorder requires that the patient have non-bizarre delusions.

- Three Psychotic Disorders form a continuum based on the duration of the episode: Brief Psychotic Disorder (duration 1 day to 1 month), Schizophreniform Disorder (duration 1 month to 6 months), and Schizophrenia (duration more than 6 months).

- The delusions or auditory hallucinations associated with the diagnosis of Schizophrenia, Paranoid Type, are not required to have a paranoid content.

Common Questions in Making a Diagnosis

1. A young man walks into a restaurant several times over a 2-day period and begins pointing at customers and talking in an excited voice. His speech seems confused and does not make any sense. As he talks, he waves his arms, makes bizarre gestures, and periodically appears to be listening to something. Can this individual be given a diagnosis of Schizophrenia? If not, what diagnosis, if any, can the patient be given with this information?

Answer: The first part of the diagnostic criteria for Schizophrenia requires that the patient have two out of the following symptoms: delusions, hallucinations, disorganized speech, disorganized or catatonic behavior, or negative symptoms. This patient is agitated, has disorganized speech, and appears to be confused. His bizarre gestures and apparent listening behavior suggest that he may also be having auditory hallucinations. However this cannot be confirmed without interviewing the patient.

The diagnosis Schizophrenia also requires evidence of significant social or occupational dysfunction, a duration of illness of at least 6 months, and the exclusion of significant mood or organic disorders that may be etiologically related to the patient's symptoms. There is no clinical evidence to confirm or deny the presence of these requirements. Therefore the patient cannot currently be given a diagnosis of Schizophrenia.

There are two other possible diagnoses, Brief Psychotic Disorder and Psychotic Disorder Not Otherwise Specified. The patient appears to have a psychosis as evidenced by his disorganized speech. The illness has also lasted for at least 1 day. This fulfills the first two requirements in the criteria set for Brief Psychotic Disorder. However, it is impossible to rule out the presence of an underlying Mood Disorder or organic etiology. Therefore, the diagnosis of Brief Psychotic Disorder cannot be made. The diagnosis of Psychotic Disorder Not Otherwise Specified does not have specific criteria. It is used to diagnose psychotic symptomatology, such as disorganized speech, when there is not sufficient information to make another, more specific, psychotic diagnosis.

2. A 23-year-old man is brought to the hospital by friends. They report that he has become increasingly suspicious over the last 2 days and communicates less and less with his friends and family. He is convinced that they are trying to hurt him. This is unusual behavior for the patient, who is generally friendly and has no previous psychiatric history. That evening he became very excited and struck one of his friends during an argument. As the patient is waiting to be examined, he keeps yelling, "Get away, don't touch me. You're trying to hurt me." He cannot be calmed by the staff. A physical examination shows an elevated pulse rate of 102 and an elevated blood pressure of 170/95. What diagnoses should be considered for this patient?

Answer: If the patient has true delusions that other people are trying to hurt him and he does not have significant mood symptoms, his symptoms fulfill the criteria for the diagnosis of Brief Psychotic Disorder. However the sudden onset of the patient's psychotic symptoms and his elevated blood pressure suggests that there may be an underlying organic basis for his disorder. The most likely diagnoses to consider would be Amphetamine Psychotic Disorder, with delusions; Cocaine Psychotic Disorder, with delusions; or Phencyclidine Psychotic Disorder, with delusions. The patient's urine and blood should be screened for these drugs. When his psychotic symptoms have resolved he may be able to provide additional information about drug use.

3. Sally is a 42-year-old woman with a 20-year history of psychiatric problems who believes that everyone is influenced by Satan. She complains, "It's getting harder and harder to trust anyone." Sally saw a private psychiatrist for many years until he moved away. Since that time she has deteriorated with increasingly frequent hospitalizations. Recently she terminated treatment with her current therapist because, "he was influenced by Satan." The patient takes antipsychotic medication but this has little effect on her concerns about Satan. She has never admitted to having hallucinations and denies feeling depressed. Despite her odd beliefs, Sally is very articulate. Recently she has become more irritable, accusing people of being Satan worshipers and of harboring evil thoughts toward her. She proclaims, "I am the avenging angel of God," and attacks them. Sally sleeps little and talks endlessly about Satan. She is noticeably eccentric in her dress. What is the appropriate differential diagnosis for this patient?

Answer: The patient's long history of bizarre delusions without symptoms of disorganized speech, disorganized behavior, or flat affect meets the criteria for Schizophrenia, Paranoid Type. However, the patient is also currently having some symptoms that are typical of a manic episode. The most notable of these are decreased sleep, increased irritability, psychomotor agitation, distractibility, and increased talkativeness. These symptoms do not quite meet the requirements for the diagnosis of a manic episode. If they did, the patient would fulfill the criteria for Schizoaffective Disorder. It would be important to check for other manic symptoms such as distractibility or increased sexual activity.

4. A 24-year-old woman begins hearing voices approximately 1 hour after she took a hallucinogen. She is aware that the voices were caused by the drug, but they still upset her. Should she receive a diagnosis of Substance-Induced Psychotic Disorder?

Answer: No. If the patient has intact reality testing and knows that the hallucinations are not real, these symptoms cannot be used to fulfill the criteria for Substance-Induced Psychotic Disorder.

5. A patient has symptoms that met the criteria for a diagnosis of Schizophrenia, Paranoid Type, 7 years ago. She had a full remission with no further symptoms. She now has developed a nonbizarre delusion that the FBI is targeting her in an investigation of drug-money laundering. She has no mood symptoms and the delusion does not markedly interfere with her functioning. Can she receive a diagnosis of Brief Psychotic Disorder?

Answer: No. Once a patient has met Criteria A for Schizophrenia, they cannot be given a diagnosis of Brief Psychotic Disorder.

6. A 25-year-old man is brought to a community mental health center by his parents. They report that he inexplicably lost his job a year ago and moved in with them. On his birthday, approximately 5 months ago, he announced that he was the Messiah. Since that time, he has maintained the delusion and continued to function at a low level. He has no other symptoms. Can this patient receive a diagnosis of Schizophrenia, Paranoid Type?

Answer: Yes. Five months of psychotic symptoms are sufficient in light of a possible prodromal period of 1 year of unemployment to make the diagnosis.

Mood Disorders

Clinical Vignettes

Vignette 1: Why Didn't I Stop Him

Elaine is a 35-year-old widowed schoolteacher with two teenage children. She was married to a successful lawyer who was part of an established firm. One day, 3 months ago, she arrived home from work and saw her husband's car in the driveway. She walked into the house and called him but there was no answer. Assuming he was busy somewhere in the house she went into the kitchen to get something to eat.

Twenty minutes later when she still had not seen or heard him she began looking through the house. As Elaine waked into the bedroom she noticed that the bathroom door was closed. She tried to go in but the door was locked. She called her husband but there was no answer. Alarmed, she used an emergency key to open the door. Inside, she found her husband lying on the floor, not breathing. A small mirror containing white powder and a razor blade lay on the sink. Elaine called the paramedics but they were unable to resuscitate her husband. Subsequently, she learned from one of her husband's partners that he had been concerned that her husband might be abusing drugs but had no proof. Her husband's death was ruled a drug overdose by the medical examiner.

Elaine was stunned by the death of her husband. She attended to the funeral arrangements and tried to help her children struggle with their feelings about their father's death. She had mixed feelings. On one hand she was enraged with her husband for using drugs. On the other hand she felt guilty that she had not recognized her husband's drug abuse in time to save him. Elaine felt sad and lonely. She reviewed their experiences together searching for any clue to when his drug problem started. Her friends and family did not want to talk about her husband's drug abuse, referring instead to his untimely death and a promising career cut short.

Four weeks after her husband's death the insurance company informed her that she might not receive any money from his policy because the company considered his death a suicide. Because he had just finished paying off loans from college and law school, the couple had little savings. Gradually she became more depressed and began to feel that she was worthless and responsible for her husband's death. She had difficulty sleeping, lying awake at night worrying about money and how she would care for her children. Elaine had little energy during the day and her friends began to comment that she looked tired and worn out most of the time. She no longer derived any pleasure from her teaching or any other activities. Her ability to concentrate diminished and the quality of her work began to deteriorate. Two months after her husband's death her school principal met with her to discuss her deteriorating work and suggested that she seek professional help.

Vignette 2: I Have a Little Poem for You

Sandra is a 43-year-old woman who has had several psychiatric hospitalizations for psychosis over the past 15 years. Six weeks ago the patient's favorite uncle died suddenly. He had helped raise her when she was a little girl and had always been supportive during periods when she was ill or under stress. Sandra was initially sad, withdrawn and mildly depressed. Her husband had some difficulty getting her out of bed in the morning before he went to work.

Approximately 3 weeks ago her behavior began to change. She became brighter and more outgoing. Unfortunately, the changes in her behavior did not stop with a reestablished optimistic outlook on life. Within 2 weeks her energy knew no bounds. She began sleeping 2–3 hours a night and then awoke to clean the house. She decided to become more involved in her 16-year-old daughter's school and called the principal early one morning to volunteer her services. Her daughter was not pleased.

One day Sandra went to the supermarket and returned with three cases of frozen orange juice, explaining, "You can never be too healthy." Sandra's behavior continued to change and she became more irritable and irrational. She talked endlessly but less and less of what she said made sense. She began to be suspicious of her family and friends. She told her husband, "I've solved the secret of aging and now they're trying to steal it from me."

This pattern of changing behavior was consistent with her past psychiatric history. In each of her previous hospitalizations the patient became overtly psychotic and delusional. She was treated with electroconvulsive therapy (ECT), responded well, and was discharged with a diagnosis of Schizophrenia on low doses of antipsychotic medication. She still had some delusions but these generally remitted after 2–3 months and the medication was discontinued. The patient had recurring episodes of illness every 3–5 years. The onset of active illness was often correlated with the loss or separation from a loved one. The last episode occurred shortly after the death of her mother 5 years before. Between episodes, the patient returned to her usual activities and remained functional, without psychiatric symptoms. However, she stopped working as a nurse after her second hospitalization.

The patient's current psychotic delusions and irritability continued and increased. She took offense at the slightest comment and started yelling at her husband. He, in turn, tried to get her to see a psychiatrist but she refused. Finally, in desperation, he took his wife to the emergency room of a nearby hospital where she was admitted to the psychiatric ward. In the hospital the patient continued to be irritable, delusional, paranoid, and critical of everyone around her. She left bizarre poems and notes for her physician each morning: "$E = MC^2$ = love makes the world go round and Jet power build strong minds and bodies." The poems were decorated with chains of daisies drawn along the edges. The psychiatrist started the patient on antipsychotic medication and, after hearing her history, contemplated beginning ECT treatments.

Core Concept of the Diagnostic Group

The core concept of the Mood Disorders diagnostic group is the development of an abnormal mood characterized by depression, mania, or both symptoms in alternating fashion. The abnormal mood may or may not impair the patient's social or occupational functioning. Depression is distinguished by an unusually sad, gloomy, and dejected mood or a markedly diminished interest and pleasure in everyday activities that is distinctly different than the patient's nondepressed state. Mania is distinguished by an unusually and persistently elevated, expansive, or irritable mood that is distinctly different than the patient's nonmanic state. Hypomania is a less severe variant of mania. The various Mood Disorder diagnoses are distinguished by the intensity of the abnormal mood; its duration; the impairment it produces; and the accompanying behavioral, cognitive, or physical symptoms.

Criteria Applicable to Multiple Disorders

The Mood Disorders category contains two groups of criteria that are applicable to multiple diagnoses. The first group contains the criteria sets for the four Mood Disorder syndromes (Major Depressive Episode, Manic Episode, Hypomanic Episode, and Mixed Episode). The second group includes criteria sets for specifiers that describe the most recent mood episode (severity/psychotic/remission, chronic, melancholic features, atypical features, catatonic features, postpartum onset) and criteria sets for specifiers that describe recurrent episodes (longitudinal course, seasonal pattern, rapid cycling). See Table 7–2 later in this chapter for a summary of the recent and recurrent mood episode specifiers applicable to each coded Mood Disorder.

Criteria for a Major Depressive Episode

A Major Depressive Episode is the core syndrome of severe depression. Many of the individual diagnoses in the Mood Disorders group (e.g., Major Depressive Disorder, Single Episode, Bipolar I Disorder, Most Recent Episode Depressed, etc.) require that the patient first fulfill the criteria for a Major Depressive Episode. These specific diagnoses are subsequently distinguished by the number of Major Depressive Episodes the patient has had and the presence or absence of manic or hypomanic episodes. The criteria for a Major Depressive Episode includes the following:

A. Five (or more) of the following symptoms have been present during the same 2-week period and represent a change from previous functioning; at least one of the symptoms is either (1) depressed mood or (2) loss of interest or pleasure.

   Note: Do not include symptoms that are clearly due to a general medical condition, or mood-incongruent delusions or hallucinations.

   (1)   depressed mood most of the day, nearly every day, as indicated by either subjective report (e.g., feels sad or empty) or observation made by others (e.g., appears tearful).   **Note:** In children and adolescents, can be irritable mood.
   (2)   markedly diminished interest or pleasure in all, or almost all, activities most of the day, nearly every day (as indicated either by subjective account or observation made by others)
   (3)   significant weight loss or weight gain when not dieting (e.g., more than 5% of body weight in a month), or decrease or increase in appetite nearly every day.   **Note:** In children, consider failure to make expected weight gains.
   (4)   insomnia or hypersomnia nearly every day
   (5)   psychomotor agitation or retardation nearly every day (observable by others, not merely subjective feelings of restlessness or being slowed down)
   (6)   fatigue or loss of energy nearly every day
   (7)   feelings of worthlessness or excessive or inappropriate guilt (which may be delusional) nearly every day (not merely self-reproach or guilt about being sick)
   (8)   diminished ability to think or concentrate, or indecisiveness, nearly every day (either by subjective account or as observed by others)
   (9)   recurrent thoughts of death (not just fear of dying), recurrent suicidal ideation without a specific plan, or a suicide attempt or a specific plan for committing suicide

B. The symptoms do not meet criteria for a Mixed Episode.

C. The symptoms cause clinically significant distress or impairment in social, occupational, or other important areas of functioning.

D. The symptoms are not due to the direct physiological effects of a substance (e.g., a drug of abuse, a medication) or a general medical condition (e.g., hypothyroidism).

E. The symptoms are not better accounted for by Bereavement, i.e., after the loss of a loved one, the symptoms persist for longer than 2 months or are characterized by marked functional impairment, morbid preoccupation with worthlessness, suicidal ideation, psychotic symptoms, or psychomotor retardation.

Criteria for a Manic Episode

A Manic Episode is the core syndrome of a Bipolar I Disorder. All Bipolar I Disorders require that the patient currently meets the criteria for a Manic Episode or has done so in the past. The disorders are further distinguished by the presence or absence of a current or previous Major Depressive Episode. The criteria for a Manic Episode includes the following:

A. A distinct period of abnormally and persistently elevated, expansive, or irritable mood, lasting at least 1 week (or any duration if hospitalization is necessary).

B. During the period of mood disturbance, three (or more) of the following symptoms have persisted (four if the mood is only irritable) and have been present to a significant degree:

(1) inflated self-esteem or grandiosity
(2) decreased need for sleep (e.g., feels rested after only 3 hours of sleep)
(3) more talkative than usual or pressure to keep talking
(4) flight of ideas or subjective experience that thoughts are racing
(5) distractibility (i.e., attention too easily drawn to unimportant or irrelevant external stimuli)
(6) increase in goal-directed activity (either socially, at work or school, or sexually) or psychomotor agitation
(7) excessive involvement in pleasurable activities that have a high potential for painful consequences (e.g., engaging in unrestrained buying sprees, sexual indiscretions, or foolish business investments)

C. The symptoms do not meet criteria for a Mixed Episode.

D. The mood disturbance is sufficiently severe to cause marked impairment in occupational functioning or in usual social activities or relationships with others, or to necessitate hospitalization to prevent harm to self or others, or there are psychotic features.

E. The symptoms are not due to the direct physiological effects of a substance (e.g., a drug of abuse, a medication, or other treatment) or a general medical condition (e.g., hyperthyroidism).

Note: Manic-like episodes that are clearly caused by somatic antidepressant treatment (e.g., medication, electroconvulsive therapy, light therapy) should not count toward a diagnosis of Bipolar I Disorder.

Criteria for a Mixed Episode

A. The criteria are met both for a Manic Episode and for a Major Depressive Episode (except for duration) nearly every day during at least a 1-week period.

B. The mood disturbance is sufficiently severe to cause marked impairment in occupational functioning or in usual social activities or relationships with others, or to necessitate hospitalization to prevent harm to self or others, or there are psychotic features.

C. The symptoms are not due to the direct physiological effects of a substance (e.g., a drug of abuse, medication, or other treatment) or a general medical condition (e.g., hyperthyroidism).

Note: Mixed-like episodes that are clearly caused by somatic antidepressant treatment (e.g., medication, electroconvulsive therapy, light therapy) should not count toward a diagnosis of Bipolar I Disorder.

Criteria for a Hypomanic Episode

A Hypomanic Episode is the core syndrome of a Bipolar II Disorder and is part of the criteria for some Bipolar I Disorders. The criteria for a Hypomanic Episode includes the following:

A. A distinct period of persistently elevated, expansive, or irritable mood, lasting throughout at least 4 days, that is clearly different from the usual nondepressed mood.

B. During the period of mood disturbance, three (or more) of the following symptoms have persisted (four if the mood is only irritable) and have been present to a significant degree:

   (1)   inflated self-esteem or grandiosity
   (2)   decreased need for sleep (e.g., feels rested after only 3 hours of sleep)

(3) more talkative than usual or pressure to keep talking

(4) flight of ideas or subjective experience that thoughts are racing

(5) distractibility (i.e., attention too easily drawn to unimportant or irrelevant external stimuli)

(6) increase in goal-directed activity (either socially, at work or school, or sexually) or psychomotor agitation

(7) excessive involvement in pleasurable activities that have a high potential for painful consequences (e.g., the person engages in unrestrained buying sprees, sexual indiscretions, or foolish business investments)

C. The episode is associated with an unequivocal change in functioning that is uncharacteristic of the person when not symptomatic.

D. The disturbance in mood and the change in functioning are observable by others.

E. The episode is not severe enough to cause marked impairment in social or occupational functioning, or to necessitate hospitalization, and there are no psychotic features.

F. The symptoms are not due to the direct physiological effects of a substance (e.g., a drug of abuse, a medication, or other treatment) or a general medical condition (e.g., hyperthyroidism).

Note: Hypomanic-like episodes that are clearly caused by somatic antidepressant treatment (e.g., medication, electroconvulsive therapy, light therapy) should not count toward a diagnosis of Bipolar II Disorder.

Specifiers Describing the Most Recent Episode

The specifiers that describe the most recent mood episode include the following: the severity/psychotic/remission specifiers, the chronic specifier, the melancholic features specifier, the atypical features specifier, the catatonic features specifier, and the postpartum onset specifier.

Criteria for Severity/Psychotic/Remission Specifiers for Major Depressive Episode

The diagnoses of Major Depressive Disorder, Single Episode, and Major Depressive Disorder, Recurrent, use the following fifth digits in DSM-IV code to specify the severity of the Major Depressive Episode.

Note: Code in fifth digit. Can be applied to the most recent Major Depressive Episode in Major Depressive Disorder and to a Major Depressive Episode in Bipolar I or II Disorder only if it is the most recent type of mood episode.

.x1—Mild: Few, if any, symptoms in excess of those required to make the diagnosis and symptoms result in only minor impairment in occupational functioning or in usual social activities or relationships with others.

.x2—Moderate: Symptoms or functional impairment between "mild" and "severe."

.x3—Severe Without Psychotic Features: Several symptoms in excess of those required to make the diagnosis, **and** symptoms markedly interfere with occupational functioning or with usual social activities or relationships with others.

.x4—Severe With Psychotic Features: Delusions or hallucinations. If possible, specify whether the psychotic features are mood-congruent or mood-incongruent:

> **Mood-Congruent Psychotic Features:**   Delusions or hallucinations whose content is entirely consistent with the typical depressive themes of personal inadequacy, guilt, disease, death, nihilism, or deserved punishment.

> **Mood-Incongruent Psychotic Features:**   Delusions or hallucinations whose content does not involve typical depressive themes of personal inadequacy, guilt, disease, death, nihilism, or deserved punishment. Included are such symptoms as persecutory delusions (not directly related to depressive themes), thought insertion, thought broadcasting, and delusions of control.

.x5—In Partial Remission: Symptoms of a Major Depressive Episode are present but full criteria are not met, or there is a period without any significant symptoms of a Major Depressive Episode lasting less than 2 months following the end of the Major Depressive Episode. (If the Major Depressive Episode was superimposed on Dysthymic Disorder, the diagnosis of Dysthymic Disorder alone is given once the full criteria for a Major Depressive Episode are no longer met.)

.x6—In Full Remission: During the past 2 months, no significant signs or symptoms of the disturbance were present.

.x0—Unspecified.

Criteria for Severity/Psychotic/Remission Specifiers for Manic Episode
The diagnoses of all Bipolar I Disorders except Bipolar I Disorder, Most Recent Episode Unspecified use the following fifth digits in DSM-IV code to specify the severity of the Manic Episode.

Note: Code in fifth digit. Can be applied to a Manic Episode in Bipolar I Disorder only if it is the most recent type of mood episode.

.x1—Mild: Meets minimum symptom criteria for a Manic Episode.

.x2—Moderate: Extreme increase in activity or impairment in judgment.

.x3—Severe Without Psychotic Features: Almost continual supervision required to prevent physical harm to self or others.

.x4—Severe With Psychotic Features: Delusions or hallucinations. If possible, specify whether the psychotic features are mood-congruent or mood-incongruent:

> **Mood-Congruent Psychotic Features:** Delusions or hallucinations whose content is entirely consistent with the typical manic themes of inflated worth, power, knowledge, identity, or special relationship to a deity or famous person.

> **Mood-Incongruent Psychotic Features:** Delusions or hallucinations whose content does not involve typical manic themes of inflated worth, power, knowledge, identity, or special relationship to a deity or famous person. Included are such symptoms as persecutory delusions (not directly related to grandiose ideas or themes), thought insertion, and delusions of being controlled.

.x5—In Partial Remission: Symptoms of a Manic Episode are present but full criteria are not met, or there is a period without any significant symptoms of a Manic Episode lasting less than 2 months following the end of the Manic Episode.

.x6— In Full Remission: During the past 2 months no significant signs or symptoms of the disturbance were present.

.x0—Unspecified.

Criteria for Severity/Psychotic/Remission Specifiers for Current (or Most Recent) Mixed Episode

Note: Code in fifth digit. Can be applied to a Mixed Episode in Bipolar I Disorder only if it is the most recent type of mood episode.

.x1—Mild: Meets no more than minimum symptom criteria for both a Manic Episode and a Major Depressive Episode.

.x2—Moderate: Symptoms or functional impairment between "mild" and "severe."

.x3—Severe Without Psychotic Features: Almost continual supervision required to prevent physical harm to self or others.

.x4—Severe With Psychotic Features: Delusions or hallucinations. If possible, specify whether the psychotic features are mood-congruent or mood-incongruent:

> **Mood-Congruent Psychotic Features:** Delusions or hallucinations whose content is entirely consistent with the typical manic or depressive themes.

Mood-Incongruent Psychotic Features: Delusions or hallucinations whose content does not involve typical manic or depressive themes. Included are such symptoms as persecutory delusions (not directly related to grandiose or depressive themes), thought insertion, and delusions of being controlled.

.x5—In Partial Remission: Symptoms of a Mixed Episode are present but full criteria are not met, or there is a period without any significant symptoms of a Mixed Episode lasting less than 2 months following the end of the Mixed Episode.
.x6—In Full Remission: During the past 2 months, no significant signs or symptoms of the disturbance were present.
.x0—Unspecified.

Chronic Specifier
The Chronic specifier can be applied to the most recent Major Depressive Episode occurring in Major Depressive Disorder, Bipolar I Disorder, or Bipolar II Disorder. This specifier should be used if the full criteria for a Major Depressive Episode have been met continuously for at least the past 2 years.

Catatonic Features Specifier
This specification can be applied to the current or most recent Major Depressive Episode, Manic Episode, or Mixed Episode in Major Depressive Disorder, Bipolar I Disorder, or Bipolar II Disorder.

The clinical picture is dominated by at least two of the following:

(1) motoric immobility as evidenced by catalepsy (including waxy flexibility) or stupor
(2) excessive motor activity (that is apparently purposeless and not influenced by external stimuli)
(3) extreme negativism (an apparently motiveless resistance to all instructions or maintenance of a rigid posture against attempts to be moved) or mutism
(4) peculiarities of voluntary movement as evidenced by posturing (voluntary assumption of inappropriate or bizarre postures), stereotyped movements, prominent mannerisms, or prominent grimacing
(5) echolalia or echopraxia

Melancholic Features Specifier
This specification can be applied to the current or most recent Major Depressive Episode in Major Depressive Disorder and to a Major Depressive Episode in Bipolar I or Bipolar II Disorder only if it is the most recent type of mood episode.

A. Either of the following, occurring during the most severe period of the current episode:

    (1)   loss of pleasure in all, or almost all, activities
    (2)   lack of reactivity to usually pleasurable stimuli (does not feel much better, even temporarily, when something good happens)

B. Three (or more) of the following:

    (1)   distinct quality of depressed mood (i.e., the depressed mood is experienced as distinctly different from the kind of feeling experienced after the death of a loved one)
    (2)   depression regularly worse in the morning
    (3)   early morning awakening (at least 2 hours before usual time of awakening)
    (4)   marked psychomotor retardation or agitation
    (5)   significant anorexia or weight loss
    (6)   excessive or inappropriate guilt

Atypical Features Specifier

This specification can be applied when these features predominate during the most recent 2 weeks of a Major Depressive Episode in Major Depressive Disorder or in Bipolar I or Bipolar II Disorder when the Major Depressive Episode is the most recent type of mood episode, or when these features predominate during the most recent 2 years of Dysthymic Disorder)

A. Mood reactivity (i.e., mood brightens in response to actual or potential positive events)

B. Two (or more) of the following features:

    (1)   significant weight gain or increase in appetite
    (2)   hypersomnia
    (3)   leaden paralysis (i.e., heavy, leaden feelings in arms or legs)
    (4)   long-standing pattern of interpersonal rejection sensitivity (not limited to episodes of mood disturbance) that results in significant social or occupational impairment

C. Criteria are not met for With Melancholic Features or With Catatonic Features during the same episode.

Postpartum Onset Specifier

This specification can be applied to the current or most recent Major Depressive, Manic, or Mixed Episode in Major Depressive Disorder, Bipolar I

Disorder, or Bipolar II Disorder; or to Brief Psychotic Disorder.

Onset of episode within 4 weeks postpartum.

Specifiers Describing the Course of Recurrent Episodes

The symptom features discussed above provide a static snapshot of the patient's symptoms at a specific point in time. However, they do not differentiate between patients based on the course of their illnesses. The Mood Disorder course specifiers serve this function by providing a standardized method of describing the progression of the patient's illness. They include specifiers for Rapid Cycling, Seasonal Pattern, and Longitudinal Course.

Rapid Cycling Specifier
This specification can be applied to Bipolar I Disorder or Bipolar II Disorder.

At least four episodes of a mood disturbance in the previous 12 months that meet criteria for a Major Depressive, Manic, Mixed, or Hypomanic Episode.

Note: Episodes are demarcated either by partial or full remission for at least 2 months or a switch to an episode of opposite polarity (e.g., Major Depressive Episode to Manic Episode).

Seasonal Pattern Specifier
This specification can be applied to the pattern of Major Depressive Episodes in Bipolar I Disorder, Bipolar II Disorder, or Major Depressive Disorder, Recurrent)

A. There has been a regular temporal relationship between the onset of Major Depressive Episodes in Bipolar I or Bipolar II Disorder or Major Depressive Disorder, Recurrent, and a particular time of the year (e.g., regular appearance of the Major Depressive Episode in the fall or winter).

   Note: Do not include cases in which there is an obvious effect of seasonal-related psychosocial stressors (e.g., regularly being unemployed every winter).

B. Full remissions (or a change from depression to mania or hypomania) also occur at a characteristic time of the year (e.g., depression disappears in the spring).

C. In the last 2 years, two Major Depressive Episodes have occurred that demonstrate the temporal seasonal relationships defined in Criteria A and B, and no nonseasonal Major Depressive Episodes have occurred during that same period.

D. Seasonal Major Depressive Episodes (as described above) substantially out-number the nonseasonal Major Depressive Episodes that may have occurred over the individual's lifetime.

Longitudinal Course Specifier

The longitudinal course of a Mood Disorder can be specified by three parameters: 1) whether the patient has recurrent Major Depressive Episodes or Manic Episodes, 2) whether the patient has had a full recovery between successive episodes (with full interepisode recovery or without full interepisode recovery), and 3) whether the Major Depressive Episode is superimposed on a Dysthymic Disorder (e.g., no Dysthymic Disorder or superimposed on Dysthymic Disorder). The general formula for specifying the longitudinal course of a Mood Disorder is:

1. specific recurrent Mood Disorder *plus*
2. with or without full interepisode recovery *plus*
3. superimposed or not superimposed on Dysthymic Disorder

The following two examples illustrate the use of the longitudinal course specifiers:

1. The diagnosis for a patient who develops a Dysthymic Disorder, 3 years later becomes ill with a Major Depressive Disorder, Single Episode, fully recovers and then a year later again has a Major Depressive Episode would be: Major Depressive Disorder, Recurrent, with full interepisode recovery superimposed on Dysthymic Disorder. The patient would also receive the comorbid diagnosis of Dysthymic Disorder.
2. The diagnosis for a patient who develops a Bipolar I Disorder, does not fully recover and then develops another Manic Episode would be: Bipolar I Disorder, Most Recent Episode Manic, Recurrent, without full interepisode recovery.

Definitions

anhedonia   Loss of interest or pleasure in everyday activities that the individual usually enjoys.

anorexia   Loss or decrease in appetite.

catalepsy   A condition of diminished responsiveness and continually maintained immobile position.

cataplexy   A loss of muscle tone with accompanying weakness.

catatonia A psychotic syndrome that is characterized by muscular rigidity and a lack of response to outside stimuli. Catatonic patients may also have periods of acute agitation.

hypersomnia Sleeping for significantly longer than the usual length of time.

insomnia Difficulty falling asleep and staying asleep.

leaden paralysis Heavy, leaden feeling in the arms and legs.

mood A pervasive and sustained emotion.

mood-congruent psychotic features Include delusions or hallucinations whose content is consistent with typical depressive themes (e.g., worthlessness, guilt, death, nihilism, or punishment) or typical manic themes (e.g., inflated worth, unusual powers, power).

mood-incongruent psychotic features Delusions or hallucinations whose content is not consistent with typical depressive or manic themes including: thought insertion, thought broadcasting, ideas of reference, and delusions of control, etc.

psychomotor agitation An abnormal increase in physical and emotional activity.

psychomotor retardation An abnormal slowing of physical and emotional responses that is commonly seen in depression.

Synopses and Diagnostic Prototypes of the Individual Disorders

The brief synopses in this section include the specific requirements or criteria that must be fulfilled for each of the diagnostic categories. Following each synopsis is a vignette that provides a clinical example of the diagnoses. Each vignette is a prototype in the sense that it represents a typical patient from that specific diagnostic category. The prototypes provide a more lifelike portrayal of the diagnosis than the criteria alone. They also provide a clinical baseline that can be used in the discussion of problems associated with the diagnosis of these disorders and as a standard for comparison even if they do not exhaust all the possibilities for the clinical presentation of a specific diagnosis.

The Mood Disorders group is unusual in the sense that many of the diagnoses in the group are based on the three main Mood Disorder syndromes: Major Depressive Episode, Manic Episode, or Hypomanic Episode. The specific diagnoses are differentiated according to whether the patient is currently experiencing or has previously experienced one or more of the episodes. Some patients may also experience a Mixed Episode with alternating Depression and Mania.

296.2x Major Depressive Disorder, Single Episode. Patients with this disorder have had a Major Depressive Episode but have never had a Manic Episode, Mixed Episode, or Hypomanic episode and do not have a current nondepressive psychotic disorder. (Use the Severity/Psychotic/Remission specifiers for a Major Depressive Episode for the fifth digit.)

> A 25-year-old woman had her first baby 3 weeks ago. The pregnancy and birth were uneventful. The day after the delivery the patient felt a sense of "letdown." The nurse told her, "It's common to feel that way after the delivery, honey. I'm sure you will feel better soon. You have a beautiful baby. Enjoy him." Two days later the patient was discharged. Her mother came to visit and help with the new baby. The patient waited, hoping she would feel better. Instead she began to feel more and more depressed. She began to lose interest in her son and felt guilty that she wasn't a good mother.
>
> During the next 2 weeks the patient felt increasingly tired, had difficulty sleeping, and had little appetite. Her mother and husband noticed that she seemed withdrawn and told her, "Cheer up, you have a lovely baby." Their comments only served to make her feel more guilty about neglecting her son. She felt less energy each day and had to drag herself out of bed each morning. Her mother and husband became worried and tried to help her but their support had little effect on her spiraling depression. The patient has no previous history of a Major Depressive Episode or a Manic Episode.

296.3x Major Depressive Disorder, Recurrent. Patients with this disorder have had two or more previous Major Depressive Episodes that are not due to the effects of a substance or general medical condition; have never had a Manic Episode, Mixed Episode, or Hypomanic Episode; and do not have a current nondepressive psychotic disorder. (Use the Severity/Psychotic/Remission specifiers for a Major Depressive Episode for the fifth digit.)

> A 67-year-old widow was brought to the hospital by her family. They were concerned about her for several weeks because she seems unhappy and cries much of the day. The patient's appetite is decreased and she has lost some weight. The family has tried to cheer her up but she doesn't seem to respond. She has little interest in her usual day-to-day activities with her friends or her grandchildren.
>
> The patient is often agitated and constantly complains that she is destitute despite the fact that her husband left her with a reasonable amount of money. She feels very guilty about "wasting" her dead husband's money and thinks she has nothing left to leave to her grandchildren. In an attempt to correct her mother's misconcep-

tion about her financial status, the daughter confronted the patient with her bank book that showed a balance of several thousand dollars. The patient looked at the bank book and said, "I don't have any money. What will I do?"

300.4   Dysthymic Disorder.   Individuals with this disorder have had persistent depression for at least 2 years, have not had a Major Depressive Episode during the first 2 years of the disorder, and have never had a Manic Episode, Mixed Episode, Hypomanic Episode, or met the criteria for Cyclothymic Disorder. During the depression the patient has experienced at least two of the following:

1. poor appetite or overeating
2. insomnia or hypersomnia
3. low energy or fatigue
4. low self-esteem
5. poor concentration or difficulty making decisions
6. feelings of hopelessness

A 33-year-old woman attorney confided to a friend that she is upset about breaking up with her boyfriend. The two had been going together for 5 years and she thought that they would get married. The patient blamed herself for the breakup. She explained that the boyfriend complained about constantly needing to reassure her that he still cared for her. Despite her accomplishments she still felt inadequate, especially in relationships with men.

   The patient admitted that she had been chronically depressed for several years and often felt hopeless about the future. She worked hard and covered up these feelings at work but often became irritable and angry because she felt the firm and some of her fellow workers took advantage of her. The patient has no previous history of a Major Depressive Episode or a Manic Episode.

311   Depressive Disorder Not Otherwise Specified.   This disorder includes syndromes with depressive symptomatology that do not meet the criteria for Major Depressive Disorder, Dysthymic Disorder, Adjustment Disorder with Depressed Mood, or Adjustment Disorder with Mixed Anxiety and Depressed Mood.

A 22-year-old, fourth-year college student is watching television with his girlfriend when she comments that he seems distant. The student begins crying and says, "I feel depressed. How am I going to get a job when I graduate? Everything I do seems worthless." He describes waking up in the middle of the night and worrying about the future.

   The patient states that he first felt depressed approximately 2 weeks ago when he did poorly on an examination in his major field of study. When he saw the grade he began to worry that his professor would not give him a recommendation and he would not be able to get a good job after graduation.

296.0x Bipolar I Disorder, Single Manic Episode. Patients with this disorder are currently (or recently) in their first Manic Episode and have had no previous Major Depressive Episodes. (Use the Severity/ Psychotic/Remission specifiers for a Manic Episode for the fifth digit.)

> A 28-year-old single man is an associate in a large law firm where he specializes in corporate litigation. He has always been conservative and modest, going quietly about his business. Recently, his colleagues have noticed a significant change in his behavior. During the last few weeks he has become more effusive and outspoken with his friends. He talks continuously about new ideas that he has that will revolutionize American business. Most of his ideas make no sense to his colleagues. Nevertheless, the patient has tried to contact the presidents of several large corporations to explain his ideas to them.
>
> His work at the firm has significantly deteriorated during the same period of time. The secretaries have sarcastically nicknamed him "Don Juan" because of his flirting. He was involved in sexual liaisons with at least two of them before the word of his activities spread around the firm. Recently one of the senior partners in the firm met with him to discuss allegations by two women attorneys that he has repeatedly pestered them to have sex with him. The patient did not deny the charges and stated that the women did not know what they were missing. The patient has no previous history of similar behavior.

296.40 Bipolar I Disorder, Most Recent Episode Hypomanic. Patients with this disorder are currently (or recently) in a Hypomanic Episode and have had at least one previous Manic Episode or Mixed Episode.

> A 36-year-old married woman with two preteen children has become increasingly irritable over the 4 or 5 days. Although she is generally tolerant of her childrens' behavior, she now becomes annoyed whenever they ask her a question and seems easily distracted. The children have told their father, "Mom's taking off again." The patient's husband reports that his wife sleeps only 2 or 3 hours each night and then gets up to work on the household bills or plans for a party she wants to give.
>
> When the couple talk the conversation is usually one-sided because the patient doesn't pause long enough to allow him to speak. During these monologues he sometimes has difficulty understanding what his wife is saying because she jumps rapidly from topic to topic. Despite this, the patient has been able to maintain the house and take care of the children. Her husband is concerned about his wife because she has had three previous manic episodes in the past 10 years. During each of these previous episodes she became increasingly irritable, developed frank delusions, and required hospitalization.

296.4x Bipolar I Disorder, Most Recent Episode Manic. Patients with this disorder are currently (or recently) in a Manic Episode and have had at least one previous Major Depressive Episode, Manic Episode, or Mixed Episode. (Use the Severity/Psychotic/Remission specifiers for a Manic Episode for the fifth digit.)

A 42-year-old business man owns a small clothing store that he runs with his wife. She reports that several days ago he began to talk about a new theory he had developed to make money in the stock market. He tried, unsuccessfully, to explain the theory to his wife. When she told him that it didn't make any sense, he began screaming, "I'm a genius. You don't know what you're talking about. I'm going to make a fortune."

He slept little and spent most of his time working on his investment theory and rearranging the merchandise in their store. A few days later he began buying large amounts of stocks on margin. The patient's wife reports that he has had a number of similar episodes in the past during which he became grandiose and developed several "sure-fire" investment schemes. During one episode he tried to corner the egg futures market and the couple ended up taking delivery on a railroad boxcar full of eggs worth $50,000. In the past his episodes have occurred when he stopped taking his medication.

296.6x   Bipolar I Disorder, Most Recent Episode Mixed.   Patients with this disorder are currently (or recently) in a Mixed Episode and have had at least one previous Major Depressive Episode, Manic Episode, or Mixed Episode. (Use the Severity/Psychotic/Remission specifiers for a Mixed Episode for the fifth digit.)

A 31-year-old woman has a history of several previous Major Depressive Episodes and Manic Episodes. She is currently in treatment with a psychiatrist who has prescribed lithium. The patient stopped taking her medication when her psychiatrist went on a 2-week vacation.

When he returned the patient reported that she had been very upset while he was away. She told him, "I feel like I've been on a roller coaster since you left. One minute I feel irritable and depressed or worthless. An hour later I feel great like I could conquer the world or do anything I set my mind to." The patient continued, "Sometimes I can't sit still or concentrate on anything. Everything distracts me." She reported that the problems started a few days after she stopped taking her medication. Since that time she has been unable to sleep more than a few hours a night because thoughts keep racing through her head.

296.5x   Bipolar I Disorder, Most Recent Episode Depressed.   Patients with this disorder are currently (or recently) in a Major Depressive Episode and have previously had at least one previous Manic Episode or Mixed Episode. (Use the Severity/Psychotic/Remission specifiers for a Major Depressive Episode for the fifth digit.)

A 40-year-old man has been unemployed for 2 months ever since he was fired from his position as an assistant administrator of a large nursing home. During the last month he reports that he has become depressed and experiences little pleasure from his usual daily activities. He has difficulty getting to sleep and wakes up periodically throughout the night obsessing about what he did wrong. During the day he has little energy and feels like he can barely move. His wife has told him, "Stop moping around! Get out and find another job."

The patient feels likes he is worthless and will never find another job again. He reports that he has had this experience before. Over the last 20 years he has had multiple periods of depression interspersed with periods when he reports that he is "on top of the world" and "everything is going great." After several weeks of elated feelings he plunges into a depression. His depressions usually last 3–4 months and then remit spontaneously. When the depression begins to lift he has more energy and starts looking for a job. He speaks well and is convincing when he isn't depressed so he commonly finds a job within a few weeks. He usually does well in his work for several months.

After a few months the patient begins to feel his confidence return. He describes it as a feeling that "I can conquer the world." He works harder, spends more time at his job. and devises new plans to improve productivity. His superiors are initially pleased but soon become concerned because the patient makes grandiose plans, talks endlessly, and never completes a project. Finally, after a few weeks of this activity he is fired. His boss is frequently apologetic, explaining that he has never run into this problem before and says, "I'm sorry but I have to let you go." The patient typically becomes depressed a few weeks later.

296.7   Bipolar I Disorder, Most Recent Episode Unspecified.   Patients with this disorder currently (or recently) meet the criteria for a Manic Episode, Hypomanic Episode, Mixed Episode, or Major Depressive Episode except for duration and have had at least one previous Manic Episode or Mixed Episode.

A 27-year-old construction worker has been depressed for the last week. His fellow workers have complained that he seems indecisive and isn't carrying his share of the work. The patient has little energy during the day. He reports that he isn't sleeping well and his appetite has decreased.

His current behavior is in sharp contrast to a period 3 years before when he seemed to have inexhaustible energy, was excessively self-confident, and needed no more than 3–4 hours of sleep a night. During that time he took out a large loan to renovate his house and another large business loan to start a contracting business. The business failed because he did not adequately manage his costs. He was eventually forced to take his current job as a construction worker to pay back his loans and support his family.

296.89   Bipolar II Disorder.   (Recurrent major depressive episodes with hypomanic episodes): Patients with this disorder have had at least one Major Depressive Episode, at least one Hypomanic Episode, and no Manic Episodes or Mixed Episodes. Specify current or most recent episode: *Hypomanic* or *Depressed*.

A 27-year-old single unmarried mother of two young children was referred by a friend to her local community mental health center. The patient reports that she has been feeling depressed and tired most of the day for the last month. She currently works as a cashier in a supermarket and frequently finds it difficult to concentrate on her work. Her supervisor has spoken to her twice in the last week because she made mistakes by either undercharging or overcharging customers. At night the patient often wakes up and worries about keeping her job and taking care of her children. She is obsessed with the thought that she might die and leave her two children alone.

The patient has had two previous similar episodes of depression. This episode began differently from the others. For the first few days the patient felt terrific. She had inexhaustible energy despite little sleep at night. She stayed long hours at work and was convinced that the manager would soon see how effective she was and promote her to his assistant or even step aside and make her the new manager. At the same time she said, "I spent more money than I could really afford on new furniture and toys for the children because I thought things were finally turning around for us." After a few days she awoke one morning feeling depressed.

301.13   Cyclothymic Disorder.   Patients with this disorder have had many periods of hypomanic symptoms and many periods of depressive symptoms for at least 2 years but have not met the criteria for a Major Depressive Episode, Manic Episode, or Mixed Episode in the first 2 years of the disturbance.

A 31-year-old woman who owns a small gourmet restaurant complains that her life feels like it is in a state of constant flux. "Some days I feel like I'm on top of the world. I can design a new dish in the afternoon and whip up thirty meals and ten soufflés an hour in the evening. My kitchen staff barely have time to wash the dishes." "On other days," she continues, "I feel depressed and can barely get out of bed and go into the restaurant."

The patient reports that she gets her work done even though it is difficult. During these periods she wonders why she even bothers running a restaurant. Everything seems to be a problem. The periods of depressed mood last a few days and then pass. Sometimes her friends and employees at work comment that her mood changes a lot and they don't know how she will be acting from one day to the next. The patient reports that her moods often do change from one extreme to another in a few days. "I feel like a ping pong ball: up, down, up, down." The patient has never had a Major Depressive Episode or a Manic Episode.

296.80   Bipolar Disorder Not Otherwise Specified.   Patients with this disorder have bipolar features but do not meet the criteria for and specific bipolar disorder.

A 36-year-old used car salesman describes himself in the following terms. "I'm an up kind of guy." He is the most productive salesman in his agency. Periodically he experiences what he calls a "selling frenzy" when he is effusive, expansive, and self-confident to the point of being obnoxious. Nevertheless, during these periods he sells substantially more cars than his fellow salesman. He won't take no for an answer and pursues customers until they get irritated or finally buy a car. One of his fellow workers says, "He just keeps on talking." His colleagues steer the most resistant customers to him. Often he is called in as the "closer" to finally persuade the customer to buy.

During these periods he works late and then spends most of the night dancing in local nightclubs and pursuing women for one-night sexual encounters. After a few weeks he settles down to what he calls his "quiet time" that lasts until another "selling frenzy" begins.

293.83   Mood Disorder Due to . . . *[Indicate the General Medical Condition].* This disorder includes a persistent and prominent disturbance of mood characterized by symptoms of depression (depressed mood, anhedonia) or mania (elevated, expansive or irritable mood) that appear to be caused by an underlying non-psychiatric medical condition and do not occur exclusively during the course of Delirium.

A 47-year-old conservative businessman began acting strangely over a period of a week or two. His business decisions became somewhat erratic and he seemed euphoric, expansive, and somewhat uninhibited. The patient made sexual overtures and inappropriate sexual comments to a secretary and the wife of one of his partners. He seemed forgetful and started missing appointments.

His wife convinced him to see the family physician. The patient's physical examination was unremarkable with the exception of some mild memory impairment noted by the physician. A subsequent Magnetic Resonance Imaging scan (MRI) disclosed a lesion in the frontal lobe area of the patient's brain that was determined at surgery to be a malignant tumor.

29x.xx   Substance-Induced Mood Disorder.   The disorder includes a persistent and prominent disturbance of mood characterized by symptoms of depression (depressed mood, anhedonia) or mania (elevated, expansive, or irritable mood) associated with evidence that the symptoms developed within 1 month of significant substance intoxication or withdrawal are etiologically related to medication use or toxin exposure.

The specific codes for (Specific Substance)-Induced Mood Disorder are determined by the specific substance: 291.8 alcohol; and 292.84 amphetamines; cocaine; hallucinogens; inhalants; opioids; phencyclidine; sedatives, hypnotics, or anxiolytics; other (or unknown) substances.

A 27-year-old taxi driver arrived in a hospital emergency room one evening complaining of depression. She explained that she had been feeling depressed with thoughts of suicide for the last 3 days. In the past month the patient reported losing

10 pounds, although her appetite had increased in the last few days. She told the physician, "I want some medicine for my depression. I know you can give me something. Xanax worked before." The patient's urine toxicology screen showed trace amounts of cocaine. The specific diagnosis was Cocaine Mood Disorder with depressive features and onset during withdrawal (292.84).

296.90   Mood Disorder Not Otherwise Specified: This disorder includes mood symptoms that do not meet the criteria for any specific Mood Disorder including Depressive Disorder Not Otherwise Specified and Bipolar Disorder Not Otherwise Specified.

A 33-year-old waitress is brought to her local community mental health center by her boyfriend. He reports that she has been very upset for the last 3 days. The patient is agitated, crying, and complains of feeling depressed and being a failure. This is followed by outburst of elevated self-esteem and assertions that she can overcome all the obstacles. She doesn't sleep well and complains of feeling tired yet she can't sit down and constantly talks about feeling depressed.

Necessary Clinical Information

The accurate diagnosis of a Mood Disorder requires the following clinical information.

- History of financial difficulties or failed business investments

- History of increased sexual activity and sexual indiscretions

- History of previous depression, hypomania, or mania

- History of rapid switches in mood

- History of substance abuse

- History of medical illness

- Current mood

- Patient's guilty feelings, quality of self-esteem, or sense of worth

- Current hallucinations or delusions

- Current and previous suicide ideation or attempts

- Change in the patient's level of energy or fatigue

- Change in the patient's pattern of sleep

Making a Diagnosis

Everyone has experienced some degree of depression and euphoria in their lives. The distinction between usual fluctuations in mood and a Mood Disorder is described in the core concept of the diagnostic group. Briefly, the diagnosis of a Mood Disorder depends on the intensity and duration of the mood disturbance, its accompanying symptoms, and the degree to which it interferes with the individual's social and occupational functioning.

The Mood Disorders diagnostic group is organized in two main categories, depressive illnesses and bipolar illnesses. Each category contains diagnoses for severe disorders (Major Depressive Disorder, Single Episode; Bipolar I Disorder, Single Manic Episode; etc.); less severe, more chronic disorders (Dysthymic Disorder, Cyclothymic Disorder, etc.); and nonspecific disorders (Depressive Disorder Not Otherwise Specified, Bipolar Disorder Not Otherwise Specified, and Mood Disorder Not Otherwise Specified). Patients may have more than one Mood Disorder at the same time. For example, a Major Depressive Disorder, Single Episode may be superimposed on a Dysthymic Disorder. Diagnoses within a category are further distinguished by the patient's current symptoms, the etiology of the disorder, and the patient's past history of psychiatric illness.

The most important diagnostic decision in the Mood Disorders groups is usually the determination of whether the patient fulfills the criteria for one or more of the four main syndromes, Major Depressive Episode, Manic Episode, Hypomanic Episode, or Mixed Episode. Once this diagnostic question is answered, the range of possible diagnoses is considerably narrowed.

The questions in this section provide a step-by-step method for processing the clinical information necessary to make the diagnosis of a typical Mood Disorder. Table 7–1 provides a summary of the relationship between current and past Major Depressive, Manic, Hypomanic, and Mixed Episodes in the diagnosis of the various Mood Disorders. Table 7–2 provides a summary of the current or recent episode and recurrent mood episode specifiers applicable to each coded Mood Disorder. Specific problems in the diagnosis of these disorders will be discussed in the next section.

1. Is the patient's mood abnormal?

The patient or another person must identify that the patient's mood is abnormal to begin the diagnostic process for a Mood Disorder. Because mood is a personal and subjective experience, it is often the patient who asks for help by telling someone that he feels depressed, sad, irritable, elated, or otherwise different from normal. This self-referral is probably more common for patients with depression than those who are manic or hypomanic. Other people may suspect that the patient has a mood disturbance if they observe typical depressed or manic behaviors such as crying, withdrawal, or pressured speech. The first step

Table 7–1 Current and past major depressive, manic, hypomanic, and mixed episodes in the diagnosis of Mood Disorders

Diagnosis	Current episode				Past episode			
	Major Depressive	Manic	Hypomanic	Mixed	Major Depressive	Manic	Hypomanic	Mixed
Major Depressive Disorder, Single Episode	●				Never	Never	Never	Never
Major Depressive Disorder, Recurrent	●				●	Never	Never	Never
Dysthymic Disorder					Not in first 2 years	Never	Never	Never
Bipolar I Disorder, Single Manic Episode		●			Never		Never	
Bipolar I Disorder, Most Recent Episode Hypomanic			●			■		■
Bipolar I Disorder, Most Recent Episode Manic		●			■	■		■
Bipolar I Disorder, Most Recent Episode Mixed				●	■	■		■
Bipolar I Disorder, Most Recent Episode Depressed	●					■		■
Bipolar I Disorder, Most Recent Episode Unspecified	▲■	▲■	▲■	▲■		■		■
Bipolar II Disorder (Major Depression with hypomania)	■		■		●	Never	●	Never
Cyclothymic Disorder	▲		■		▲●	Not in first 2 years	●	Not in first 2 years

Note. ● = Required episode(s) for diagnosis of a disorder. ■ = Alternate episode choices, only one type of episode is necessary to satisfy criteria for diagnosis. ▲ = Patient has mood symptoms but does not meet the full criteria for a Major Depressive, Manic, Hypomanic, or Mixed Episode. *Never* = Patient has never fulfilled criteria for a specific episode. *Not in first 2 years* = Episode may not occur within first 2 years of disorder but may occur thereafter.

Table 7-2 Specifiers for current or most recent episode and recurrent episodes

Diagnosis	Current or recent episode			Recurrent episode		
	Severity, Psychotic, and Remission	Chronic, Melancholic, and Atypical	Catatonic, and Postpartum	Longitudinal Course	Seasonal Pattern	Rapid Cycling
Major Depressive Disorder, Single Episode	X	X	X			
Major Depressive Disorder, Recurrent	X	X	X	X	X	
Dysthymic Disorder		X*				
Bipolar I Disorder, Single Manic Episode	X		X			
Bipolar I Disorder, Most Recent Episode Hypomanic				X	X	X
Bipolar I Disorder, Most Recent Episode Manic	X		X	X	X	X
Bipolar I Disorder, Most Recent Episode Mixed	X		X	X	X	X
Bipolar I Disorder, Most Recent Episode Depressed	X	X	X	X	X	X
Bipolar I Disorder, Most Recent Episode Unspecified			X	X	X	X
Bipolar II Disorder (Major Depression with hypomania)	X	X	X		X	X

*Only Atypical Features Specifier applies to Dysthymic Disorder.

in diagnosis is to identify which abnormal symptoms of a Mood Disorder the patient is currently experiencing.

2. Could the patient's symptoms be produced by drugs or a nonpsychiatric medical illness?

Determine whether the patient has any current nonpsychiatric medical illnesses or substance-related problems. If so, deciding the relationship between these problems and the patient's psychiatric symptoms should be the first step in the diagnostic process. The presence of nonpsychiatric medical illnesses or substance-related problem in conjunction with psychiatric symptoms does not imply the former caused the latter.

The occurrence of psychiatric symptoms before the onset of a medical illness or use of a substance suggests that they have an independent etiology. Similarly, the persistence of the psychiatric symptoms after adequate treatment of the medical illness or cessation of substance use implies that the two are unrelated. Generally, symptoms that occur more than a month after an episode of drug intoxication or withdrawal are not considered to be due to the drug. The diagnoses of Mood Disorder Due to a General Medical Condition and Substance-Induced Mood Disorder can be excluded if there is no evidence that a nonpsychiatric medical disorder or drugs have produced the patient's symptoms.

Note: Assume that an organic etiology for the patient's symptoms has been ruled out for the remaining questions in this section.

3. Does the patient have symptoms of psychosis (e.g., delusions, hallucinations, thought insertion, thought broadcasting)?

- If the patient does not currently (or did not recently) have symptoms of psychosis, the following diagnoses can be excluded: Schizoaffective Disorder, Schizophrenia, Schizophreniform Disorder, Delusional Disorder, and Psychotic Disorder Not Otherwise Specified.

- If the patient has psychotic symptoms (or did recently) but they have not occurred for at least 2 weeks in the absence of the mood symptoms, the diagnosis of Schizoaffective Disorder can be excluded.

- If the patient has psychotic symptoms that only occur in the presence of the mood symptoms, the diagnosis is either Major Depressive Disorder, Depressive Disorder Not Otherwise Specified, Bipolar I Disorder, or Bipolar Disorder Not Otherwise Specified.

4. Has the patient ever had a manic, hypomanic, or mixed episode?

- If the patient currently or in the past has met the criteria for a Manic, Mixed, or Hypomanic Episode, all of the depressive disorders may be excluded.

- If the patient currently does not have a current Manic, Hypomanic, or Mixed Episode, the following diagnoses are excluded: Bipolar I Disorder Single Manic Episode; Bipolar I Disorder, Most Recent Episode Hypomanic; Bipolar I Disorder, Most Recent Episode Manic; and Bipolar I Disorder, Most Recent Episode Mixed.

- If the patient has never had a previous Manic or Mixed Episode, the following diagnoses are excluded: Bipolar I Disorder Most Recent Episode Depressed and Bipolar I Disorder Most Recent Episode Unspecified.

5. Is the patient's current mood depressed?

- If the patient fulfills the criteria for a Major Depressive Episode and there have been no previous Manic Episodes, the diagnosis is Major Depressive Disorder.

- If the patient fulfills the criteria for a Major Depressive Episode and there has been a previous Manic or Hypomanic Disorder, all of the depressive diagnoses can be excluded.

- If the patient fulfills the criteria for a Major Depressive Disorder and also fulfills the criteria for a Dysthymic Disorder, he can receive both diagnoses if he did not have a Major Depressive Episode within the first 2 years of the Dysthymic Disorder. In other words, a Major Depressive Disorder can be superimposed on a Dysthymic Disorder if the latter diagnosis has been independently established.

Common Problems in Making a Diagnosis

There are three main areas of uncertainty in the differential diagnosis of Mood Disorders.

1. Some patients initially come close but don't actually fulfill the criteria for a specific diagnosis. More information or a further consideration of the diagnostic criteria may or may not resolve the problem.
2. Some patients fulfill the diagnostic criteria for more than one, mutually exclusive, Mood Disorder during the course of their illness.
3. Some patients have isolated symptoms of depression or mania associated with other psychiatric disorders but do not fulfill the criteria for a specific Mood Disorder.

Patients Who Almost Fulfill the Diagnostic Criteria

Most people have felt depressed or euphoric at one or more periods in their life. A portion of these have a diagnosable Mood Disorder. Unfortunately, it is not always easy to determine when an individual has passed over the line separating normal mood fluctuations from mood pathology. Patient's who almost fulfill the diagnostic criteria fall into this borderline area. The patient may present complaints that are consistent with a Mood Disorder but do not completely fulfill the criteria for a specific diagnosis.

Frequently, further inquiry will elicit the necessary additional clinical information. At other times it may be impossible to obtain the necessary information to determine whether the patient fulfills the required criteria for a Mood Disorder. For example, a patient may have a distinctly elevated mood and other manic symptoms but still not fulfill all the criteria required for a Bipolar I Disorder. Most of the diagnoses in the Mood Disorders group depend on whether the patient has currently or previously experienced one or more of the three main mood syndromes: Major Depressive Episode, Manic Episode, and Hypomanic Episode.

Similarly, many of the problems in diagnosis of these disorders relate to decisions of whether the patient has fulfilled the criteria for these syndromes and what diagnosis to use if they have not. Problems in fulfilling the criteria usually revolve around questions of the duration, number, and type of symptoms the patient has experienced. For example, a patient may have all of the symptoms of a Dysthymic Disorder but the disorder has lasted less than 2 years. In situations like this it is often useful to refer back to the core concept of the diagnostic group as well as the diagnostic criteria and remember that DSM-IV is a set of guidelines rather than rigid rules. The clinician has considerable leeway in deciding how to interpret the patient's symptoms to fulfill the criteria for a specific diagnosis.

Example 1

A 28-year-old woman reports that she feels very depressed, worthless, and hopeless for periods of up to a week several times a year. During these periods she sleeps poorly, is tired most of the day, and has recurrent thoughts of death. What diagnosis can be made with this clinical information?

The patient's illness can be summarized as recurrent, brief episodes of depression. The episodes meet the criteria for a Major Depressive Episode except for the duration requirement of 2 weeks or more. Therefore, the diagnosis of Major Depressive Disorder, Recurrent cannot be made. The patient's symptoms do not meet the criteria for a Dysthymic Disorder because the required number and type of symptoms are not present and the duration of symptoms is less than two years. She can be given a diagnosis of Depressive Disorder Not Otherwise

Specified with the information provided. This is essentially a wastebasket diagnosis for patients who have depression but don't meet the criteria for any other specific depression diagnosis.

Clearly the requirement for a symptom duration of 2 weeks or more in the diagnosis of a Major Depressive Episode is an arbitrary choice. A clinician could probably justify making a diagnosis of Major Depressive Disorder, Single Episode if the patient had symptoms for only 11 or 12 days. In this patient it would probably be useful for the clinician to question the patient further about the duration of symptoms because she may be underestimating them.

A more important question is whether a patient who had repeated episodes of severe depression separated by brief periods without depression that do not fulfill the duration criterion, should be treated any differently than a patient with a severe depression that just meets the duration criterion for a Major Depressive Disorder, Recurrent. Most clinicians would probably treat them the same. Unfortunately, a diagnostic system based on specific criteria includes distinct limits that may not always make clinical sense.

Example 2

A 37-year-old woman has felt very depressed, worthless, and has had difficulty sleeping for several weeks. She also reports having repeated thoughts of death and dying, some suicidal ideation, and has often envisioned herself lying in a coffin. The symptoms have significantly interfered with her ability to work. The patient has no previous history of depression or mania. What diagnosis can be given to this patient based on this information?

The criteria for a Major Depressive Episode requires that the patient have five of the nine symptoms in part A of the criteria set for at least 2 weeks. This patient has met the duration criteria by experiencing symptoms for several weeks. However, she reports only four symptoms: depression, feelings of worthlessness, insomnia, and recurrent thoughts of death with suicidal ideation. Therefore by a strict interpretation of the criteria, the patient has not experienced a Major Depressive Episode and cannot receive a diagnosis of Major Depressive Disorder, Single Episode.

Because she has had no previous history of depression and the symptoms have lasted less than 2 years, she cannot receive a diagnosis of Dysthymic Disorder. The only remaining diagnosis is a Depressive Disorder Not Otherwise Specified. A minor Depressive Disorder is an unofficial subcategory of this diagnosis. It includes patients who fulfill most of the criteria for a Major Depressive Disorder, Single Episode but do not have the five symptoms required for the diagnosis.

Many clinicians would find the diagnosis of Depressive Disorder Not Otherwise Specified for this patient unsettling. The patient is very depressed and potentially suicidal. This diagnosis does not adequately communicate the severity or nature of the patient's illness. Therefore, it could be argued that the patient should receive a diagnosis of Major Depressive Disorder, Single Episode even though she demonstrates only four of the required five items for a Major Depressive Episode. Further interview or clinical observation may identify a fifth item at a later time.

Example 3

A 31-year-old electrician who works for a small electrical contracting company reports that he has felt elated and almost "high" for the last 2 weeks. People have commented that he seems different and more cheerful than usual. He talks incessantly, sleeps only a few hours each night, and works long hours. His boss has praised him, commenting that the patient is a changed man and now does the work of two men. The patient says, "My boss is a jerk. I could run things better than him and make twice as much money. I have a million ideas about how to improve the company. He should make me a partner." The patient presented some of his ideas to his boss and got angry when the man seemed uninterested. The patient has had one previous Major Depressive Episode but no previous Manic or Hypomanic Episodes. What diagnosis (es), if any, should this patient receive?

This patient's mood change suggests that he may have Bipolar Disorder. He meets the duration and symptom criteria for both a Manic and Hypomanic Episode. The disturbance has lasted more than 1 week and he has an elevated mood, grandiosity, decreased need for sleep, increased talking, and increased goal-directed activities at work. All of these symptoms are significantly different from his usual behavior. The changes in his behavior have also been noticed and commented on by others.

The major diagnostic question is whether the patient is currently having a Manic or a Hypomanic Episode. The patient has had a previous Major Depressive Episode. Therefore, his present diagnosis would be Bipolar I Disorder, Most Recent Episode Manic if he is currently having a Manic Episode and Bipolar II Disorder (recurrent major depressive episodes with hypomania) if he currently has a Hypomanic Episode. Manic and Hypomanic Episodes are mainly differentiated by their duration and the degree of impairment they produce in occupational functioning, social activities, or relationships with others. This patient's disturbance has lasted for 2 weeks, which exceeds the requirements for both episodes. The patient's productivity at work has improved rather than declined since the onset of the disturbance. However, there is some suggestion that his grandiosity, increased irritability, and confrontation with his boss could be considered an impairment of his occupational functioning and could lead to his dismissal.

The differential diagnosis of Manic versus Hypomanic Episode rests on the interpretation of the patient's functionality. This decision is based on the physician's judgment. An equally important question is whether the patient should be given medication. It could be argued that treatment is necessary because the patient is currently in a Manic Episode or because he will progress to one if not treated.

Example 4

A 43-year-old woman reports that she has been feeling very depressed on and off for the last 3 months. During these periods she feels worthless and has suicidal preoccupations, although she has no suicidal intent. The depression usually lasts for several days, lifting for a few days when the patient has something positive like a party or trip she is anticipating. After the event she becomes depressed again within a day or two.

   During the periods of depression the patient goes to bed early in the evening, sleeps through the night, and has difficulty waking up in the morning. She feels tired most of the day and frequently takes a nap during the afternoon. The patient also complains that she has gained approximately 7 pounds during the 3 months because her appetite has increased. She has no previous history of a Major Depressive Episode or a Manic or Hypomanic Episode. Can this patient receive a diagnosis of Major Depressive Disorder, Single Episode?

This patient is similar in one way to the patient in Example 1. She appears to have repeated periods of severe depression that last an indeterminate length of time. Therefore, it is difficult to decide whether she meets the duration criteria of 2 weeks necessary for the diagnosis of a Major Depressive Episode. She has two other typical symptoms of depression, feelings of worthlessness and suicidal preoccupations. Her other symptoms of hypersomnia, increased appetite, and weight gain are atypical. As a result, she does not fit the criteria for a standard Major Depressive Episode. However, her symptoms are consistent with a Major Depressive Episode with Atypical Features. The problem of her apparent separate periods of depression could be resolved by interpreting them as a continuous depression broken by periods of mood reactivity to positive events with subsequent reversion to depressed mood. The diagnosis would be Major Depressive Disorder, Single Episode With Atypical Features.

Example 5

A 32-year-old man has had numerous Hypomanic Episodes interspersed with intervals of severe depression over several years. The periods of depression last several days during which the patient has difficulty sleeping, suicidal ruminations, and a sense of worthlessness or significantly diminished self-esteem. The patient has never had a Manic Episode. What diagnosis(es) should this patient receive?

There are only two diagnoses in the Mood Disorders group that include hypomanic and depressive symptoms and exclude a Manic Episode. The diagnosis of Bipolar II Disorder (recurrent major depressive episodes with hypomania), requires the presence of at least one Hypomanic Episode and one or more Major Depressive Episodes. There is no specific duration requirement other than those implicit in the criteria for the Hypomanic and Major Depressive Episodes. The diagnosis of Cyclothymic Disorder requires numerous periods of hypomanic symptoms and numerous periods of depressed mood occurring over a period of at least 2 years. A Manic Episode may occur after this initial 2-year period.

The Cyclothymic Disorder is considered a less serious disorder than a Bipolar II Disorder and is similar to the distinction between a Dysthymic Disorder and a Major Depressive Disorder, Single Episode. In this case the patient has a Hypomanic Episode and a severely depressed mood. However, he does not quite meet the criteria for a Major Depressive Episode because he has only four instead of five symptoms and there is some uncertainty about whether the symptoms have lasted at least 2 weeks.

Officially the patient should receive a diagnosis of Cyclothymic Disorder. However, the severity of his symptoms should influence the physician to probe for additional clinical information that might confirm a Major Depressive Episode at some time in the past. Symptoms such as fatigue and indecisiveness are subjective enough that further discussion might confirm their presence and thereby fulfill the criteria for a Bipolar II Disorder.

Patients Who Fulfill the Diagnostic Criteria for More Than One Mood Disorder

A patient may fulfill the criteria for more than one Mood Disorder diagnosis at the same time. Usually when this occurs the rules for the precedence of diagnosis (see section on The Precedence of Diagnosis) or the general criteria will determine which diagnosis to use. Sometimes the patient may actually have two comorbid Mood Disorders superimposed on each other or overlapping in time.

In some circumstances, if the patient fulfills the criteria for both disorders he should be given both diagnoses. For example, a patient who develops an initial Major Depressive Episode 2 years after the development of a Dysthymic Disorder should receive an additional diagnosis of a Major Depressive Disorder, Single Episode at that time. However, if the Major Depressive Episode occurs less than 2 years after the onset of the Dysthymic Disorder, the diagnosis of Major Depressive Disorder, Single Episode or Recurrent Episode would take precedence.

A different type of diagnostic problem occurs when a patient develops a Mood Disorder that could have more than one etiology. For example, a patient who has a history of a Major Depressive Disorder develops another Major Depressive Episode at the same time that she stops using cocaine. Is her diagnosis Major Depressive Disorder, Recurrent or Cocaine Mood Disorder with onset during withdrawal? Although there are some guidelines for distinguishing between these diagnoses, frequently the distinction is based on the clinician's judgment.

Example 6

A 35-year-old man has experienced periods of elevated mood accompanied by increases in self-esteem, work productivity, and casual unsafe sex with multiple partners for the last 18 months. These periods have alternated with brief periods when he is depressed and feels guilty about his sexual escapades. His sleeping has been diminished most of the time.

Recently the patient experienced a 2-week period during which he had an intensification of his elevated mood accompanied by pressured speech and a sense that his thoughts were racing too fast to allow him to communicate his ideas. The patient has never had a Major Depressive Episode. What diagnosis should this patient receive?

This patient's problem is analogous to that of the patient described above who developed a Major Depressive Episode while having Dysthymic Disorder. The current patient has had Hypomanic Episodes alternating with depressed mood for 18 months. Recently he has fulfilled the criteria for a Manic Episode. The criteria for Cyclothymic Disorder requires that the patient experience Hypomanic Episodes and depressed mood for at least 2 years before the occurrence of a Manic Episode. Therefore, he does not meet the criteria for Cyclothymic Disorder.

The occurrence of a single Manic Episode without a previous Major Depressive Episode fulfills the criteria for a diagnosis of Bipolar 1 Disorder, Single Manic Episode. If the patient had met the duration criteria for a Cyclothymic Disorder before the onset of the Manic Episode, he would receive both diagnoses.

Example 7

A 40-year-old woman who was recently diagnosed with systemic lupus erythematosus has been depressed for the last month. She has lost 5 pounds, has little energy or interest in life, sleeps poorly, feels worthless and hopeless about her life, and has thoughts of death and suicide. The patient's husband reports that her thinking and physical activity are markedly slowed down and she has difficulty concentrating.

The patient has been taking 80 mg of prednisone per day for the last month. Her husband also reports that her present mood and behavior are similar to the way they were 3 years before when she was hospitalized with a Major Depressive Disorder, Single Episode. What is this patient's current psychiatric diagnosis?

This patient presents a complex clinical picture that is not unusual for patients having a serious medical illness. The patient is severely depressed and exceeds the minimal psychological criteria for a Major Depressive Episode. However, these criteria stipulate that the symptoms are not due to the direct effects of a substance (e.g., medication) or a general medical condition. In fact, this patient has at least four possible etiologies for her depression.

1. She has had a previous Major Depressive Disorder, Single Episode, so this could be a recurrence of that disorder.
2. She has recently been diagnosed with a serious medical illness so her depression could be a psychological reaction to her lupus erythematosus (i.e., Adjustment Reaction With Depressed Mood).
3. The systemic lupus erythematosus may involve her central nervous system, producing a Mood Disorder Due to a General Medical Condition With Depressive Features.
4. She may have a depression as a side effect of a high dose of a corticosteroid (i.e., Substance-Induced Mood Disorder With Depressive Features). Although corticosteroids generally produce an elevated or manic type mood, they can produce a depressed mood.

There is no investigative approach that will always identify the single correct diagnosis. However, there is a general line of reasoning that may help identify the most likely diagnosis. If the patient's depression continues after the acute episode of systemic lupus erythematosus is brought under control, the depression is probably not caused by the organic effects of the patient's physical illness and the diagnosis of Mood Disorder Due to a General Medical Condition can be excluded.

If the depression began before the patient started prednisone or if it continues after the prednisone is substantially reduced or discontinued, the depression is probably not caused by the medication and the diagnosis of Substance-Induced Mood Disorder can be excluded. Finally, the diagnosis of Major Depressive Disorder, Recurrent takes precedence over the diagnosis of an Adjustment Disorder With Depressed Mood. It may be difficult to wait until the patient's systemic lupus erythematosus is under control and the prednisone discontinued before beginning treatment. Therefore, the clinician should identify a working diagnosis to guide treatment. The most useful working diagnosis is Major Depressive Disorder, Recurrent.

Mood Symptoms Associated With Other Psychiatric Disorders

Depression, mania, and hypomania are frequently found in conjunction with a number of other psychiatric disturbances including Substance-Related Disorders, Psychotic Disorders, Adjustment Disorders, and Personality Disorders.

When this occurs, rules of diagnostic precedence are applied to determine the primary disorder. For example, a patient may have a Major Depressive Episode superimposed over an existing Schizophrenia. In this case there are several choices: 1) the patient could receive either a Mood Disorder or Psychotic Disorder diagnosis; 2) the patient could receive both diagnoses (dual diagnoses); or 3) the patient could receive a third diagnosis such as Schizoaffective Disorder. The diagnosis would depend on the timing and relative frequency of mood symptoms to psychotic symptoms even though the main criteria for both diagnoses are met.

Example 8

A 36-year-old man has been convinced, for the last 3 years, that he has a human immunodeficiency virus (HIV) infection. Repeated negative blood tests for HIV have not convinced him that he is wrong. In each case he has insisted that his test was performed incorrectly or that his results were mixed up with those from other healthy people.

The patient has never had any of the symptoms in Criterion A for Schizophrenia (delusions, hallucinations, disorganized speech or behavior, negative symptoms). Three weeks ago his mood became increasingly elevated and expansive. He started talking incessantly, jumping from one idea to the next without finishing a thought. He began sleeping 3–4 hours a night and his colleagues noticed that his work was deteriorating. His delusions continued. What is this patient's diagnosis(es)?

This patient has a 3-year history of a Psychotic Disorder characterized by a nonbizarre somatic type delusion that he has an HIV infection. Because he has never had symptoms that meet Criterion A for Schizophrenia, he meets the criteria for the diagnosis of a Delusional Disorder. Recently he developed a Manic Episode superimposed on the Psychotic Disorder.

The main diagnostic question is whether the patient's current symptoms constitute a single disorder or two separate disorders. There are several possibilities among the Mood and Psychotic Disorders. Schizoaffective Disorder combines both psychotic and mood symptoms. However, the criteria for this disorder requires that the patient's mood symptoms be concurrent with symptoms that meet Criterion A for Schizophrenia. Because the patient has never experienced any of the symptoms in Criterion A, the diagnosis of Schizoaffective Disorder is excluded.

No other Psychotic Disorder combines mood and psychotic symptoms. The criteria for a Delusional Disorder stipulate that if mood episodes do occur concurrently with delusions, the total duration of the mood symptoms must be brief relative to the duration of the delusional periods. In this patient the mood symptoms have lasted 3 weeks. If the clinician considers this brief relative to the 3-year history of delusions, the patient can still be given a diagnosis of Delusional Disorder to account for the psychotic symptoms.

The remaining question is how to diagnose the patient's mood symptoms. The patient cannot receive a diagnosis of Bipolar I Disorder, Bipolar II Disorder, or Cyclothymic Disorder because these diagnoses are excluded if the patient's mood symptoms are superimposed over Delusional Disorder. He cannot receive a diagnosis of Mood Disorder Due to a General Medical Condition or Substance-Induced Mood Disorder because there is no evidence of a discernible organic basis for the patient's symptoms. The patient can be given a diagnosis of Bipolar Disorder Not Otherwise Specified because it includes all disorders with bipolar features that do not meet the criteria for any specific bipolar disorder. If the patient's mood symptoms persist or recur the diagnosis may have to be re-evaluated. For example, the diagnosis might change to Bipolar I Disorder, Most Recent Episode Manic With Mood-Incongruent Psychotic Features.

Example 9

A 28-year-old woman with a diagnosis of Schizophrenia, Paranoid Type reports a history of several years of hearing voices that tell her to hurt herself and continually comment on her behavior and thoughts. She has been hospitalized twice and treated each time with medication, producing a full remission. Five weeks ago the patient again described hearing voices. Three weeks later she reported feeling depressed and also complained of difficulty sleeping, decreased appetite, excessive fatigue, and feeling guilty that she caused the death of her mother from cancer. What is the most appropriate diagnosis for this patient?

This patient had a previous diagnosis of Schizophrenia, Paranoid Type that was episodic with complete remissions between psychotic episodes. Five weeks ago she began to experience an exacerbation of her Schizophrenia characterized by the reappearance of auditory hallucinations. Three weeks later she reported the development of symptoms that fulfill the criteria for a Major Depressive Episode. If the patient's depression had developed while she was still in full remission from Schizophrenia, she would have fulfilled the criteria for a Major Depressive Disorder, Single Episode.

However, the exacerbation of the patient's Schizophrenia produces a diagnostic problem. The diagnosis of Major Depressive Disorder, Single Episode is excluded if the patient's disorder can be better accounted for by a Schizoaffective Disorder or if her symptoms are superimposed on Schizophrenia. The criteria for the diagnosis of a Schizoaffective Disorder requires an uninterrupted period of illness during which the patient experiences a Major Depressive Episode or Manic Episode concurrent with symptoms that meet Criterion A for Schizophrenia. The mood symptoms must be present for a substantial portion of the total duration of the illness, although the psychotic symptoms must occur for at least 2 weeks in absence of prominent mood symptoms.

The main diagnostic question is whether this single episode of depression in conjunction with an episode of Schizophrenia can justify a switch to a diagnosis of Schizoaffective Disorder. The alternative is to give the patient two separate diagnoses: Schizophrenia, Paranoid Type and Depressive Disorder Not Otherwise Specified. A compromise solution is to give the patient the latter two diagnoses for this episode and continue to follow the patient. If the patient develops a second similar episode of psychotic and depressive symptoms the diagnosis can be switched to Schizoaffective Disorder. This approach emphasizes the importance of determining that the patient's symptoms are reproducible and stable before changing a diagnosis.

Precedence of Diagnosis

Many of the cases in preceding sections discuss diagnostic dilemmas that arise when patients have symptoms consistent with more than one diagnosis. The diagnoses may belong to the same diagnostic group (e.g., Mood Disorders) or different groups (e.g., Mood Disorders and Schizophrenia and Other Psychotic Disorders). When these conflicts occur they are often resolved using the rules of diagnostic precedence that are included in the criteria for many diagnoses. However, these rules are not infallible and in some circumstances we have seen that they are mutually exclusive. Therefore, the rules of diagnostic precedence, rather than taken as hard and firm, should be seen as guidelines. They suggest those other diagnoses that should be considered before a specific diagnosis is made and they indicate the circumstances under which the diagnosis in question may be excluded if the patient fulfills the criteria for other diagnoses.

Mood Disorders frequently appear in conjunction with another psychiatric disorder. Table 7–3 presents a list of disorders that may take precedence over various Mood Disorders. Two examples of this problem were discussed in the last section. Usually, the criteria for the respective disorders include rules that indicate how the conflict should be resolved. The most common example of this problem is the simultaneous occurrence of a Mood Disorder such as a Major Depressive Disorder and Schizophrenia or another psychotic disorder. As discussed above, the primary diagnosis usually depends on the duration of mood symptoms relative to psychotic symptoms.

Another potential conflict occurs around the precedence of organic diagnoses (e.g., Substance-Induced Mood Disorder) over nonorganic diagnoses (e.g., Major Depressive Disorders, Bipolar I Disorders) and vice versa. This reciprocal relationship appears contradictory. However, it serves the purpose of emphasizing that the co-occurrence of mood symptoms and organic factors is not necessarily a cause-and-effect relationship. At the same time it emphasizes the importance of ruling out a possible organic etiology in every Mood Disorder. Table 7–3 should be used as a reminder of those diagnoses that must be considered and excluded before a specific Mood Disorder diagnosis can be made.

Table 7–3 Precedence of diagnosis for mood disorders

Mood disorder	Disorders taking precedence
Major Depressive Disorder, Single Episode Major Depressive Disorder, Recurrent	Has never met criteria for Manic Episode, Hypomanic, or Mixed Episode Does not occur exclusively during Schizophrenia, Schizophreniform Disorder, Delusional Disorder, Psychotic Disorder NOS Not better accounted for by Schizoaffective Disorder Not due to effects of a substance or general medical condition
Dysthymic Disorder	Has never met criteria for Manic Episode, Hypomanic, or Mixed Episode; Cyclothymic Disorder Does not occur exclusively during Schizophrenia, Delusional Disorder Not better accounted for by Major Depressive Disorder Not due to effects of a substance or general medical condition
Depressive Disorder NOS	Does not meet criteria for any specific Depressive Disorder, Adjustment Disorder With Depressed Mood, Adjustment Disorder With Mixed Anxiety and Depressive mood
Bipolar I Disorder Single Manic Episode	Has never met criteria for Major Depressive Episode Does not occur exclusively during Schizophrenia, Schizophreniform Disorder, Delusional Disorder, Psychotic Disorder NOS Not better accounted for by Schizoaffective Disorder Not due to effects of a substance or general medical condition

Bipolar I Disorder
  Most Recent Episode Hypomanic
  Most Recent Episode Manic
  Most Recent Episode Mixed
  Most Recent Episode Depressed
  Most Recent Episode Unspecified
Bipolar II Disorder
Cyclothymic Disorder
	Does not occur exclusively during Schizophrenia, Schizophreniform Disorder, Delusional Disorder, Psychotic Disorder NOS
	Not better accounted for by Schizoaffective Disorder
	Not due to effects of a substance or general medical condition

Bipolar Disorder NOS	Does not meet criteria for any other specific bipolar disorder

Table 7–3 Precedence of diagnosis for mood disorders *(continued)*	
Mood disorder	**Disorders taking precedence**
Mood Disorder Due to a General Medical Condition	Does not occur exclusively during Delirium Not better accounted for by another mental disorder
Substance-Induced Mood Disorder	Does not occur exclusively during Delirium Not better accounted for by Mood Disorder that is not substance-induced
Mood Disorder NOS	Does not meet criteria for any other non-substance-induced specific Mood Disorder

Note.   NOS = Not Otherwise Specified.

Discussion of Clinical Vignettes

Vignette 1: Why Didn't I Stop Him

Elaine's initial sadness and loneliness appeared to be part of a common mourning reaction to the death of her husband. However, the circumstances and consequence of his death were not usual. She was angry that he deceived her about using drugs and died leaving her with responsibility for the children and few financial resources. Gradually, she became depressed and began to feel guilty about her husband's death and her anger.

The main diagnostic question for this patient is distinguishing between a common mourning reaction and a clinical depression. Because the predominant mood in mourning is one of sadness or depression, it is difficult to make a specific diagnosis of depression during the period of mourning if the patient's only symptoms are depressed mood. In accordance with this observation, the criteria for a Major Depressive Episode specifies that the diagnosis not be made if the patient's symptoms occur within 2 months of the loss of a loved one. The only exceptions are when the patient has other relevant symptoms in addition to depressed mood. Specifically, the presence of significant functional impairment, morose preoccupations with worthlessness, suicidal ideation, psychomotor retardation, or symptoms of psychosis allow the diagnosis of a Major Depressive Episode to be made within the first 2 months of a period of mourning.

Elaine fulfills all of the criteria for a Major Depressive Episode. She has been depressed for more than 2 weeks and has a diminished interest in usual daily activities, insomnia, feelings of worthlessness and excessive guilt, fatigue and loss of energy, diminished ability to concentrate, and a significant impairment of her performance at work. The symptoms do not appear to be caused by a drug or medication or by a general medical condition. If she has not had any previous psychotic symptoms and has never had a manic or hypomanic episode, her diagnosis is Major Depressive Disorder, Single Episode. If she has had a previous Major Depressive Episode the diagnosis is Major Depressive Disorder, Recurrent.

Vignette 2: I Have a Little Poem for You

Sandra has had multiple episodes of illness characterized by symptoms of irritability, grandiosity, pressured speech, paranoia, psychotic delusions, and a thought disorder. These episodes occur in 3- to 5-year intervals and appear to be correlated with the loss or separation from a loved one. The patient has fulfilled the criteria for a Manic Episode with symptoms of grandiosity, elevated and irritable mood, decreased need for sleep, pressured speech, and increased goal-directed activity during the initial stages of the episode. However, the patient also has prominent signs of psychosis with disorganized speech and thought and delusions. The main diagnostic question is which, if any, of these symptoms take precedence. The initial differential diagnosis includes Schizophrenia; Schizophreniform Disorder; Brief Psychotic Disorder; Schizoaffective Disorder; and Bipolar I Disorder, Most Recent Episode Manic.

The diagnosis of Schizophrenia can be excluded for two reasons. The patient has had a Manic Episode and she has not had continuous signs of a disturbance for 6 months that include at least 1 month of psychotic symptoms found in part A of the general criteria set for Schizophrenia. The presence of a Manic Episode also excludes the diagnosis of Schizophreniform Disorder and Brief Psychotic Disorder. The two remaining diagnoses, Schizoaffective Disorder and Bipolar I Disorder, Most Recent Episode Manic, are mainly distinguished by the relationship of the psychotic symptoms to the mood symptoms. In a Schizoaffective Disorder the psychotic symptoms take priority and must be present for at least 2 weeks in absence of prominent mood symptoms. Sandra does not fulfill these requirements because her delusions appeared after the onset of the her mood symptoms and did not occur independent of these symptoms. Therefore, her diagnosis is Bipolar I Disorder, Most Recent Episode Manic because she is currently in a Manic Episode and has had at least one previous Manic Episode.

Key Diagnostic Points

- A Hypomanic Episode differs from a Manic Episode because it lasts less than 1 week, has no psychotic features, and is not severe enough to cause marked impairment in social or occupational functioning, or to necessitate hospitalization.

- A Bipolar I Disorder with psychotic symptoms can be distinguished from a Schizoaffective Disorder because the latter requires delusions or hallucinations for at least 2 weeks in absence of the mood symptoms.

- The diagnosis of a Bipolar II Disorder cannot be made if the patient has ever had a Manic Episode.

- Rapid cycling is the occurrence of at least four episodes of a mood disturbance in the previous 12 months that meet the criteria for a Manic, Hypomanic, or Major Depressive Episode. The episodes are demarcated by a switch to an episode of opposite polarity.

- Patients with an abnormally elevated or expansive mood require three additional symptoms for the diagnosis of a Manic or Hypomanic Episode. Patients with abnormally increased irritability require four additional symptoms for either diagnosis.

- A Cyclothymic Disorder is distinguished from a Bipolar II Disorder because patients with a Cyclothymic Disorder have experienced symptoms for at least 2 years and have never experienced a Major Depressive Episode.

Common Questions in Making a Diagnosis

1. A 32-year-old woman complains that she has been feeling somewhat down or mildly depressed for several years. She also feels pessimistic, has low self-esteem, and is chronically irritable. She has had no previous Major Depressive Episode or Manic Episode. What diagnosis, if any, should this patient receive?

   Answer: The patient's depression is chronic but mild. The duration of the depression, her pessimism, low self-esteem, and irritability fulfill the criteria for a Dysthymic Disorder. However, these latter three symptoms are quite general and could be found in many people without Depressive Disorder. The nature of the patient's depressed mood should be investigated further to determine whether she is actually having clinical depression or whether she is describing a general outlook or attitude toward life. The mild nature of her symptoms could as easily justify not giving her a diagnosis of Dysthymic Disorder.

2. A 42-year-old woman currently has symptoms of a Manic Episode. Her family relates that she has had a 3-year history of periods of hypomanic symptoms alternating with depressed mood. She has never had a Major Depressive Episode and has not experienced more than a few weeks without symptoms during the 3 years. What diagnosis(es) should the patient receive?

   Answer: The diagnosis of Cyclothymic Disorder requires that the patient have numerous periods with hypomanic symptoms and numerous periods with depressed mood within a 2-year period. During this 2-year period the patient cannot have a Manic Episode. This patient has experienced 3 years of alternating hypomanic and depressed symptoms followed by a Manic Episode. Therefore, she meets the criteria for Cyclothymic Disorder. The occurrence of a Manic Episode in the absence of previous Manic or Major Depressive Episodes and in the presence of a current Cyclothymic Disorder fulfills the criteria for a Bipolar I Disorder, Single Manic Episode, superimposed on Cyclothymic Disorder.

3. Three weeks ago a 42-year-old man lost the job he had held for 15 years. Since that time he reports feeling depressed and worthless. He is having difficulty sleeping, difficulty concentrating, and feels like he has no energy. The patient states that he is trying to adjust to the loss of his job and he is sure that his depression will pass as soon as he finds another job. He denies suicidal ideation and has never had a similar episode of depression. What is the best diagnosis for this patient?

   Answer: There are two possible diagnoses for this patient: Adjustment Disorder With Depressed Mood and Major Depressive Disorder, Single Episode. His depression is a reaction to losing his job and he meets the criteria for a Major Depressive Episode. The diagnosis of Adjustment Disorder With Depressed Mood is excluded if the patient meets the criteria for any other Axis I diagnosis. Therefore, his diagnosis is Major Depressive Disorder, Single Episode.

4. A 37-year-old man had a previous diagnosis of Schizophreniform Disorder in full remission 3 years previously. During that episode he heard voices telling him that he was diseased. Three weeks ago he became severely depressed with insomnia, psychomotor agitation, indecisiveness, and recurrent thoughts of death. At the same time he again began to hear voices that continually commented on his behavior and told him that he was evil and diseased. He has never had a previous Major Depressive Episode. What is the patient's diagnosis?

   Answer: The patient is currently experiencing a Major Depressive Episode. The diagnosis of a Schizoaffective Disorder requires that the patient have either a Manic or Major Depressive Episode concurrent with symptoms that meet Criterion A for Schizophrenia. In addition, the patient's psychotic symptoms must occur for at least 2 weeks in the absence of the mood symptoms. This patient's auditory hallucinations fulfill Criterion A. However, they began at the same time as the depression. Therefore, the diagnosis of Schizoaffective Disorder is excluded at this time. The appropriate current diagnosis is Major Depressive Disorder, Single Episode with mood-congruent Psychotic Features.

5. A 29-year-old man reports that he has been moderately depressed for more than a year. He feels hopeless, inadequate, guilty about his relationship with his parents, and experiences little pleasure in his current life. What is the appropriate diagnosis for the patient based on this clinical information?

Answer: A patient who has these symptoms for a period of 2 years fulfills the criteria for the diagnosis of a Dysthymic Disorder. This patient reports having the symptoms for more than a year. The clinician should try to pin down the patient's estimate of the duration of his symptoms. He may be able to do this by asking the patient whether he was depressed on specific holidays in the past or on past birthdays. The core concept of a Dysthymic Disorder is the presence of a long-term depressed mood that is not severe enough to meet the criteria for a Major Depressive Episode. If the patient reports that the depression has lasted for significantly more than a year, the clinician may chose to make a diagnosis of Dysthymic Disorder. If the duration of the mood disturbance remains uncertain or the patient indicates that it has lasted for substantially less than 2 years, the diagnosis is Depressive Disorder Not Otherwise Specified.

6. A 37-year-old woman currently fulfills the criteria for a Hypomanic Episode. She has previously had alternating Major Depressive Episodes and Hypomanic Episodes and at least one previous Manic Episode. What is her diagnosis?

Answer: Patients with alternating depressive episodes and Hypomanic episodes can be given a diagnosis of Bipolar II Disorder if they have never had a Manic Episode. Because this patient has had a prior Manic Episode, this diagnosis is excluded. Because the patient is currently having a Hypomanic Episode, the diagnosis is Bipolar I Disorder, Most Recent Episode Hypomanic.

7. A 28-year-old woman reports that she has felt very depressed for the last 4 weeks. However, her mood is reactive and she feels less depressed when she anticipates a positive event, such as dinner at a fancy restaurant. During the time the patient has been depressed she reports feeling worthless, having recurrent suicidal ideation, gaining several pounds, and sleeping several hours longer than she does when she is not depressed. She has never had a previous Major Depressive Episode. What is this patient's diagnosis?

Answer: The common symptoms associated with a Major Depressive Episode usually includes persistent depression, weight loss, and insomnia. However, some patients do have mood reactivity, weight gain, and hypersomnia. This patient's diagnosis is Major Depressive Disorder, Single Episode With Atypical Features.

Anxiety Disorders

Clinical Vignettes

Vignette 1: I'm Not Safe in My Own Home

Nancy, a 25-year-old woman, moved from the small town where she had been born to a large city to take a new job. Because she did not have a car, she found a small apartment within walking distance of her job. Soon after moving into her apartment she began to notice some aspects of the neighborhood that she had not noticed before. Each afternoon and evening small groups of young men gathered on the street corners. They often made suggestive comments to her as she walked by. Nancy found the comments uncomfortable but decided that they were part of living in a large city.

One hot summer night she returned home after work to discover that her air conditioner did not work. It was too late to call a repair man that evening so she opened the window in her bedroom to get some air and went to sleep. In the middle of the night she suddenly awoke, feeling a heavy weight on top of her. A hand grabbed her throat and a man's voice said, "Take your nightgown off. Don't yell and you won't get hurt. If you make any noise I'll kill you." The man pulled off her nightgown and began to have sex with her. Although scared and feeling helpless, Nancy was able to ask the man if he would use a condom. Her attacker agreed, put on a condom, and proceeded to rape her. When he had finished, he told her not to tell anyone what had happened or he would come back and kill her.

When she heard him leave, Nancy jumped up and locked the door and window. She felt in a daze and was uncertain what to do next. Finally she called one of her co-workers in the office to ask for help. The woman immediately came over to Nancy's apartment and took her to a local hospital emergency room. The police were called by the hospital and they interviewed her after the physician's examination. She could not describe her assailant because the room had been dark during the attack.

Following the interview with the police, Nancy went to her friend's home and stayed until moving into a new apartment a few days later. The night of her move she checked the door and windows several times to see if they were locked and prepared to go to sleep alone for the first time since the rape. She lay in bed trying to sleep but began to think about the attack. After a few restless hours she finally drifted off to sleep only to wake up in the middle of the night with a distressing dream of the attack.

Nancy continued to have dreams of the attack and difficulty sleeping for several weeks. She also developed a set of rituals that she felt compelled to perform each night. As it began to get dark she would look out her front and back windows, turn on a light in each room, and check each of the doors and windows several times to make sure they were locked. She slept with the light on. Nancy realized that her checking routine was excessive but she became anxious when she omitted it. If she heard an unusual noise during the night, she checked each door and window again.

During the day Nancy found it difficult to concentrate on her work. She felt anxious and somehow detached from her co-workers and friends, almost as if there was a physical space separating them from her. Little problems at work and at home irritated her to the point that she would make snide and overtly angry comments to her co-workers. Several friends commented that she had become unusually touchy. She found it difficult to come to work because the neighborhood reminded her of the attack.

Nancy became increasingly dissatisfied with her job, blaming her employers for not warning her about the neighborhood before she moved into the first apartment. When she heard about a job opportunity in another company, she quit her first job and moved to the new company, which was located in a better part of the city.

Vignette 2: It Hit Me Like a Ton of Bricks

Sharon is a 31-year-old physician in private practice who recently finished her training and moved to a new city to join 10 other physicians in an established group practice. Over the last few months she had been feeling a significant amount of stress related to finishing her training, moving, buying a house, beginning a new job, and making school and day-care arrangements for her two young children. Her husband was also busy overseeing the renovation of their house and starting a new job as a junior partner in a local law firm.

One morning Sharon left her house late, in a hurry to drive to work. As she turned a corner a few blocks from her office she suddenly began to feel afraid that something dreadful was about to happen and that she might die. Her heart began to pound, she felt nauseated, dizzy, and short of breath. She pulled the car over to the side of the road and held the steering wheel tightly to try and calm herself. The feelings increased in intensity for a few minutes and then began to decrease. When they had finally subsided she felt drained and noticed that she had been sweating profusely. She started the car and continued to the office.

When she arrived at her office she immediately went to see one of the senior doctors in the group, an experienced internist. Sharon described the episode and told her colleague, "It hit me like a ton of bricks." After listening to Sharon's story the physician gave her a brief physical examination, including an electrocardiogram, but found no evidence of any medical problems. Following the exam she asked Sharon about her family and her experiences moving and starting a new practice. Sharon admitted that she felt under a great deal of stress. Her colleague suggested that she might have experienced a "stress attack" and advised Sharon to try and learn some stress reduction techniques.

Sharon worked through the day without any further distress. However, at the end of the workday she began to become anxious at the thought of driving home, fearing she might experience another attack. She asked one of her colleagues to ride with her. Although she did not experience any further attacks over the next 2 weeks, she became increasingly fearful about driving. Five weeks after the initial episode, Sharon experienced another attack as she was getting out of her car in a shopping mall. After this second attack subsided she telephoned her husband and asked him to come drive her home.

Following this episode Sharon found it impossible to drive her car. She became anxious when she thought about driving and experienced another attack one day when she tried to drive to work. Subsequently she refused to drive and her husband had to take her to work each morning and pick her up in the evening. Sharon tried treating the anxiety by taking diazepam (Valium) but it was not effective. Finally, in desperation, she asked one of her colleagues for a referral to a psychiatrist.

Core Concept of the Diagnostic Group

The core concept of the Anxiety Disorders group includes: 1) the frequent experience of anxiety, worry, and apprehension that is more intense and lasts for a longer period of time than the anxiety experienced by the average person in everyday life; and 2) the frequent development of avoidance, ritual acts, or repetitive thoughts as a means of protecting the sufferer from experiencing the anxiety.

Criteria Applicable to Multiple Disorders

There is a significant amount of overlap between the specific diagnoses within the Anxiety Disorders group because they often share similar criteria. There are two types of common criteria. The first is composed of relatively general criteria that apply to many of the disorders in the diagnostic group. The second comprises the cluster of symptoms that define a panic attack.

General Criteria

The general criteria including the following:

1. The disorder is not due to an abused substance or a known nonpsychiatric medical disorder. (This is not a member of the criteria set for Specific Phobia, Posttraumatic Stress Disorder, Anxiety Disorder Due to a General Medical Condition, or Substance-Induced Anxiety Disorder.)
2. The symptoms associated with the disorder are not better accounted for by another psychiatric disorder.
3. The disorder produces significant impairment of social or occupational functioning or causes the patient marked distress. (This is not a member of the criteria set for following disorders: Panic Disorder Without Agoraphobia, Panic Disorder With Agoraphobia, Agoraphobia Without History of Panic Disorder, and Anxiety Disorder Not Otherwise Specified.)

The first requirement above does not apply to the diagnosis of Specific Phobia or Posttraumatic Stress Disorder. Presumably the authors of the criteria sets decided that the possibility of an organic etiology for these disorders was very low. Nevertheless, it is always important to inquire about the possibility of an underlying detectable, organic etiology in the onset of any disorder even if it seems unlikely. What appears at first to be Specific Phobia or Posttraumatic Stress Disorder could turn out to be substance-related.

The second general criterion implies that certain psychiatric diagnoses take priority over others in the Anxiety Disorders group. This is similar to the case in many diagnostic groups when the patient fulfills the criteria for more than one specific diagnosis. The problem is discussed in detail for the Anxiety Disorders in the section on Precedence of Diagnosis below.

The third criterion above was discussed in a general sense in the first chapter. The exclusion of Panic Disorder Without Agoraphobia, Panic Disorder With Agoraphobia, and Agoraphobia Without History of Panic Disorder from compliance with this criterion suggests that significant impairment of social and occupational functioning and marked distress are implicit in these diagnoses. It is difficult to envision how a patient's symptoms could meet the criteria for panic disorder or agoraphobia without experiencing significant impairment or distress.

The exclusion of Anxiety Disorder Not Otherwise Specified from compliance with the third criterion is related to its status as a "catchall" or "wastebasket" diagnosis that can be used for patients who do not fit any of the other specific diagnoses in the Anxiety Disorders group. The requirement of significant impairment or marked distress might not be present in patients who have mild Anxiety Disorders.

Criteria for Panic Attack

A panic attack is a syndrome or reproducible cluster of symptoms that can occur in several different Anxiety Disorders including Panic Disorder, Social Phobia, simple phobia, and Posttraumatic Stress Disorder. It is not, in itself, a specific diagnosis. Panic attacks in different patients may display diverse characteristics. The essential feature of a panic attack is the occurrence of a discrete period of intense fear or discomfort, usually lasting for several minutes, and accompanied by at least four of the following symptoms, which develop abruptly and reach a peak of intensity within 10 minutes.

1. Palpitations, pounding, or accelerated heart rate
2. Sweating
3. Trembling or shaking
4. Sensations of shortness of breath or smothering
5. Feeling of choking
6. Chest pain or discomfort
7. Nausea or abdominal distress
8. Feeling dizzy, unsteady, lightheaded, or faint
9. Derealization (feelings of unreality) or depersonalization (being detached from oneself)
10. Fear of losing control or going crazy
11. Fear of dying
12. Paresthesias (numbness or tingling sensations)
13. Chills or hot flushes

There are two general categories of panic attacks. Unexpected (uncued) panic attacks occur without any obvious external trigger. The diagnosis of Panic Disorder requires the occurrence of unexpected panic attacks. Situationally bound (cued) panic attacks occur immediately after exposure to a situational trigger or in anticipation of such an exposure. Social Phobia and Specific Phobia are commonly accompanied by situationally bound panic attacks.

Criteria for Agoraphobia

Patients may experience agoraphobia independently or in the context of other Anxiety Disorders. The criteria for agoraphobia include the following:

Note: Agoraphobia is not a codable disorder. Code the specific disorder in which the agoraphobia occurs (e.g., 300.21 Panic Disorder With Agoraphobia or 300.22 Agoraphobia Without History of Panic Disorder.

A. Anxiety about being in places or situations from which escape might be difficult (or embarrassing) or in which help may not be available in the event of having an unexpected or situationally predisposed Panic Attack or panic-like symptoms. Agoraphobic fears typically involve characteristic clusters of situations that include being outside the home alone; being in a crowd or standing in a line; being on a bridge; and traveling in a bus, train, or automobile.

Note: Consider the diagnosis of Specific Phobia if the avoidance is limited to one or only a few specific situations, or Social Phobia if the avoidance is limited to social situations.

B. The situations are avoided (e.g., travel is restricted) or else are endured with marked distress or with anxiety about having a Panic Attack or panic-like symptoms, or require the presence of a companion.
C. The anxiety or phobic avoidance is not better accounted for by another mental disorder, such as Social Phobia (e.g., avoidance limited to social situations because of fear of embarrassment), Specific Phobia (e.g., avoidance limited to a single situation like elevators), Obsessive-Compulsive Disorder (e.g., avoidance of dirt in someone with an obsession about contamination), Posttraumatic Stress Disorder (e.g., avoidance of stimuli associated with a severe stressor), or Separation Anxiety Disorder (e.g., avoidance of leaving home or relatives).

Definitions

phobia   A persistent and irrational fear of an object or situation that leads to attempts to avoid it.

obsessions   Recurrent, intrusive, and anxiety-provoking thoughts, impulses, or images.

compulsions   Repetitive behaviors or mental acts that a person feels driven to perform.

Synopses and Diagnostic Prototypes of the Individual Disorders

The brief synopses in this section summarize the specific requirements or criteria that must be fulfilled for each of the diagnostic categories. Each synopsis includes a brief vignette that provides a clinical examples of the diagnoses. Each vignette is a prototype in the sense that it represents a typical patient from a specific diagnostic category. The prototypes provide a more lifelike portrayal of the diagnosis than the criteria alone. They also provide a clinical baseline that can be used in the discussion of problems associated with the diagnosis of these disorders and as a standard for comparison even if they do not exhaust all the possibilities for the clinical presentation of a specific diagnosis.

300.01 Panic Disorder Without Agoraphobia. Individuals with this disorder experience recurrent, unexpected panic attacks without agoraphobia that are followed by at least a month of worry about having additional attacks, concern about the implications of attacks, or a change in behavior related to the attacks

> A 35-year-old clothing salesman was showing a particularly fussy customer a suit 2 months ago and suddenly began to sweat profusely. His heart started to pound, he felt dizzy, and became fearful that he was about to die. The customer didn't notice his condition and continued to question him about the suit in minute detail. The patient, feeling faint, abruptly left the customer and went to lie down in the back of the store. The customer became insulted, complained to the manager, and left. When the manager found the patient he was slumped in a chair in the back room trembling.
>
> Approximately 10 minutes later the patient's symptoms began to subside. He saw his physician the next day who found no evidence of any medical problems. Two weeks later he had another similar unexpected attack. Since that time he has worried continuously about having another attack. His friends and colleagues have noticed that he is no longer as spontaneous and outgoing as he had been in the past.

300.21 Panic Disorder With Agoraphobia. Individuals with this disorder experience recurrent, unexpected panic attacks with agoraphobia that are followed by at least a month of worry about having additional attacks, concern about the implications of the attacks, or a change in behavior related to the attacks.

> A 28-year-old woman was walking through her local shopping mall when she began to feel intensely anxious. The anxiety was accompanied by sensations of choking, smothering, and a sudden sense that the people and stores around her were unreal. She began to fear that she was going crazy and the more she worried about this the more anxious she became. A guard, seeing that she was in distress, brought her to the mall office where she was able to lie down. A few minutes later the symptoms began to subside. She went home after leaving the mall but she did not tell her husband what had happened.
>
> A week later she had a similar attack while she was walking down the street. She was able to reach her house where she lay down until the attack ended. In the following 3 weeks she had two more attacks. Between attacks she was constantly worried about having another attack. The patient was finally forced to tell her husband about the problem because she was so fearful of not being able to get help if an attack occurred that she would not leave her house alone or travel on public transportation.

300.22 Agoraphobia Without History of Panic Disorder. Individuals with this disorder experience agoraphobia related to the fear of developing panic-like symptoms but have never met the criteria for Panic Disorder.

A 36-year-old woman experienced several episodes of feeling dizzy and faint over a 3-month period. A full medical examination did not reveal any physical problems. Her physician told her, "The problem's all in your head. You don't have any medical problems." This reassuring advice did not lessen her concerns that she might experience the symptoms in a situation where she could not obtain help. Her fears led to a significant constriction of her previously active lifestyle. She would not leave the house without a friend, walk in a crowd, drive by herself, or wait in the line at a supermarket for fear that she would have an attack.

300.29   Specific Phobia.   Individuals with this disorder have an excessive and unreasonable fear of exposure to a specific object or situation that provokes an immediate anxiety response that may take the form of a panic attack. The object or situation is avoided by the person or endured with intense distress. The person recognizes that the fear is unreasonable.

A 27-year-old, athletic young man has an intense fear of needles. He tries to rationalize his fear by explaining that he is just being cautious and protecting himself from acquired immunodeficiency disease syndrome (AIDS). He realizes that his fear is irrational but is unable to control it. The patient has fainted twice in the past when his blood was drawn during a physical examination. He becomes extremely anxious at the sight of a needle and worries for days before an appointment with his physician or dentist.

300.23   Social Phobia.   Individuals with this disorder fear one or more social or performance situations in which they are exposed to scrutiny by others and fear that they will act in a way that will be humiliating or embarrassing. Exposure to the feared situation almost invariably provokes anxiety that may take the form of a panic attack. The feared situations are avoided or endured with intense anxiety or distress. The individual recognizes that the fear is unreasonable.

A 28-year-old woman is a rising junior executive in her investment company. Her increasing duties require her to make periodic formal presentations to the senior management of the company. However, she becomes intensely anxious at the thought of speaking in public. When she is forced to give a presentation she begins to feel anxious days in advance of the talk and the anxiety increases as the time for the talk approaches. She is concerned that her anxiety will become noticeable during the talk or that she will do something to embarrass herself.

300.3   Obsessive-Compulsive Disorder.   Individuals with this disorder have either obsessions (i.e., recurrent, persistent, and intrusive thoughts that cause anxiety or distress) that they try to suppress and neutralize or compulsions (i.e., repetitive behaviors) that they feel driven to perform in an attempt to prevent distress or some dreaded event. The person has recognized at some point that the obsessions or compulsions are excessive and unreasonable.

A 26-year-old man is very concerned about cleanliness and hygiene. He spends a significant amount of time each day washing his hands or showering, especially after touching a toilet seat, doorknob, or any other item he thinks may be dirty or contaminated. The patient explains that he is concerned about becoming infected or sick from touching these objects. He periodically acknowledges that the washing is excessive but explains that he becomes very anxious when he tries to avoid washing and eventually feels compelled to wash even more to make up for the omission.

309.81   Posttraumatic Stress Disorder.   Individuals with this disorder have been exposed to a traumatic event in which they or others were threatened with death or serious injury. During the event they responded with fear, helplessness, or horror and since the event they have had the following symptoms for more than 1 month.

Reexperiencing of the trauma: The traumatic event is persistently reexperienced in at least one of the following ways:

1. Recurrent and intrusive distressing recollections of the event
2. Recurrent distressing dreams of the event
3. Acting or feeling as if the traumatic event were recurring
4. Intense psychological distress at exposure to cues that symbolize or resemble aspects of the event
5. Physiological reactivity on exposure to cues that symbolize or resemble aspects of the event

Avoidance and numbing: Persistent avoidance of stimuli associated with the trauma and numbing of general responsiveness as indicated by at least three of the following:

1. Efforts to avoid thoughts, feelings, or conversations associated with the trauma
2. Efforts to avoid activities, places, or people that arouse recollections of the trauma
3. Inability to recall an important aspect of the trauma
4. Diminished interest or participation in significant activities
5. Feeling of detachment or estrangement from others
6. Restricted range of affect
7. Sense of foreshortened future

Arousal: Persistent symptoms of arousal as indicated by at least two of the following:

1. Difficulty falling or staying asleep
2. Irritability or outbursts of anger

3. Difficulty concentrating
4. Hypervigilance
5. Exaggerated startle response

> A 36-year-old man and his young son were driving through an intersection when another car ran through a red traffic light and struck them. The two were trapped in the car until a fire department rescue team freed them. The patient was bruised but not seriously hurt. His son had a broken leg.
>
> The first few days after the accident the patient was preoccupied with arranging care for his son and getting the car repaired. A few days later he began having recurrent distressing thoughts and images of the accident. These symptoms lasted for several weeks. The memory of his son's screams after the car was struck seemed particularly vivid. The patient became irritable, had difficulty concentrating, and avoided talking about the accident. He went out of his way to avoid driving down the street where the accident occurred. As time went on he could no longer remember whether the traffic light was red or green when he approached it.

308.3   Acute Stress Disorder.   Individuals with this disorder have been exposed to a traumatic event in which they or others were threatened with death or serious injury. During the event they responded with fear, helplessness, or horror and since the event they have had the following symptoms for a minimum of 2 days and a maximum of 4 weeks. The symptoms occurred within 4 weeks of the traumatic event.

Dissociative symptoms: Either while experiencing, or immediately after experiencing the distressing event, the individual has at least three of the following dissociative symptoms:

1. Subjective sense of numbing, detachment, or absence of emotional responsiveness
2. A reduction in awareness of one's surroundings
3. Derealization
4. Depersonalization
5. Dissociative amnesia

Reexperience of the trauma: The traumatic event is persistently reexperienced in one of the following ways: recurrent images, thoughts, dreams, illusions, flashback episodes, or a sense of reliving the experience; or distress on exposure to reminders of the traumatic event.

Avoidance: Marked avoidance of stimuli that arouse recollections of the trauma (e.g., thoughts, feelings, conversations, activities, places, or people).

Arousal: Marked symptoms of anxiety or increased arousal (e.g., difficulty sleeping, irritability, poor concentration, hypervigilance, exaggerated startle response, and motor restlessness).

A 20-year-old woman and her girlfriend were walking through their college campus one night when a man jumped out of the bushes, pointed a gun at them, and ordered them to give him their money. The friend protested and the gunman knocked her to the ground, grabbed both women's purses, and ran off. The friend was shaken but unhurt. The two women immediately went to the campus security office to report the robbery. The patient found it difficult to describe what had happened. She felt numb and dazed as if she had experienced a dream. The entire event seemed unreal and she had difficulty remembering what the gunman looked like.

During the next few days she had recurrent thoughts of the episode and difficulty sleeping. Every little noise seemed to startle her. She avoided walking near the site of the robbery because it made her anxious.

300.02 Generalized Anxiety Disorder. Individuals with this disorder have excessive anxiety and worry that they cannot control a number of events or activities. The anxiety lasts for at least 6 months and the focus of the anxiety is not confined to the features of another Axis I disorder. The anxiety and worry are associated with at least three of the following symptoms:

1. Restlessness or feeling "keyed up" or on edge
2. Being easily fatigued
3. Difficulty concentrating or mind going blank
4. Irritability
5. Muscle tension
6. Sleep disturbance (difficulty falling or staying asleep, or restless unsatisfying sleep)

A 38-year-old man has been increasingly anxious about his job in a large manufacturing company. He feels that he has been passed over for a promotion several times. The patient is preoccupied with many small events and conversations that have occurred at work during the year and worries how his superiors will interpret them. He finds it difficult to control his worrying. During the day at work he feels restless and edgy. At home he is irritable and has difficulty sleeping. His wife asks him about work but he doesn't want to talk about it.

293.89 Anxiety Disorder Due to . . . *[Indicate the General Medical Condition].* Individuals with this disorder have prominent anxiety, panic attacks, obsessions, or compulsions that appear to be caused by the direct physiological consequences of a general medical condition.

A 68-year-old man has chronic obstructive pulmonary disease caused by 45 years of smoking. During the last year he has had several periods of intense anxiety, often associated with mild to moderate hypoxia. The hypoxia has progressed to the stage that he now requires continuous oxygen delivered through a nasal cannula.

29x.xx   Substance-Induced Anxiety Disorder.   Individuals with this disorder have prominent anxiety, panic attacks, obsessions, or compulsions associated with evidence that the symptoms developed within 1 month of significant substance intoxication or withdrawal or are etiologically related to medication use or toxin exposure.

The specific codes for (Specific Substance)-Induced Anxiety Disorder are determined by the specific substance: 291.8 alcohol; 292.89 amphetamines; caffeine; cannabis; cocaine; hallucinogens; inhalants; phencyclidine; sedative, hypnotics, or anxiolytics; other (or unknown) substances.

> A 26-year-old woman reports that she becomes very anxious each morning at work. The anxiety usually subsides by lunch time. The anxiety is accompanied by restlessness, muscle twitching, increased urination, and some stomach distress. Further questioning reveals that the patient drinks four to five cups of coffee each morning. When she reduces her coffee consumption to one cup a day the symptoms disappear.

300.00   Anxiety Disorder Not Otherwise Specified.   Individuals with this disorder have prominent anxiety or phobic avoidance that does not meet the criteria for any other specific anxiety disorder.

> A 35-year-old man with psoriasis avoids going to parties or social occasions because of his skin disease. He is convinced that other people are disgusted with his appearance. When he is forced to attend a social function because of his work, he becomes anxious and fearful that someone will make fun of his appearance.

Necessary Clinical Information

- Current and past history of anxiety

- Feelings of derealization, depersonalization, or emotional numbing

- Fears of losing control or going crazy

- Sleep disturbance, bad dreams

- Medical illnesses

- Physical symptoms

- Previous and current psychiatric illnesses

- Current medications and abused substances

- Current or past traumatic events or stress

- Compulsive behaviors or rituals

- Obsessive, intrusive thoughts

- Phobic fears and the context within which they occur

Making a Diagnosis

Anxiety is ubiquitous in every aspect of human health and illness. As a result, it is often difficult to judge whether a patient is having the usual anxiety of everyday life or whether the anxiety is intense enough to be considered a symptom of a psychiatric illness. The core concept of the diagnostic group is the best guide in making this decision.

Briefly, this concept specifies that all Anxiety Disorders have two common characteristics. First, patients with these disorders usually experience anxiety, worry, and apprehension that is more intense and lasts for a longer period of time than the anxiety experienced by the average person in everyday life. Second, patients often develop avoidance mechanisms, ritual acts, or repetitive thoughts as a means of protecting themselves from the anxiety.

Anxiety Disorders are categorized according to the presence or absence of external stimuli, the etiology of the disorder, and the nature of the symptoms. The following questions provide an organized approach to the diagnosis of the typical Anxiety Disorder. Specific problems in the diagnosis of these disorders will be discussed in the next section.

1. Could the patient's symptoms be produced by drugs or a nonpsychiatric medical illness?

Determine whether the patient has any current nonpsychiatric medical illnesses or substance-related problems. If so, deciding the relationship between these problems and the patient's psychiatric symptoms should be the first step in the diagnostic process.

The presence of nonpsychiatric medical illnesses or substance-relat 'd problem in conjunction with psychiatric symptoms does not imply the former caused the latter. The occurrence of psychiatric symptoms before the onset of a medical illness or use of a substance suggests that they have an independent etiology. Similarly, the persistence of the psychiatric symptoms after adequate treatment of the medical illness or cessation of substance use implies that the two are unrelated. Generally, symptoms that occur more than a month after an episode of drug intoxication or withdrawal are not considered to be due to the drug. The diagnoses of Anxiety Disorder Due to a General Medical Condition and Substance-Induced Anxiety Disorder can be excluded if there is no evidence that a nonpsychiatric medical disorder or drugs have produced the patient's symptoms.

Note: Assume that an organic etiology for the patient's symptoms has been ruled out for the remaining questions in this section.

2. Is the onset of the patient's anxiety linked to a specific situational trigger ("cue") or is it unexpected?

- If the patient's anxiety is triggered by a specific cue, the diagnoses of Panic Disorder With Agoraphobia and Panic Disorder Without Agoraphobia can be excluded.

- If the patient's anxiety is unexpected, the diagnoses of Panic Disorder With Agoraphobia and Panic Disorder Without Agoraphobia can be made if the patient fulfills the criteria for panic attacks.

- If the anxiety is unexpected and the patient does not fulfill the criteria for panic attacks, there are two possibilities. Either there is an external situational trigger that the patient has not or will not identify or the diagnosis is one of the following: Obsessive-Compulsive Disorder, Generalized Anxiety Disorder, or Anxiety Disorder Not Otherwise Specified.

3. If the patient's anxiety is cued, what types of external situational triggers precipitate it?

- If the patient's anxiety is triggered by a specific object or situation (e.g., animals, lightening, water, heights, etc.), the diagnosis is Specific Phobia.

- If the anxiety is triggered by the patient's involvement or anticipation of involvement in a social or performance situation in which the patient will be exposed to unfamiliar people or be under the scrutiny of others, the diagnosis is Social Phobia.

- If the patient's anxiety is triggered by a traumatic event or reminders of a traumatic event, the diagnoses may be Posttraumatic Stress Disorder or Acute Stress Disorder if the other criteria for these disorders are fulfilled.

4. Does the patient experience long-term anxiety that is neither unexpected nor situationally triggered?

- If the patient experiences recurrent, intrusive and distressing thoughts, impulses, or images or if the patient is driven to perform repetitive behaviors or mental acts to reduce the anxiety, the diagnosis is Obsessive-Compulsive Disorder.

- If the patient experiences excessive anxiety associated with everyday events and activities, the diagnosis is Generalized Anxiety Disorder if the other criteria for the diagnosis are fulfilled.

Common Problems in Making a Diagnosis

There are three main areas of uncertainty in the differential diagnosis of Anxiety Disorders.

1. Some patients initially come close but don't actually fulfill the criteria for a specific diagnosis. More information or a further consideration of the diagnostic criteria may or may not resolve the problem.
2. Some patients fulfill the diagnostic criteria for more than one, mutually exclusive, Anxiety Disorder during the course of their illness.
3. Some patients have isolated symptoms of anxiety associated with other psychiatric disorders but do not fulfill the criteria for a specific Anxiety Disorder.

Patients Who Almost Fulfill the Diagnostic Criteria

The differential diagnosis of Anxiety Disorders commonly depends on difficult clinical decisions about the presence, nature, etiology, and duration of anxiety symptoms such as panic attacks, obsessive thoughts, compulsive behavior, and specific fears. Diagnostic problems develop when patients come close or appear to fulfill the criteria for a diagnosis without actually fulfilling them. Under these circumstances the clinician may be convinced that the patient has Anxiety Disorder even though the criteria are not fully met. When this happens he is forced to account for the discrepancy between the diagnostic criteria and the patient's symptoms. Because there is usually a fair amount of latitude in the interpretation of the patient's symptoms, the clinician may choose to magnify or minimize the discrepancy.

There are three types of situations in which a patient almost fulfills the diagnostic criteria. First and most common, the patient may present complaints that are consistent with Anxiety Disorder but do not completely fulfill the criteria for a specific diagnosis. Frequently, further inquiry will elicit the necessary additional clinical information. At other times it may be impossible to obtain the necessary information to determine whether the patient fulfills the required criteria for Anxiety Disorder. For example, a patient may not be able to provide an accurate account of when his symptoms began.

Second, a patient can have symptoms of anxiety without having a diagnosable Anxiety Disorder. For example, students who become anxious during examinations do not necessarily have Anxiety Disorder. Third, a patient may focus on or be aware of only the physiological symptoms that accompany anxiety rather than the anxiety itself. For example, the patient may concentrate on the cardiovascular symptoms of Anxiety Disorders such as tachycardia or chest discomfort and not experience the anxiety.

Example 1

Valerie is a 26-year-old woman who complains of that she often feels in a "panic" when she is home alone at night. What diagnosis(es), if any, should Valerie receive?

The patient who complains of feeling "panicky" does not necessarily have a panic attack or Panic Disorder. The term "panicky" is often used in a general, exaggerated sense by patients to describe feeling stressed or overwhelmed. The diagnosis of Panic Disorder (With or Without Agoraphobia) requires that the patient meet the criteria for recurrent unexpected panic attacks as described above.

This is a common problem in the diagnosis of the Anxiety Disorders because there are so many lay terms used to describe varying degrees of anxiety and its accompanying physical symptoms. Furthermore, patients may use terms to express their anxiety in a way that is very different from the way that the term is used by clinicians. The clinician cannot take a patient's description at face value but must probe to translate the patient's experience into diagnostically acceptable signs and symptoms. In some patients further information will confirm a specific diagnosis. In other cases the patient's obvious symptoms of anxiety may still not fulfill the diagnostic criteria for the diagnosis of Anxiety Disorder.

Example 2

Lewis is a 47-year-old man who is short of breath and having chest discomfort. He is afraid that he is having a "heart attack." What diagnosis(es), if any, should Lewis receive?

Panic attacks have historically been confused with cardiac disorders because of their prominent cardiovascular symptoms including: palpitations, chest pain, shortness of breath, and dizziness. This misconception is evident in early diagnoses such as "irritable heart" and "cardiac neurosis" that were applied to patients with these symptoms. In fact, many patients are more aware of the physiological symptoms of their attacks than the anxiety symptoms. The similarity of the symptoms explains why patients who are experiencing an initial panic attack might think that they are having a heart attack. This similarity also makes it important to give patients having an initial attack a physical examination to make certain they do not have an underlying cardiac disorder.

Example 3

Mark is a 33-year-old man who is afraid to leave his house during the day and has not gone outside for several weeks. What diagnosis(es), if any, should Mark receive?

The major diagnostic question is whether the patient has agoraphobia, Specific Phobia, Social Phobia, or a realistic fear associated with leaving his home. In the latter case the patient might be afraid to leave his home because someone is after him (e.g., drug dealers, etc.). If there is no rational reason for the fear, the patient might have a Specific Phobia such as a fear of cars or of catching an infection from another person if he leaves the house. The patient could also have Social Phobia if he or she is embarrassed about bodily functions such as eating or blushing in public.

These two phobias should be distinguished from agoraphobia; a fear of being in a situation in which it would be difficult or impossible to obtain help if the patient became ill or incapacitated. These situations typically include being in crowds, in an elevator, on a bus, etc. If the patient has agoraphobia, it may or may not be associated with panic attacks. Agoraphobia commonly develops after one or more unexpected panic attacks. In these situations the patient is fearful of being in a place where he cannot obtain help if he has a panic attack. If the patient has had previous panic attacks, the diagnosis is Panic Disorder With Agoraphobia. If the agoraphobia develops without previous panic attacks, the diagnosis is Agoraphobia Without History of Panic Disorder.

Example 4

Gwen is a 25-year-old woman who has been afraid of snakes for many years and will not take her children to see the snakes at the zoo. What diagnosis(es), if any, should Gwen receive?

The fear or dislike of snakes is not necessarily a phobia. The feature that distinguishes a mundane fear or dislike of snakes from a Specific Phobia is the intensity of the anxiety provoked by snakes. It is realistic for an individual who is exposed to dangerous or poisonous snakes to develop a healthy fear or respect for the animals. Patients who have a snake phobia have an extreme fear of the animal that is generalized to all snakes, dangerous or not. Exposure to a snake may provoke a severe anxiety response or panic attack. Despite their fear most phobic patients recognize that their fear is excessive and unreasonable.

Example 5

Lance is a 30-year-old man who complains of intense discomfort that he finds difficult to describe. He does not complain of feeling nervous or anxious. Lance has been examined by his internist who did not find any physical basis for his discomfort. What diagnosis(es), if any, should Lance receive?

A panic attack usually includes the sudden onset of severe anxiety, fear, or apprehension accompanied by physiological symptoms that produce intense discomfort. Occasionally, a patient will not be aware of the anxiety and will experience the attack as intense discomfort. In fact, the criteria for a panic attack can be fulfilled even if the patient does not complain of fear or anxiety.

Example 6

Anita is a 21-year-old woman who repeatedly refuses to go out to dinner with her boyfriend because she is afraid to eat. What diagnosis(es), if any, should Anita receive?

Fear of eating is a true Social Phobia that must be differentiated from Anorexia Nervosa. Patients who have an eating phobia may be fearful of eating in front of other people or may even be fearful of eating alone. This phobia can be distinguished from Anorexia Nervosa because it is not the fear of getting fat and altered body image associated with the latter.

Example 7

Dana is a 45-year-old woman who became very anxious after she was in a serious automobile accident. What diagnosis(es), if any, should Dana receive?

The two Anxiety Disorders that commonly occur after a traumatic or stressful experience are Acute Stress Disorder and Posttraumatic Stress Disorder. They are differentiated by their duration and symptomatology. Acute Stress Disorder requires the presence of several dissociative symptoms such as amnesia, derealization, or depersonalization during or immediately after the traumatic event. These are not required for the diagnosis of Posttraumatic Stress Disorder. In addition, the former disorder has a duration of less that 4 weeks, whereas the latter has a duration of more than 4 weeks.

If the symptoms developed before the accident, neither diagnosis would be appropriate unless there was evidence of a separate traumatic event preceding the onset of the anxiety. There are two remaining possibilities. The patient might fulfill the criteria for a different Anxiety Disorder that is independent of the accident or the patient's anxiety may be related to the accident but not fulfill the necessary criteria for any disorder. In the latter case the patient might fulfill the criteria for a diagnosis of Anxiety Disorder Not Otherwise Specified.

Example 8

Herbert is a 39-year-old man who reports that he has periodically felt anxious for several years. What diagnosis(es), if any, should Herbert receive?

Patients who report feeling anxious for months or years should be asked to elaborate on the duration, intensity and circumstances of the episodes of anxiety. The patient may initially say she is anxious all the time but more detailed questioning may indicate that her anxiety occurs in certain settings (e.g., Specific Phobia, Social Phobia), during circumscribed periods of time (e.g., Panic Disorder With Agoraphobia, Panic Disorder Without Agoraphobia), or in association with the use of abused substances (e.g., Cocaine-Induced Anxiety Disorder). If the criteria for these specific diagnoses are not met, the patient may have Generalized Anxiety Disorder.

Example 9

James is a 30-year-old man who has been anxious and had difficulty sleeping since he saw someone assaulted. What diagnosis(es), if any, should James receive?

Witnessing a traumatic event that involves the death or serious injury of another person is sufficient to produce significant psychiatric symptoms. It is not necessary for an individual to personally experience the traumatic event. Sleep disturbances, including recurrent distressing dreams, is a common symptom of Posttraumatic Stress Disorder or Acute Stress Disorder.

The distinction between the two diagnoses depends on the type of symptoms the patient experiences and the length of time the symptoms are experienced. If the patient does not meet the criteria for either of the above two diagnoses, he could be given a diagnosis of Anxiety Disorder Not Otherwise Specified. The patient might also receive a diagnosis of Adjustment Disorder with Anxiety if it could be determined that the distress is in excess of what would normally be expected from exposure to a stressor such as the assault of another person. This judgment would depend on the nature of the assault, the patient's past experience, and other factors.

Example 10

Sean is a 38-year-old man who initially had unexpected panic attacks. These panic attacks are more likely to occur when he is flying in a plane. What diagnosis(es), if any, should Sean receive?

The diagnosis of Panic Disorder requires that the panic attacks are recurrent and unexpected. The diagnosis of a Specific Phobia requires that exposure to the phobic stimuli always provokes intense anxiety. In this case the patient falls in between the two diagnoses. Because he does not always experience a panic attack during flying, the diagnosis of a Specific Phobia would not be appropriate. However, because some of his panic attacks are cued, he no longer completely fulfills the criteria for Panic Disorder. He is experiencing situationally predisposed panic attacks. These attacks more likely, but do not inevitably, occur when he is exposed to a potentially phobic stimulus. Because many of the attacks remain unexpected, the most appropriate diagnosis would remain Panic Disorder Without Agoraphobia. This case is different than that of a patient in the next section whose initially uncued panic attacks subsequently all became associated with a specific cue.

Example 11

Vern is a 36-year-old man who has dissociative symptoms of Acute Stress Disorder that have lasted for more than 4 weeks. What diagnosis(es), if any, should Vern receive?

Acute Stress Disorder and Posttraumatic Stress Disorder differ in the duration of the disorder and the nature of some of the symptoms. Acute Stress Disorder lasts for less than 4 weeks, whereas Posttraumatic Stress Disorder lasts more than 4 weeks. The criteria for the former includes mainly dissociative symptoms, whereas the latter includes symptoms of avoidance.

However, a closer examination of the criteria for the two disorders suggests that the distinction between dissociation and avoidance is subtle and that the respective symptoms tend to overlap. The dissociation relates more to a sense of detachment from one's self, whereas avoidance refers to a detachment from other people, activities, and places related to the traumatic event.

The clinician should be alert to these differences. In most cases it is assumed that the dissociative symptoms of Acute Stress Disorder will resolve over time or gradually transform into the symptoms of avoidance. If the dissociative symptoms begin to dominate the patient's clinical presentation, the clinician should investigate the possibility of a Dissociative Disorder. However, if the disorder becomes chronic, and the patient fulfills most of the criteria for a stress-related disorder, even with lingering dissociative symptoms, the appropriate diagnosis would be Posttraumatic Stress Disorder.

Example 12

Maud is a 27-year-old woman who has panic attacks that are triggered when she is in various locations that provoke memories of very painful experiences of abuse that occurred when she was a child. What diagnosis(es), if any, should Maud receive?

This patient has panic attacks that are triggered by unusual cues that do not fit the typical cues associated with a diagnosis of Agoraphobia Without History of Panic Disorder, Specific Phobia, or Social Phobia. Agoraphobia is anxiety about being in a situation from which escape would be difficult or help would not be readily available if the patient experienced panic-like symptoms. This patient's panic attacks are produced by the memories of previous abuse, not the inability to obtain help. The anxiety associated with Specific Phobia is usually triggered by exposure or anticipation of exposure to a feared object (e.g., animal, knife) or a situation (e.g., flying, riding in an elevator). In this patient's case any location that stimulates the memories will produce the panic attacks.

Social Phobia requires that the patient fear exposure to unfamiliar people or scrutiny by others because he or she may act in a way that is humiliating or embarrassing. None of these cues are applicable to the patient's panic attacks. A final possibility is that the patient's panic attacks are a symptom of Posttraumatic Stress Disorder. Panic attacks are not specifically defined as a part of this disorder, however, they can fulfill the criteria for "intense psychological distress" at exposure to external cues that symbolize an aspect of the trauma.

Patients Who Fulfill Diagnostic Criteria for More Than One Anxiety Disorder

Periodically a patient will fulfill the diagnostic criteria for the more than one Anxiety Disorder. In most cases, the DSM-IV rules of diagnostic precedence determine which diagnosis should be selected. However, in some circumstances the decision is not covered by the rules of precedence. The most common example of this problem occurs when the psychiatric symptoms associated with an illness change over time. When this happens a patient who initially fulfilled the criteria for one Anxiety Disorder may now fulfill the criteria for a different mutually exclusive disorder. In another situation a patient may fulfill the criteria for two Anxiety Disorders that are not mutually exclusive.

Example 13

Trudy is a 28-year-old woman who develops panic attacks that are initially unexpected and then are triggered only when she has to attend a business party or reception. What diagnosis(es), if any, should Trudy receive?

Panic attacks may occur in many Anxiety Disorders. When they occur, the distinction between the various Anxiety Disorders depends, among other things, on whether the panic attacks were cued or uncued. However, during the course of the illness a patient's symptoms may change. Patients who initially experience uncued panic attacks may find that the attacks eventually become cued. Therefore, they initially fulfill the criteria for a Panic Disorder (uncued) and subsequently fulfill the criteria for another cued Anxiety Disorder such as Specific Phobia or Social Phobia.

In this example the patient's panic attacks gradually shift to become associated with social occasions. If the patient now meets the criteria for Social Phobia, the clinician must make a decision to emphasize either the initial unexpected panic attacks or the later cued panic attacks in the diagnosis. Because the patient is now only experiencing panic attacks associated with social occasions, it is reasonable to make a diagnosis of Social Phobia. If the patient is treated for Social Phobia and subsequently begins to again experience unexpected panic attacks, the diagnosis can be revised.

Example 14

Graham is a 34-year-old man who complains of intrusive thoughts of exposing himself to women that he passes on the street. He has developed an elaborate mental ritual, taking several minutes, that involves counting the number of cars on the street and the number of cracks in the pavement when he has these impulses. Graham also has periodic, unexpected panic attacks. What diagnosis(es), if any, should Graham receive?

This patient appears to have two different Anxiety Disorders, Obsessive-Compulsive Disorder and Panic Disorder Without Agoraphobia. The initial diagnostic question is whether one of these two diagnoses takes precedence over the other. The first step is to determine whether the patient's panic attacks are actually unexpected. For example, the patient might not be aware that the attacks only occur when he becomes fearful that he might actually act on his impulses. If this is the case the diagnosis of Obsessive-Compulsive Disorder would take precedence because the attacks are associated with the content of the obsessions. If, however, the panic attacks are independent of the patient's obsessions or rituals, it would be appropriate to give the patient both diagnoses.

Anxiety Symptoms Associated With Other Psychiatric Disorders

The various forms of anxiety may appear as symptoms associated with several different psychiatric disorders. When phobias, obsessive thoughts, compulsive behavior, anxiety, fear, or apprehension occur in conjunction with Psychotic, Mood, or Cognitive Disorders, it is often difficult to determine whether one disorder predominates or whether they represent comorbid disorders. The following examples illustrate some of these problems.

Example 15

Shirley is a 42-year-old woman who is depressed and complains about feeling anxious. What diagnosis(es), if any, should Shirley receive?

Patients who are depressed commonly have symptoms of anxiety. Psychomotor agitation, a form of anxiety characterized by increased motor activity (e.g., pacing, hand wringing) associated with internal tension and discomfort, is one of the criteria for the diagnosis of Major Depressive Disorder (Single Episode or Recurrent). Anxiety also occurs with other Depressive Disorders. The important distinction is whether the patient has only anxiety symptoms or Anxiety Disorder.

The presence of anxiety alone is not sufficient for the diagnosis of Anxiety Disorder. If a patient meets the criteria for Anxiety Disorder and the criteria for Mood Disorder, he should receive a dual diagnosis of both disorders. If he does not meet the criteria for Anxiety Disorder, he should receive only the Mood Disorder diagnosis with a notation that there is accompanying anxiety.

Example 16

Lamont is a 22-year-old man who routinely abuses illegal drugs and complains of feeling anxious. What diagnosis(es), if any, should Lamont receive?

The anxiety experienced by a patient with Substance-Related Disorder may be a symptom of intoxication (Cocaine-Induced Anxiety Disorder, Caffeine-Induced Anxiety Disorder, etc.) or withdrawal (Alcohol Withdrawal Anxiety Disorder, Nicotine Withdrawal Anxiety Disorder, etc.) syndrome associated with the abused substance, or it may be a symptom of comorbid Anxiety Disorder. The patient should be questioned carefully about the temporal relationship between the use of the substance and the onset, duration, and intensity of the anxiety. The anxiety is likely to be independent of the abused substance if the symptoms of anxiety preceded the onset of substance use, are more intense than would be expected by the substance in question, or have lasted more than 1 month after the cessation of substance use.

Example 17

Travis is a 26-year-old man who frequently hears voices and states that he feels anxious. What diagnosis(es), if any, should Travis receive?

Anxiety is a common symptom in many psychiatric disorders. This was noted above in the discussion about the relationship between anxiety and depression. Similarly, it is not unusual for a patient to become anxious when experiencing auditory hallucinations. The co-occurrence of anxiety and auditory hallucinations raises several diagnostic questions. Does the patient meet the criteria for a specific Anxiety Disorder? Posttraumatic Stress Disorder is the only Anxiety Disorder that includes hallucinations in the diagnostic criteria. The hallucinations generally arise during a flashback experience when the patient feels that the traumatic event is recurring. The auditory hallucinations usually have a content related to the traumatic event. The symptoms of anxiety and auditory hallucinations could also be caused by an abused substance taken by the patient.

In this case the patient should receive two diagnoses, Substance-Induced Anxiety Disorder and Substance-Induced Psychotic Disorder. It is conceivable that the patient could meet the criteria for Generalized Anxiety Disorder in the early prodromal stages of Schizophrenia or another Psychotic Disorder. However, the presence of active Psychotic Disorder precludes the diagnosis of Generalized Anxiety Disorder. Finally, the anxiety could be a comorbid symptom occurring in a patient with active Psychotic Disorder such as Schizophrenia or one of its subtypes. The patient could be anxious because the voices command him to commit some violent, inappropriate, or illegal act that he feels he may not be able to resist performing. It is also possible that he is startled by the voices, even if they do not command him to perform an inappropriate act, because he has had no previous experience with auditory hallucinations.

Example 18

Vincent is a 33-year-old man who is hypervigilant, paranoid, and complains of feeling anxious. What diagnosis(es), if any, should Vincent receive?

The relationship between anxiety, worry, apprehension, hypervigilance, and paranoia is not always clear. The first three generally imply that a patient is fearful of some future trouble or the occurrence of an undesirable event. The object of the fear may be vague or uncertain. Patients who are hypervigilant or paranoid fear that some other person or omniscient agent is attempting to harm them. Hypervigilance and paranoia often include, but are not limited to, anxiety and apprehension. Neither of these symptoms are an explicit part of the criteria for any specific nonorganic-based Anxiety Disorder. Hypervigilance and paranoia associated with anxiety or agitation do occur in patients who have stimulant intoxication Anxiety Disorder such as Amphetamine-Induced Anxiety Disorder or Cocaine-Induced Anxiety Disorder. When these symptoms occur in the absence of a history of substance abuse, the clinician should consider a diagnosis of Paranoid Schizophrenia if the patient fulfills the other criteria for this disorder.

Precedence of Diagnosis

Anxiety is a common human experience for healthy individuals and psychiatrically ill patients. Some element of anxiety occurs in almost every psychiatric illness. As a result, there are patients who meet the criteria for two diagnoses. These may both be within the Anxiety Disorders group or one may be in another diagnostic group. Under some circumstances it may be appropriate to give the patient a dual diagnosis. In other situations one of the Anxiety Disorders or the nonanxiety disorder may take precedence over the primary Anxiety Disorder. Table 8–1 shows the disorders that take diagnostic precedence over specific Anxiety Disorders. The list of disorders taking precedence for a specific Anxiety Disorder should be applied with some discretion. The example of a patient who had symptoms of Panic Disorder Without Agoraphobia and Obsessive-Compulsive Disorder was discussed in a previous section. In this case the diagnosis of Obsessive-Compulsive Disorder would only take precedence if the panic attacks were better explained by the patient's obsessions or compulsive rituals. If there is no relationship between the two syndromes, the patient could

Table 8–1 Precedence of diagnosis for Anxiety Disorders	
Anxiety Disorder	**Disorders taking precedence**
Panic Disorder Without Agoraphobia Panic Disorder With Agoraphobia	Not better accounted for by Obsessive-Compulsive Disorder, Posttraumatic Stress Disorder, Separation Anxiety Disorder, Specific Phobia, Social Phobia Not due to effects of a substance or general medical condition
Agoraphobia Without History of Panic Disorder	Has never met criteria for Panic Disorder Not due to effects of a substance or general medical condition
Specific Phobia	Not better accounted for by Obsessive-Compulsive Disorder, Posttraumatic Stress Disorder, Separation Anxiety Disorder, Social Phobia, Panic Disorder With Agoraphobia, Agoraphobia Without History of Panic Disorder
Social Phobia	Not better accounted for by Panic Disorder With Agoraphobia, Panic Disorder Without Agoraphobia, Separation Anxiety Disorder, Body Dysmorphic Disorder, Pervasive Developmental Disorder, Schizoid Personality Disorder Not due to effects of a substance or general medical condition
Obsessive-Compulsive Disorder	Not better accounted for by Eating Disorder, Trichotillomania, Body Dysmorphic Disorder, Substance Use Disorder, Hypochondriasis, Paraphilia, Major Depressive Disorder Not due to effects of a substance or general medical condition
Posttraumatic Stress Disorder	None
Acute Stress Disorder	Not better accounted for by Brief Psychotic Disorder Not due to effects of a substance or general medical condition
Generalized Anxiety Disorder	Does not occur exclusively during Mood Disorder, Psychotic Disorder, Pervasive Developmental Disorder Not better accounted for by Panic Disorder, Social Phobia, Obsessive-Compulsive Disorder, Separation Anxiety Disorder, Anorexia Nervosa, Hypochondriasis, Posttraumatic Stress Disorder Not due to effects of a substance or general medical condition

(continued)

Table 8–1 Precedence of diagnosis for Anxiety Disorders (continued)	
Anxiety Disorder	**Disorders taking precedence**
Anxiety Disorder Due to a General Medical Condition	Does not occur exclusively during Delirium Not better accounted for by another mental disorder in which stressor is a serious medical illness
Substance-Induced Anxiety Disorder	Does not occur exclusively during Delirium Not better accounted for by Anxiety Disorder that is not substance-induced
Anxiety Disorder NOS	Does not meet criteria for any specific Anxiety Disorder, Adjustment Disorder With Anxiety, Adjustment Disorder With Mixed Anxiety and Depressed Mood

Note. NOS = Not Otherwise Specified.

be given both diagnoses. Therefore, the precedence list is not inflexible. Rather, it is a guideline that should remind the clinician of other possible diagnoses that are consistent with the patient's symptoms.

Discussion of Clinical Vignettes

Vignette 1: I'm Not Safe in My Own Home

Nancy developed several distressing psychiatric symptoms after her rape. The most likely diagnoses for these symptoms are Posttraumatic Stress Disorder and Acute Stress Disorder. The appearance of ritual behavior also suggests the possibility of a diagnosis of Obsessive-Compulsive Disorder. The first two criteria for Posttraumatic Stress Disorder and Acute Stress Disorder require that the patient experience or witness a traumatic event that involved actual or threatened death or serious injury, or a threat to the physical integrity of the patient or others. Furthermore, the patient's response must involve intense fear or helplessness.

Nancy also fulfills other common criteria of these two disorders. She felt helpless during the rape and was fearful that she might be killed. After the rape she reported feeling "in a daze." Nancy also has repeated dreams about the attack, difficulty sleeping, increased irritability, difficulty concentrating, a sense of detachment from others, diminished participation in social activities, and avoidance of the neighborhood where she lived and continued to work after the attack.

The main distinction between the two disorders is based on the patient's experience of dissociative symptoms during or immediately after the event and the length of time the symptoms last. Although Nancy reports some sense of detachment from other people in the days following the event, she experienced no other dissociative symptoms. The symptoms continued for a "few weeks" after the event. The dividing line between Acute Stress Disorder and Posttraumatic Stress Disorder, with regard to duration of the syndrome, is 4 weeks. The former lasts less than 4 weeks and the latter syndrome lasts at least 4 weeks. Nancy reports that her symptoms have continued for "several weeks." Therefore, the appropriate diagnosis is Posttraumatic Stress Disorder. Nancy also developed a set of nightly ritual behaviors after the attack. They included turning on a light in each room and checking each of the doors and windows several times to make sure they were locked. These behaviors could be considered compulsions and therefore they raise the possibility that the patient also has Obsessive-Compulsive Disorder. Compulsions are defined as repetitive behaviors that the person feels compelled to perform in response to obsessive thoughts or according to a rigid set of rules. These behaviors are aimed at reducing the person's distress or preventing some dreaded event. However, the behaviors are not realistically connected with the events they are designed to prevent, or they are clearly excessive.

The criteria for the diagnosis of Obsessive-Compulsive Disorder also requires that the rituals take a significant amount of the patient's time or interfere with her usual activities. In addition, the patient must recognize, at some point, that the compulsive behaviors are excessive. Finally, if another Axis I disorder is present, the compulsions cannot be restricted to the content or themes of that disorder.

Nancy fits some of these diagnostic criteria but not all. The compulsive checking behavior is a reaction to her assault and an attempt to protect herself from additional attack. In that sense the behavior is not unreasonable. However, there is a question about whether it is excessive. Nancy recognizes that the repeated checking is silly but she is unable to stop it without becoming anxious. These symptoms are consistent with the diagnosis of Obsessive-Compulsive Disorder. However, the content of Nancy's compulsions, namely the repetitive checking, is clearly restricted to experience of being raped and the subsequent Posttraumatic Stress Disorder. Therefore, this diagnosis takes precedence over the diagnosis of Obsessive-Compulsive Disorder.

Vignette 2: It Hit Me Like a Ton of Bricks

Sharon describes experiencing a typical unexpected panic attack while driving to work. The attack consisted of a sudden unexpected episode of intense fear that something dreadful was about to happen associated with several physiological symptoms. A subsequent physical examination revealed no underlying medical problems. Despite the fact that the panic attack subsided with no obvious sequela, Sharon became anxious about driving and began to worry about another attack. A second attack occurred 5 weeks later as she was getting out of her car. The third attack occurred several weeks after the first when she tried to drive to work despite her anxiety. Subsequently she was unable to drive.

Sharon's symptoms illustrate a common problem in the diagnosis of Panic

Disorder. Her first two panic attacks were unexpected and not associated with ago-raphobia so she meets the criteria for a diagnosis of Panic Disorder Without Agora-phobia. Subsequent panic attacks became associated with a specific cue, driving. Sharon's fear of driving might be considered agoraphobia if her concern is that she would not be able to obtain help if she had a panic attack while driving. However, her case is atypical for agoraphobia because patients with this disorder commonly have anxiety associated with a cluster of everyday experiences such as riding in a bus, standing in a crowd, or leaving home alone. Therefore, her current diagnosis remains Panic Disorder Without Agoraphobia. However, if her panic attacks remain specifically associated with the driving and do not generalize to other situations it would be reasonable to consider a diagnosis of Specific Phobia in the future.

Key Diagnostic Points

- Panic attacks can occur in number of Anxiety Disorders in addition to Panic Disorder.

- The diagnosis of Panic Disorder requires the presence of recurrent unexpected (uncued) panic attacks.

- The uncued panic attacks of Panic Disorder can progress, over time, to the cued attacks of Specific Phobia or Social Phobia.

Common Questions in Making a Diagnosis

1. Jane, a 29-year-old housewife, was driving on the highway after taking her children to school. Suddenly a car crossed the center strip approximately 100 feet ahead of her and smashed into a tree. The driver of a second car im-mediately pulled up to the crash scene to help the victim. Jane also stopped and ran over to the crashed car to help. She felt helpless as she saw the driver's bloody head sticking through the car's windshield. The driver of the second car asked her to call for an ambulance. Jane got back into her car and drove to the nearest telephone to call the police and emergency units. When she returned to the crash the police were there and she was not needed. She continued on home.

   Over the next few days Jane began to experience recurrent images of the victim's bloody head. She found herself driving a different route home after taking her children to school. Sometimes the memory of the accident made it difficult for her to fall asleep or concentrate on her work. After 3 or 4 weeks the feelings subsided, although she still preferred to drive a different route. Should Jane receive a diagnosis of Posttraumatic Stress Disorder? What di-agnosis(es), if any, should she receive?

Answer: Symptoms must be present for more than 4 weeks for a diagnosis of Posttraumatic Stress Disorder. Furthermore, this patient's symptoms do not fulfill the criteria for Acute Stress Disorder. Her response might be considered a common reaction to a very stressful experience. It is not pathological.

2. A 25-year-old young man comes to a hospital emergency department complaining that he feels very nervous. He is irritated that he has to wait before seeing the physician and begins to argue with the clerk. When he is told that he will have to wait his turn he begins to pace around the waiting room and seems to be closely watching the other patients and staff. When he is seen an initial physical examination reveals that he has a heart rate of 104 and a blood pressure of 165/100. There are no other positive physical findings. The patient states that he has had episodes of "nervousness" on and off for several days. What diagnosis(es), if any, should he receive?

Answer: The staff should be suspicious that the patient is intoxicated with a substance. A urine drug screen should be obtained. The patient's symptoms are consistent with Cocaine Intoxication but there is insufficient data to make this diagnosis without laboratory evidence of cocaine in the patient's urine.

3. A 27-year-old woman has dissociative symptoms accompanied by nightmares, hypervigilance, and anger that continue 6 weeks after being a victim of an armed robbery and assault. What diagnosis, if any, should she receive?

Answer: The diagnostic decision is between Acute Stress Disorder and Posttraumatic Stress Disorder. Acute Stress Disorder lasts for less than 4 weeks, whereas Posttraumatic Stress Disorder lasts more than 4 weeks. The criteria for the former includes more dissociative symptoms, whereas the latter includes symptoms of avoidance. The diagnostician seems to be forced to decide whether to emphasize the type of symptoms or the duration of the symptoms in making a diagnosis. However, a closer examination of the criteria for the two disorders suggests that the distinction between dissociation and avoidance is subtle and that the respective symptoms tend to overlap as discussed above. Even if some of the dissociative symptoms remain, the crucial concept is that the patient is experiencing a more chronic stress disorder. The appropriate diagnosis would be Posttraumatic Stress Disorder.

4. A patient had an initial unexpected panic attack while riding in an elevator and subsequently had additional panic attacks in the same situation. He now becomes anxious at the thought of riding in a elevator and always uses the stairs.

Answer: The criteria for Panic Disorder Without Agoraphobia are met in this example because the initial attack was unexpected. However, subsequent attacks are clearly associated with a specific stimuli (i.e., riding in an elevator). In addition, the patient has developed a phobia focused on elevators. This is Panic Disorder that changed into Specific Phobia over time.

5. A patient reports that he has been excessively anxious and worried for several years. He also admits that has been routinely using cocaine for the last year. What diagnosis(es), if any, should he receive?

Answer: Anxiety is a symptom of intoxication or withdrawal with many abused substances. Cocaine is a classic example of a drug that produces anxiety, psychomotor agitation, and stereotypic activity that may appear to be compulsive behavior. The main question in this example is whether the patient's anxiety is a product of preexisting Anxiety Disorder, the current use of cocaine, or a combination of the two. However, the diagnosis of Substance-Related Disorder takes precedence over the diagnosis of other Anxiety Disorder. Therefore, if the patient fulfills the criteria for a Cocaine-Induced Anxiety Disorder, he cannot be given a diagnosis of Generalized Anxiety Disorder even if he previously or currently meets the criteria for this disorder. Despite this restriction the clinician should be aware of the possibility of preexisting Anxiety Disorder that might reappear once the patient has stopped using cocaine.

6. A 35-year-old woman was assaulted in the local movie theater when she was 21 years old. Since that time she has had a phobia about theaters. She becomes extremely anxious when approaching a theater and frequently experiences a panic attack if she is forced to go inside. She does not have severe anxiety in other situations. What diagnosis(es), if any, should she receive?

Answer: The major diagnostic distinction in this case is between Specific Phobia cued by exposure to a movie theater or Posttraumatic Stress Disorder related to the assault. Because the latter diagnosis takes precedence over the former, it would be important to establish whether the patient fulfilled the other criteria for the diagnosis of Posttraumatic Stress Disorder. The patient reports intense distress at exposure to an external cue (a movie theater) that resembles the location of the original assault. The remaining criteria for the diagnosis include persistent avoidance of stimuli associated with the trauma, a general numbing of responsiveness, and symptoms of increased arousal. The patient's clinical presentation is deceptive because it is somewhat atypical for Posttraumatic Stress Disorder. The symptoms have persisted for an unusually long period of time and they appear to be primarily focused on movie theaters rather than other cues that might symbolize the attack. In that sense the disorder appears to be a phobia. In fact, if the criteria for the diagnosis of Posttraumatic Stress Disorder are not completely met, the diagnosis of Specific Phobia could be justified. Specific Phobia can usually be differentiated from Posttraumatic Stress Disorder because it does not have the symptoms of general arousal associated with the latter.

7. A 38-year-old depressed man is obsessed with thoughts that he is evil and guilty of being insensitive to others. He has intrusive thoughts that he should kneel down in front of his co-workers in the weekly staff meeting and ask their forgiveness. He tries to ignore these thoughts and suppress them by repeatedly counting the number of ceiling tiles in the room when the thoughts occur. Periodically, he recognizes that the concerns are excessive but he cannot control them. What diagnosis(es), if any, should he receive?

Answer: The diagnosis of Obsessive-Compulsive Disorder requires recurrent and persistent exaggerated thoughts that the person attempts to ignore or suppress and which he recognizes are the product of his own mind. At some stage in the disorder the person recognizes that the thoughts are excessive and unreasonable. This patient fulfills the criteria for this disorder. However, the diagnosis of Obsessive-Compulsive Disorder is precluded in patients who have guilty ruminations in the course of a major depression. It would be important to determine if this depressed patient met the criteria for Major Depressive Disorder. If the patient met the criteria for Major Depressive Disorder and also had intrusive thoughts or impulses that were of a sexual nature, such as propositioning women he passed on the street, he could receive a comorbid diagnosis of both the depression and Obsessive-Compulsive Disorder. In this case the impulses would not be necessarily consistent with the ruminations associated with major Depressive Disorder.

8. A patient is afraid of going out in public because she might become anxious and lose control of her bladder in front of other people before she is able to reach a bathroom. Her anxiety frequently meets the criteria for a panic attack. What diagnosis(es), if any, should she receive?

Answer: This case presents a subtle distinction between two possible diagnoses. The patient can be given a diagnosis of Agoraphobia Without History of Panic Disorder if she is fearful of becoming anxious or having a panic attack in a situation or place from which escape might be difficult or embarrassing. She can receive a diagnosis of Social Phobia if she is fearful that she may act in a way that will be humiliating in public when she becomes anxious. In this case she would be embarrassed by becoming incontinent. The diagnostic decision depends on whether the clinician decides to emphasize the patient's fear of not being able to escape or fear of incontinence.

91. A 27-year-old compulsive, organized man had two unexpected panic attacks in a period of 1 week approximately 1 year ago. He has had no further panic attacks since that time. He continues to have intrusive worries about the implications of the attacks and is preoccupied with fears that he may be "losing his mind." His concern leads him to consult a psychiatrist. What diagnosis(es), if any, should this patient receive?

Answer: The patient has had two (recurrent) panic attacks followed by at least a month or more of worry about the implications of the attacks. If there is no evidence of agoraphobia or indication that the panic attacks were due to Substance-Induced Anxiety Disorder or secondary Anxiety Disorder Due to a General Medical Condition, the patient could be given the diagnosis of Panic Disorder Without Agoraphobia. Although this patient fulfills the explicit criteria for the diagnosis of Panic Disorder, some clinicians might question whether this is the best diagnosis for the patient because it emphasizes the distant panic attacks over the patient's current state of chronic anxiety and worry. The persistent worries might be more indicative of Obsessive-Compulsive Disorder or Anxiety Disorder Not Otherwise Specified.

10. A patient has had several unexpected panic attacks and then gradually develops a fear of eating in public because he feels he might do something to embarrass himself. Subsequent panic attacks only occur when he is eating in public. The patient does not experience agoraphobia and recognizes that his fear is unreasonable. What diagnosis(es), if any, should he receive?

Answer: The initial symptom of unexpected panic attacks that are not associated with agoraphobia meets the criteria for the diagnosis of Panic Disorder Without Agoraphobia. However, subsequent panic attacks are only triggered by eating in public. This shift to cued panic attacks means that the patient no longer meets the criteria for Panic Disorder Without Agoraphobia. Eating in public is a social situation during which the patient is exposed to scrutiny by strangers. His fear of becoming embarrassed when eating in public and the accompanying anxiety fulfill the criteria for the diagnosis of Social Phobia. The clinician must decide whether to base his diagnosis on the original history of the patient's illness or the current symptoms. Unfortunately, the decision cannot be based on the precedence of one disorder over the other because the criteria of both disorders indicate that the diagnosis cannot be made if the symptoms are better accounted for by the other. A diagnostic decision to emphasize the patient's current presentation acknowledges the natural progression of the illness. However, it is not clear whether treating the patient for Social Phobia would lead to the subsequent reappearance of uncued panic attacks.

Somatoform Disorders

Clinical Vignette

Doctor, I Have a Lump

Norman is a 54-year-old man who called his internist, Stanley, for an urgent appointment, stating that he was concerned that he had breast cancer. When he saw the physician, he related the following story. Several months previously while showering, he had noted some swelling in the area of his left nipple. He had not thought much of the problem initially and continued to check the area each time he showered.

After several weeks, Norman became alarmed because he thought he could feel a distinct lump next to the nipple. The thought that he might have cancer occurred to him one day while he was watching a television news program that included a report on breast cancer in women. Norman initially dismissed the idea but soon began thinking more and more about the possibility that he might have cancer and checked the area several times a day. He read about breast cancer in men and learned that it was rare. This information didn't seem to comfort him.

He repeatedly asked his wife if she could feel the lump. Each time he asked, his wife reassured him that she couldn't feel anything. Norman persisted until she finally became irritated and said, "If you're so worried about your breast, call your doctor." Norman became frantic. He took his wife's hand and placed the fingers next to his left nipple over the area where he felt the lump. "Feel here," he said. She poked the area with her fingers and said, "Norman, I don't feel anything. Call your doctor if you're concerned about it." Norman got angry. He was convinced he had breast cancer and no one would be able to detect it until it was too late. He called his internist in a panic.

Stanley had been Norman's physician for several years. He knew that Norman frequently became concerned about having a serious illness after observing vague physical symptoms. When he examined Norman he observed that the area next to the left nipple was slightly reddened and tender but there was no evidence of a lump. Stanley finished the physical examination, asked Norman to get dressed, and left the examining room. Norman prepared for the worst. A few minutes later the doctor reappeared and sat down to talk. "Norman," he said, "I don't feel a lump in your breast. I don't think you have breast cancer. In fact, I didn't find anything wrong with you." Norman took a deep breath and said, "What am I feeling?" Stanley replied, "I don't know, but it isn't breast cancer. Stop poking at the area and it won't be so red and tender."

Norman seemed reluctantly reassured and left. However, 3 days later he called the physician again and told him that he still could feel the lump and thought it had grown larger. After some discussion, Norman seemed somewhat reassured but later told his wife, "My doctor really isn't a specialist. Maybe I should see someone who specializes in cancer."

Core Concept of the Diagnostic Group

The core concept of the Somatoform Disorders includes: 1) persistent or recurring complaints of physical symptoms that are not supported by actual physical findings, 2) persistent worry about having a physical illness that is not supported by actual physical findings, or 3) exaggerated concern about minor or imagined physical defects in an otherwise normal-appearing person. The symptoms commonly appear to be associated with psychological factors.

Definition

somatization   The expression of psychological pain through physical symptoms or concerns.

Synopses and Diagnostic Prototypes
of the Individual Disorders

The brief synopses in this section summarize the specific requirements or criteria that must be fulfilled for each of the diagnostic categories. Many of the synopses include a brief vignette that provides a clinical example of the diagnoses. Each vignette is a prototype in the sense that it represents a typical patient from a specific diagnostic category. The prototypes provide a more lifelike portrayal of the diagnosis than the criteria alone. They also provide a clinical baseline that can be used in the discussion of problems associated with the diagnosis of these disorders and as a standard for comparison even if they do not exhaust all the possibilities for the clinical presentation of a specific diagnosis.

300.81   Somatization Disorder.   Individuals with this disorder have a several-year history, beginning before age 30 years, of seeking treatment for or becoming impaired by multiple physical complaints that cannot be fully explained by a general medical condition, or are in excess of what would be expected from examination, and are not intentionally feigned. The symptoms must include all of the following symptoms:

1. Four pain symptoms in different sites
2. Two gastrointestinal symptoms without pain
3. One sexual symptom without pain
4. One pseudoneurological symptom without pain

> Lucy is a 31-year-old woman who was recently admitted to the hospital by her family physician for evaluation of persistent nausea and vomiting. She is well known to the hospital staff from her four previous hospital admissions and multiple emergency and outpatient visits over the last 10 years. Lucy has a long history of multiple medical complaints that are characterized by their endurance and resistance to treatment.
>
> Her initial problems began at age 14 years when she achieved menarche followed by several cycles of irregular and painful menses. Her mother took her to a gynecologist for evaluation, but no obvious cause was found for the problem. She continued to have problems with menstruation for many years. At age 17 years her headaches started and she periodically complained of difficulty swallowing and blurred vision. Lucy was evaluated by a neurologist for multiple sclerosis with no positive findings. She finished high school, went through a 1-year secretarial training program, and found a job as a secretary in the main office of a local factory.
>
> Her first hospital admission occurred at age 20 years when she complained of acute abdominal pain and vomiting. Despite the absence of any other signs or symptoms, she was taken to surgery and a normal appendix was removed. Lucy was discharged after 1 week. The abdominal pain and vomiting recurred periodically after that initial episode.
>
> Three additional hospitalizations followed over the next 10 years for various physical complaints including pain in her joints and extremities, chronic diarrhea, and excessive menstrual bleeding. Lucy's medical complaints seemed to increase in frequency and intensity as she grew older. She quit her job at the age of 25 to devote her energy to keeping track of her various medical symptoms and seeking appropriate treatment.

300.81   Undifferentiated Somatoform Disorder.   Individuals with this disorder have persistent (6 months) physical complaints that either 1) cannot be explained by a known general medical condition or pathophysiologic mechanism, or 2) if there is a related general medical condition, the physical complaints or impairment is grossly in excess of what would be expected from the physical findings. The symptoms are not intentionally produced.

Veronica is an attractive, 24-year-old woman who is concerned about the effect of her health on her social life. She has met eight men in the last year who have asked her out. A few hours before five of the dates she had a sudden attack of diarrhea and vomiting and had to cancel the dates. On two other dates she had an attack of nausea and vomiting in the restaurant powder room. On the eighth date she did not have any symptoms but the man turned out to be a jerk. Veronica denies any anxiety during the dates and is convinced that she has a chronic virus that periodically causes her problems. She has had at least two medical examinations that have not revealed any physical evidence of disease.

300.11   Conversion Disorder.   Individuals with this disorder have one or more symptoms or deficits affecting voluntary motor or sensory function that are not intentionally produced, yet are judged to be temporally associated with psychological factors such as stress or conflict. The symptoms cannot be fully explained by the direct effects of a substance, a neurological or general medical condition, and are not limited to pain or a sexual dysfunction. Specify one of the following four types:

With Motor Symptom or Deficit
With Seizures or Convulsions
With Sensory Symptom or Deficit
With Mixed Presentation

Sadie, a 43-year-old woman, was brought into a hospital emergency room by her family who reported that she experienced the sudden onset of blindness. The family explained that Sadie had just discovered that her husband had been having an affair with another woman. She was arguing with her husband when she suddenly stopped and announced that she could not see anything. The family was concerned that the patient might have had a stroke because she had hypertension. The patient's husband and sister brought her to the emergency room.

Sadie was examined by the emergency-room physician and the neurologist on call who found no evidence of neurological deficits. The patient's blood pressure was mildly elevated. A psychiatrist was called to see the patient. When he entered the examining room he found a concerned middle-aged woman, the sister, sitting next to the patient and holding her hand. The physician asked Sadie to tell him what had happened and she stated, "I was arguing with my husband and suddenly I couldn't see anymore, but that's OK." The patient seemed to be indifferent to her blindness. The diagnosis is Conversion Disorder With Sensory Symptom.

300.7   Hypochondriasis.   Individuals with this disorder have a persistent (6 months or more) nondelusional belief that they have a serious illness, despite medical reassurance, a lack of physical findings, and failure to develop the disease. Specify *with poor insight* if for most of the time during the current episode, the individual does not recognize that the concern is excessive.

Walt is a 46-year-old man who has been chronically worried about his health for several years. When he visited his internist for a general physical examination last year, his blood pressure was mildly elevated at 145/93 and his electrocardiogram (EKG) was normal. The physician suggested that he have his blood pressure taken every few months, but decided not to start him on any medication. Despite the reassurance Walt became convinced that he had hypertension. He also began to complain of vague chest pains.

One night he awoke to feel his pulse throbbing in his forehead and some discomfort in his chest. He became convinced that he was having an episode of acute hypertension and a possible heart attack. He became so agitated that his wife drove him to the local hospital emergency room for an evaluation. The nurse took his blood pressure and found it to be mildly elevated at 155/95. An EKG was normal.

The next day Walt made an appointment with his physician. The examination in the doctor's office again showed a mildly elevated blood pressure of 145/90. The physician reassured Walt again, prescribed a mild diuretic, and sent him home after telling him that his chest discomfort was not an indication of a heart attack. Walt felt somewhat better but began to worry again later in the evening when he became aware of his heart beat while lying quietly in bed.

300.7 Body Dysmorphic Disorder. Individuals with this disorder have a preoccupation with an imagined defect or markedly excessive concern about a minor physical anomaly.

Denny is a 21-year-old man who is concerned about his appearance. One day when he was age 13, Denny was looking in the mirror while combing his hair and noticed that his nose was slightly crooked. He examined it closely from several angles and became convinced that it was abnormal. At breakfast he asked his mother to look at his nose. "It looks fine to me," she said. Denny was not reassured. At school he asked his best friend Steve, "Does my nose look alright to you?" "You mean aside from the big zit," Steve laughed. Denny frowned, "I mean, does it look crooked to you." Steve looked at Denny with a slight smile and said, "It's a nose. What do you want from it? Let's go to lunch."

Despite reassurances from friends and family, Denny continued to be concerned about his nose. He became so self-conscious about his nose that he often held his hand up to cover it when he spoke with people. By the time he was age 18, Denny began to investigate the possibility of plastic surgery to straighten his nose. When he was age 21, he made an appointment with a plastic surgeon for an evaluation.

Pain Disorders

307.80 Pain Disorder Associated With Psychological Factors. Individuals with this disorder have pain in one or more anatomical sites that is of sufficient severity to warrant clinical attention. Psychological factors are judged to have an important role in the onset, severity, exacerbation, or maintenance of the pain. The symptom is not intentionally produced. Specify either:

Acute (duration of less than 6 months)
Chronic (duration of 6 months or more)

Jack is a 38-year-old man who injured his back at work 4 years ago. At that time he was having difficulty in his job and constant arguments with his supervisor. Jack had a long history of job trouble, usually leading to his being fired. The injury occurred when he was bending down to pick up a heavy carton at work. He suddenly felt a sharp pain in his back and was unable to stand up straight. His co-workers rushed him to the local hospital emergency room where he had X rays taken of his back and was examined by the emergency physician. The physical examination and tests did not reveal any obvious abnormalities. Jack was given a diagnosis of "paraspinal muscle spasms" and sent home with a prescription for a muscle relaxant and directions to stay in bed for several days. He was referred to an orthopedic surgeon who specialized in back problems for further evaluation.

Jack remained in bed for 3 days but the pain did not diminish. He made an appointment to see the surgeon who prescribed a conservative treatment regimen consisting of strict bed rest for 2 weeks accompanied by pain medication and additional muscle relaxants. At the end of the 2 weeks Jack's pain had decreased significantly. He returned to work with orders from his doctor not to do any heavy lifting.

Two months later Jack felt another sharp pain in his back when he stumbled while getting up from his chair. He returned to bed for 2 more weeks until the pain subsided. Jack had repeated episodes of back pain over the next 2 years despite extensive physical therapy and medication. He would tell everyone, "Everything is great in my life except for this back pain. If my doctors could only make the pain go away, I wouldn't have any problems." Unfortunately, his doctors were never able to discover any physical signs of disease in Jack's back. Finally, the orthopedist suggested surgery as a way of "stabilizing" his back and Jack agreed.

Following the Jack's surgery his mother arrived to help care for him. In conversations with Jack's wife she described her son as a sickly child who often missed school for colds, influenza, and various other childhood ailments. Jack was her only child and she did not work when he was young. When he got sick, she stayed home with him even when he was in high school. Jack's mother spoke fondly of those days when he was sick and would sit in the kitchen talking to her while she cooked meals. She looked forward to caring for him again.

Jack's surgery was not entirely successful. He continued to have moderate pain in his back. The orthopedist prescribed physical therapy and referred him to a chronic pain specialist. The pain continued and seemed refractory to treatment. Finally Jack quit his job and went on disability. He spent most of his days in bed or sitting in a chair watching television. His mother moved into his house to care for him while his wife worked.

307.89 Pain Disorder Associated With Both Psychological Factors and a General Medical Condition. Individuals with this disorder have pain in one or more anatomical sites that is of sufficient severity to warrant clinical attention. Both psychological factors and a general medical condition are judged to have an important role in the onset, severity, exacerbation, or maintenance of the pain. The symptom is not intentionally produced. Specify either:

Acute (duration of less than 6 months)
Chronic (duration of 6 months or more)

Claudia is a 28-year-old married woman who has had pain in her pelvic area for 5 years. When she was age 22, she had emergency surgery for a ruptured ovarian cyst. The surgery went well and she returned to work at a high-powered advertising agency after recuperating at home for a week.

Several months later she began to experience pain in her pelvic area. At first the pain was episodic, occurring every few days. Soon the pain occurred every day and later became constant. She had a gynecological examination that revealed no evidence of infection or other physical abnormalities. The pain was not uniquely associated with her menstrual periods. Finally, after several weeks of unremitting pain, she underwent a laparoscopy in an attempt to determine the cause of her pain. The procedure showed that she had some adhesions from her earlier surgery and mild endometriosis. However, the endometriosis was not judged to be severe enough to account for her pain.

Claudia had always been independent, self-sufficient, and an overachiever. Now she was constantly preoccupied with the pelvic pain. She took a leave of absence from her job and saw several physicians for evaluation and treatment. Some of the treatments were effective for a few weeks but eventually the pain returned. After a year, she quit her job and applied for disability. She subsequently spent most of her time at home in bed trying various remedies to cope with the pain.

xxx.xx Pain Disorder Associated With a General Medical Condition. A general medical condition has a major role in the onset, severity, exacerbation, or maintenance of the pain. Psychological factors, if present, have a minor role. Code on Axis III based on the anatomic site.

300.81 Somatoform Disorder Not Otherwise Specified. Individuals with this disorder have somatoform symptoms that do not meet the criteria for any specific Somatoform Disorder.

Necessary Clinical Information

The specific information necessary for the diagnoses of Somatoform Disorders includes the following:

- Current and past nonpsychiatric medical illnesses and surgery

- Current and past worries about illness

- Current medications and abused substances

- Physical symptoms including pain and fatigue

- Degree of distress produced by the physical symptoms

- Psychiatric symptoms

- History of stressors

- Impairment in daily functioning

- Stressors (e.g., death, divorce, separation, victimization, accidents, job loss)

- Psychological conflicts (dependence vs. independence, anger vs. love, sexual desire vs. inhibitions, etc.)

- Psychological needs (dependency, intimacy, control, etc.)

- Typical reaction to external stressors

Making a Diagnosis

Somatoform Disorders, more than any other single diagnostic group, force the clinician to address the problem of the relationship between physical and psychiatric illness in a specific patient. Clinicians are always alert to the problem of ruling out a potential organic etiology for a patient's psychiatric symptoms. In the diagnosis of Somatoform Disorders the problem is just the opposite; ruling out a potential organic etiology for the patient's physical symptoms.

The criteria for many of the diagnoses in this group require evidence of psychological factors associated with the initiation or exacerbation of the patient's symptoms. This association is almost always established as a correlation based on a close temporal relationship between psychological factors, external stressors, and internal conflicts or needs. Correlations are not cause-and-effect relationships. Therefore, the relationship between these factors and the patient's symptoms is usually impossible to prove.

As a result, there is a significant amount of leeway in the diagnosis of these disorders and the interpretation of the relevance of the various psychological factors. This weakens the underlying etiologic concept of Somatoform Disorder diagnoses, in essence making them diagnoses of exclusion that are used when all physical etiologies for the symptoms are ruled out. Realistically, the psychological factors are usually applied to the patient's symptoms in retrospect to fulfill the required criteria.

The following questions provide an organized approach to the diagnosis of the typical Somatoform Disorder. In each case, the precedence of diagnosis should be examined before the diagnosis is made. For example, the diagnosis of Hypochondriasis cannot be made if the symptoms occur exclusively in the course of a psychiatric disturbance such as Major Depressive Disorder. Specific problems in the diagnosis of these disorders will be discussed in the next section.

1. Does the individual have a substance-related problem or a general medical condition that could produce his or her symptoms?

- The diagnosis of a substance-related problem or a general medical condition takes precedence over the diagnosis of most Somatoform Disorders unless the individual's symptoms are in excess of those expected for the disorder or there are significant contributing psychological factors.

2. Does the individual have another mental disorder that could better account for his or her symptoms?

- Somatic symptoms are associated with many psychiatric disorders. Table 9-1 (see page 255) contains a list of diagnoses that take precedence over each of the Somatoform Disorders. In most cases, the diagnosis of Somatoform Disorder cannot be made if the symptoms occur exclusively during the course of another specific mental disorder. Sometimes one Somatoform Disorder takes diagnostic precedence over another.

3. Does the individual worry excessively about having a serious illness or defect in appearance despite a lack of significant physical evidence?

- If an individual has been worried that he is seriously ill for more than 6 months despite medical reassurance to the contrary, consider the diagnosis of Hypochondriasis. If the belief has lasted less than 6 months, the diagnosis is Somatoform Disorder Not Otherwise Specified.

- If an individual is preoccupied with an imagined defect in appearance or a slight physical anomaly, consider the diagnosis of Body Dysmorphic Disorder.

4. Does the individual complain exclusively of pain?

- If the individual complains exclusively of pain, the diagnosis cannot be Somatization Disorder, Conversion Disorder, Hypochondriasis, or Body Dysmorphic Disorder. The first two of these diagnoses require other physical symptoms in addition to pain. The last two do not include pain as part of the criteria.

- If an individual complains of significant pain and psychological factors are judged to have a major role in the onset, severity, exacerbation, or maintenance of the pain, consider the diagnosis of Pain Disorder Associated With Psychological Factors. If both psychological factors and a general medical condition are judged to have important roles, consider the diagnosis of Pain Disorder Associated With Both Psychological Factors and a General Medical Condition.

5. Does the individual complain exclusively of symptoms affecting voluntary motor or sensory function that are not limited to pain or sexual dysfunction?

- If the patient complains only of a symptom of sensory deficit (e.g., blindness, loss of pain sensation) or loss of voluntary motor function (e.g., paralysis, muscle weakness), consider the diagnosis of Conversion Disorder.

6. Does the individual complain of multiple physical symptoms?

- If an individual has a history of multiple physical symptoms (four pain, two gastrointestinal, one sexual, and one pseudoneurological symptom) beginning before age 30 and occurring over several years, consider the diagnosis of Somatization Disorder.

- If the patient has multiple physical symptoms, yet they are not sufficient in number, distribution, or type to fulfill the criteria for Somatization Disorder or Conversion Disorder there are two diagnostic choices. Patients complaining of significant pain that cannot be fully explained by a nonpsychiatric physical illness can receive a diagnosis of Pain Disorder, even in the presence of other physical symptoms. If the symptoms do not include pain, or if pain is not the most prominent symptom and the condition has existed for more than 6 months, the diagnosis is most likely Undifferentiated Somatoform Disorder.

Common Questions in Making a Diagnosis

There are three main areas of uncertainty in the differential diagnosis of Somatoform Disorders.

1. Some patients initially come close but don't actually fulfill the criteria for a specific diagnosis. More information or a further consideration of the diagnostic criteria may or may not resolve the problem.
2. Some patients fulfill the diagnostic criteria for more than one, mutually exclusive, Somatoform Disorder during the course of their illness. This problem mainly occurs in association with the Somatization Disorder.

3. Some patients have isolated somatic symptoms associated with other psychiatric disorders, but do not fulfill the criteria for a specific Somatoform Disorder.

Patients Who Almost Fulfill the Diagnostic Criteria

In some cases the patient has symptoms or deficits that almost, but not quite, fulfill the necessary criteria for a diagnosis. This problem usually occurs when the diagnostic criteria require the presence of multiple symptoms, a specific intensity of symptoms, or a specific duration of symptoms. In the Somatoform Disorders group this problem occurs mainly in the diagnosis of Somatization Disorder because of the large number of required symptoms. However, the problem can also occur in other disorders.

Example 1

Miriam is a 29-year-old woman who has had multiple medical problems for the last 6–7 years. She has had repeated episodes of painful menses, chronic abdominal pain, and pain in her joints. The abdominal pain has led to one exploratory laparotomy. Miriam has also had several other symptoms including chronic nausea, irregular menses, excessive menstrual bleeding, and several episodes of difficulty swallowing and a few episodes of blurred vision. The latter two symptoms were evaluated by a neurologist, but no obvious physical pathology was found. What diagnosis(es), if any, should Miriam receive?

Miriam has had three pain symptoms, one gastrointestinal symptom, two sexual symptoms, and two pseudoneurologic symptoms. This partially fulfills the criteria necessary for the diagnosis of Somatization Disorder. The clinician is faced with a decision. Should he ignore the missed criteria and make a diagnosis of Somatization Disorder, or should he rigidly adhere to the criteria and make a diagnosis of Somatoform Disorder Not Otherwise Specified or Undifferentiated Somatoform Disorder?

The best approach is to examine the underlying core concept of the specific diagnosis. The diagnosis of Somatization Disorder was created to categorize a group of patients who have multiple physical complaints that begin when they are young adults, continue for an extended period of time, and cannot be fully explained by a nonpsychiatric medical condition. The implication is that the patient's main mode of responding to stress and psychological conflict is through the development of physical symptoms. Furthermore, this process represents a pervasive and enduring element of the patient's personality.

Viewed in this sense, the question of diagnosis can be rephrased. If the clinician feels that there is enough evidence to indicate that the patient routinely responds to social and psychological problems by developing physical symptoms, he would be justified in making a diagnosis of Somatization Disorder, even if the criteria are not entirely satisfied. If he is not convinced of this, he can make an initial diagnosis of Somatoform Disorder Not Otherwise Specified or Undifferentiated Somatoform Disorder until he has gathered more information.

Example 2

Melvin is a 24-year-old man who is preoccupied with a specific problem. His left arm is 2 inches shorter than his right arm. This difference makes it very difficult for him to buy clothes. He also feels very self-conscious about his physical appearance, and often holds his left arm slightly behind his back or drapes a coat over it so no one will notice it is shorter than his right arm. What diagnosis(es), if any, should Melvin receive?

Melvin is very concerned about the difference in the length of his arms. The diagnosis of Body Dysmorphic Disorder requires that if an individual has a slight physical anomaly, the individual's concern about that defect must be markedly excessive. There are two questions in this case. Is Melvin's anomaly *slight* and is his concern *markedly excessive?* If the clinician decides that the physical anomaly is significant, the intensity of Melvin's reaction is irrelevant. If the defect is considered slight, the clinician must decide whether Melvin's reaction is markedly excessive. One element in this decision is the degree of discomfort that Melvin feels when he cannot conceal his left arm or when someone notices the discrepancy in length. If he is significantly bothered by this, the diagnosis of Body Dysmorphic Disorder would be appropriate.

Patients Who Fulfill the Criteria for More Than One Somatoform Disorder

Periodically a patient will meet the criteria for two different diagnoses in the Somatoform Disorders group. Depending on the disorders, one diagnosis may take precedence over the other or the patient may be given two comorbid diagnoses. For example, the diagnosis of Conversion Disorder cannot be made if the symptoms occur exclusively during the course of Somatization Disorder. However, Conversion Disorder and Pain Disorder Associated With Psychological Factors could conceivably be diagnosed together if the criteria for both disorders were met.

Example 3

Leslie is a 32-year-old woman who has complained of severe headaches. She describes them as throbbing in nature and occurring each morning when she leaves home to go to work. They began approximately 4 months ago. At that time Leslie was assigned to a new boss who she does not like. She denies that this has anything to do with the headaches. The headaches also occur during the weekends but they are not as severe.

Leslie has a history of multiple medical problems that have occurred over the last 10 years. She has had chronic abdominal, back, and joint pain, as well as repeated episodes of nausea and vomiting, irregular menses, and weakness of both arms. Numerous medical evaluations have not revealed any underlying physical disorder. What diagnosis(es), if any, should Leslie receive?

Leslie's symptoms meet the criteria for the diagnosis of Pain Disorder Associated With Psychological Factors. However, her symptoms also meet the criteria for the diagnosis of Somatization Disorder. This disorder takes precedence over Pain Disorder. Her current headaches should be seen as an extension of Somatization Disorder.

Somatoform Symptoms Associated With Other Psychiatric Disorders

Somatic symptoms are common in many psychiatric disorders. The diagnosis of Somatoform Disorder usually cannot be made if the somatic symptoms occur exclusively in the context of another mental disorder. For example, if an individual obsesses about a minor physical defect in the context of Obsessive-Compulsive Disorder, the diagnosis of Body Dysmorphic Disorder is excluded. If a non-Somatoform Disorder develops in the midst of a previously established Somatoform Disorder, the patient can receive both diagnoses.

Example 4

Woody is a 26-year-old man who works in the public library and shares an apartment with a friend. The roommate reports that Woody has been behaving strangely for 3 days. He has not slept for the last two nights and wanders around the apartment talking to himself. This morning he appeared at breakfast with half of his face covered with masking tape and said, "The left side of my face is all shriveled up and my left eye is much smaller than the other one. I don't want people to see it." His roommate was alarmed and took Woody to a local hospital emergency room.

In the hospital, Woody admitted to the physician that he had been hearing voices telling him that his face was going to be destroyed because he was evil. When the physician removed the masking tape, he could not find any physical abnormalities on Woody's face. He held a mirror in front of Woody, who looked at his face and said, "My face is broken. I have to cover it to stop the evil." What diagnosis(es), if any, should Woody receive?

Woody is preoccupied with an imaginary physical defect on one side of his face. Under some circumstances this preoccupation would fulfill the criteria for a diagnosis of Body Dysmorphic Disorder. However, Woody's belief in the defect is of delusional proportions and is accompanied by auditory hallucinations. It meets the criteria for Brief Psychotic Disorder. This diagnosis takes precedence over the diagnosis of Body Dysmorphic Disorder.

Example 5

Winnie is a 31-year-old woman who reports a 2-year history of chronic abdominal pain and nausea. She has seen several physicians who have been unable to discover any physical cause for her symptoms. Two months ago she became depressed about her physical problems and her empty social life. She made an appointment at a local community mental health center where she reported feeling chronically tired, sleeping poorly, having difficulty concentrating, and having recurrent thoughts of dying. What diagnosis(es), if any, should Winnie receive?

Winnie's symptoms meet the criteria for the diagnosis of both Undifferentiated Somatoform Disorder and Major Depressive Disorder, Single Episode. If her somatic symptoms had arisen exclusively during the course of the depression, they would not fulfill the criteria for Undifferentiated Somatoform Disorder. However, her somatic symptoms were well established before the onset of the depression. Therefore, they fulfill the criteria for both disorders.

Precedence of Diagnosis

In the right-hand column of Table 9–1 is a list of psychiatric disorders and general medical disorders that take precedence in the diagnosis of the patient. For example, several disorders (Generalized Anxiety Disorder, Obsessive-Compulsive Disorder, Panic Disorder, Major Depressive Disorder, Separation Anxiety Disorder, and any other Somatoform Disorder) are listed in the right-hand column next to Hypochondriasis. When a patient's symptoms meet the criteria for Hypochondriasis, the clinician should examine these disorders. If the patient's symptoms meet the criteria for any of these disorders, he should be given that diagnosis instead of the Hypochondriasis diagnosis. The clinician should note that the diagnoses listed next to each Somatoform Disorder represent the main diagnoses taking precedence over that disorder, but do not include all of the diagnoses that do so.

Discussion of Clinical Vignette

Doctor, I Have a Lump.

The patient's main symptom is his concern that he has breast cancer. This worry is not of delusional quality because he can temporarily be reassured by the physician that he does not have the illness. Because the patient has no pain and complains of only one physical symptom, the diagnosis of Somatization Disorder and Pain Disorder can be excluded. Conversion Disorder can be ruled out because the patient's physical symptom does not include an alteration in sensation or voluntary motor

Table 9–1   Precedence of diagnosis for Somatoform Disorders

Somatoform Disorder	Disorders taking precedence
Somatization Disorder	Not better accounted for by a neurological or general medical condition
Conversion Disorder	Does not meet criteria for Factitious Disorder, Malingering, Pain Disorder, Sexual Dysfunction Does not occur exclusively during Somatization Disorder Not better accounted for by a neurological or general medical condition or a mental disorder
Hypochondriasis	Does not occur exclusively during Generalized Anxiety Disorder, Obsessive-Compulsive Disorder, Panic Disorder, Major Depressive Disorder, Separation Anxiety Disorder, or any other Somatoform Disorder
Body Dysmorphic Disorder	Not better accounted for by any other mental disorder
Pain Disorder Associated with Psychological Factors	Does not meet criteria for Somatization Disorder, Dyspareunia Not better accounted for by Mood Disorder, Anxiety Disorder, Psychotic Disorder
Pain Disorder Associated with Both Psychological Factors and a General Medical Condition	Does not meet criteria for Dyspareunia Not better accounted for by Mood Disorder, Anxiety Disorder, Psychotic Disorder
Undifferentiated Somatoform Disorder	Does not occur exclusively during any other Somatoform Disorder, Sexual Dysfunction, Mood Disorder, Anxiety Disorder, Sleep Disorder, Psychotic Disorder
Somatoform Disorder NOS	Does not meet criteria for any specific Somatoform Disorder

Note.   NOS = Not Otherwise Specified.

function. Similarly, the diagnosis cannot be Body Dysmorphic Disorder because the patient's main complaint is not about the appearance of his breast. Rather, he is concerned about the imagined existence of an underlying disease process that is manifest despite the normal appearance of the breast.

The diagnosis of Undifferentiated Somatoform Disorder requires the presence of one or more physical complaints with associated psychological factors for at least 6 months. Assuming that the time criteria are fulfilled, the use of this diagnosis depends on whether the clinician decides that the patient's symptom was an actual physical complaint rather than a worry about having an illness. If the symptom is deemed to be an unreasonable worry about having an illness, the diagnosis is either Hypochondriasis or Somatoform Disorder Not Otherwise Specified. The deciding factor is whether the symptom has persisted for at least 6 months. If it has, the diagnosis is Hypochondriasis. If not, the diagnosis is Somatoform Disorder Not Otherwise Specified.

Key Diagnostic Points

- The presence of pain is part of the criteria for the diagnosis of Somatization Disorder, Pain Disorder, Undifferentiated Somatoform Disorder, and Somatoform Disorder Not Otherwise Specified. The loss of pain sensation is a more typical symptom for the diagnosis of Conversion Disorder.

- Symptoms of pain are required for the diagnosis of Somatization Disorder and Pain Disorder, but are optional for other Somatoform Disorders.

- Patients who have Body Dysmorphic Disorder do not appear to have any physical defects to the outside observer.

Common Problems in Making a Diagnosis

1. Sylvester is a 46-year-old man who recently had a violent physical argument with his wife. He now complains of pain while moving his right arm. Can he receive a diagnosis of Conversion Disorder?

   Answer: The diagnosis of Conversion Disorder requires the development of a symptom affecting sensory or voluntary motor function. Sylvester's complaints of pain fall into neither category. Therefore, the patient's symptoms do not fulfill the criteria for Conversion Disorder.

2. Perry is a 46-year-old man who has been significantly depressed for 2 months. He has been convinced that he has stomach cancer for the last several weeks. Should he receive a diagnosis of Hypochondriasis?

   Answer: The diagnosis of Major Depressive Disorder always takes precedence over the diagnosis of Hypochondriasis if the patient's concerns about illness occur exclusively during the course of the depression.

3. Margaret is a 34-year-old woman who has a delusional preoccupation that other people are offended by the shape of her legs. When she mentions this to family and friends, they tell her that her legs are shaped normally. Should she receive a diagnosis of Body Dysmorphic Disorder or Somatoform Disorder Not Otherwise Specified?

   Answer: The patient should not receive either diagnosis. Both diagnoses require that the patient's preoccupation with an imagined defect be nondelusional.

4. Anthony recently developed chest pain and discomfort 2 weeks after the death of his father from a heart attack? He has no signs of abnormal cardiac function? What diagnosis(es), if any, should Anthony receive?

   Answer: Anthony reports a physical symptom (pain) that is typical of a heart attack rather than a fear or preoccupation with having heart disease. This rules out the diagnosis of Hypochondriasis. The symptom is not related to normal sensory or motor function so the patient is not having Conversion Disorder. The psychological factor associated with the patient's symptom would presumably be the stress of his father's death and his identification with the father. Therefore, the patient fulfills the criteria for a diagnosis of Acute Pain Disorder Associated With Psychological Factors.

5. Malcolm is a 47-year-old man who has become very concerned over the last few months that he has hypertension. He has been reassured several times by his physician, but on each occasion he begins worrying again within a few days. The patient has no other psychiatric or nonpsychiatric symptoms. What diagnosis(es), if any, should Malcolm receive?

   Answer: Malcolm's symptoms meet five of the criteria for the diagnosis of Hypochondriasis. He is fearful that he has a serious illness despite repeated reassurance by his physician. The belief is not of delusional intensity, does not occur in the course of another psychiatric disorder, and causes the patient marked distress. However, the duration of the problem is uncertain. The final criteria for Hypochondriasis requires that the disturbance last for 6 months. The patient reports that he has been worried about his blood pressure for a few months but cannot be more specific about the length of time. If the clinician is willing to assume that the patient's report of a few months fulfills the requirement for 6 months duration, he can make a diagnosis of Hypochondriasis. If he feels that the duration has not been sufficiently established, he should make a diagnosis of Somatoform Disorder Not Otherwise Specified. The decision rests more on the clinician's judgment of the stability of the syndrome than the exact length of time the patient has had the symptoms.

6. Rhoda is a 23-year-old woman with a diagnosis of Anorexia Nervosa who has become preoccupied with the shape of her face. She feels it is too round and asymmetric. Can Rhoda be given a diagnosis of Body Dysmorphic Disorder?

   Answer: No. The diagnosis of Body Dysmorphic Disorder cannot be given to a patient if the patient's preoccupations could be better accounted for by another mental disorder. In this case, the patient's concerns about the shape of her face can be seen as a component of her Anorexia Nervosa.

7. Ursula is a 31-year-old woman who has complained of intermittent abdominal pain, periodic nausea, vomiting and diarrhea, irregular menses, and periodic weakness in her legs associated with a normal physical examination for the last 2–3 years. What diagnosis(es), if any, should Ursula receive?

   Answer: The diagnosis of Somatization Disorder requires a history of pain in at least four sites or functions. Because the patient has only complained of pain in one site, this criterion has not been met. The patient's symptoms do meet the criteria for a diagnosis of Undifferentiated Somatoform Disorder.

Factitious Disorders

Clinical Vignette

My Stomach Is Burning

Troy is a 32-year-old man who was brought to the emergency room one July evening after he vomited blood while eating dinner in a local restaurant and complained of an intense burning pain in his stomach. He reported that 10 years ago he first experienced a bleeding duodenal ulcer while serving in the Marine Corps. He was rushed to the base hospital and given three units of blood. A subsequent evaluation by the psychiatrist led to a medical discharge. He was told that the stress of Marine life caused his ulcer.

Troy subsequently went back to school, earned a college degree, and took a job in an advertising firm. Four years ago he had another bleeding ulcer. The physician who treated him for that episode told him that the ulcer was caused by stress at work. Troy reports that he took a less stressful job when he was discharged from the hospital. Within 2 months he met and began dating a woman who was a co-worker. They were married 3 years ago. Troy thought the marriage was going well until a year ago when he discovered that his wife was having an affair. He forgave his wife and told her that he wanted to continue the marriage, but she insisted on a divorce. Troy reported feeling depressed and under stress since the divorce became final 2 months ago.

The physician listened quietly to Troy's history while she examined him. She asked about the two old surgical scars on his abdomen. Troy explained that one scar was from his gallbladder operation and the other was from a wound he received while in the Marine Corps. He would not elaborate on the latter, stating only that it was a secret mission. Troy asked the physician if she was going to pass a nasogastric tube to drain the contents of his stomach. The physician seemed surprised and nodded. The procedure showed bright red blood in Troy's stomach. He was admitted to the hospital for further evaluation and treatment.

An emergency gastroscopy was performed that evening to look for the source of the bleeding. Blood was seen in his stomach but no active bleeding site was discovered. Troy continued to complain of burning in his stomach and demanded pain medication. The following morning he received an upper gastrointestinal barium X ray that showed no abnormalities. When the physician informed him of the results Troy said, "What's wrong with you doctors? I'm bleeding, my stomach hurts, and you can't find anything wrong. Don't you know what you're doing?"

Later that afternoon he had another episode of vomiting blood. Additional tests were unable to discover the site of the bleeding and Troy again became abusive to the physician when she asked him for more information about his past medical history. Troy was vague about the details of his previous treatments. He suggested that the doctor was incompetent and insisted on leaving the hospital against her advice.

Two months later his physician received a call from a colleague at another hospital in the city asking whether she had recently seen a male patient with gastrointestinal bleeding of undetermined origin. She told her colleague about Troy and discovered that he had recently been admitted to the other hospital with similar problems. He left the hospital abruptly after a nurse walked into his bathroom and found him drinking a small bottle of animal blood.

Core Concept of the Diagnostic Group

The core concept of Fictitious Disorders is the individual's attempt, through deception, to feign physical or emotional illness in order to assume the role of a patient.

Definition

factitious   Artificial, contrived, or deceptive.

Synopses and Diagnostic Prototypes
of the Individual Disorders

The disorders in Fictitious Disorders are differentiated based on the nature of the patient's factitious signs and symptoms: physical, psychological, or a combination of the two. The criteria are similar for all Factitious Disorders. The patient intentionally feigns physical or psychological signs and symptoms to assume a sick role. There are no external incentives for the behavior.

300.16   Factitious Disorder With Predominantly Psychological Signs and Symptoms.   Individuals with this disorder have predominantly psychological signs and symptoms.

Amy is a 27-year-old woman who was admitted to the hospital after she appeared in the emergency room complaining that she was going to kill herself. When she was interviewed, Amy stated that her husband was killed in front of her 3 months before in an abortive holdup attempt. The killer was never caught. Since that time Amy reports experiencing flashbacks of her husband's death. She is unable to sleep or concentrate on her work as a nurse.

Once admitted, Amy was reluctant to talk about her husband's death in detail and became agitated when pressed for further information. She became involved in the treatment of other patients and established a close relationship with two nurses on the ward. Eventually, the nurses and other staff began to argue about how to treat Amy. When the social worker tried to obtain information about her family, Amy refused to cooperate.

Finally, her sister was located. She revealed that Amy had never been married and, as far as she knew, had not witnessed a murder. However, Amy had been involved in several tumultuous relationships with men and had a long psychiatric history. When Amy was confronted with this information she became enraged, denied her sister's report, threatened the staff with legal action for incompetence, and immediately signed out of the hospital.

300.19   Factitious Disorder With Predominantly Physical Signs and Symptoms. Individuals with this disorder have predominantly physical signs and symptoms.

300.19   Factitious Disorder With Combined Psychological and Physical Signs and Symptoms.   Individuals with this disorder have psychological and physical signs and symptoms but neither predominate in the clinical presentation.

300.19   Factitious Disorder Not Otherwise Specified.   Individuals with this disorder do not meet the criteria for a specific Factitious Disorder.

Gwen is a little girl 18 months of age who was rushed to the emergency room with seizures. When the seizures subsided, she remained semicomatose. Her laboratory tests showed an abnormally low blood glucose level. She was given an intravenous injection of glucose and rapidly regained consciousness. Gwen was admitted for further evaluation and treatment with a working diagnosis of idiopathic hypoglycemia.

The social worker spent an hour talking to Gwen's distraught mother and offering psychological support. The mother insisted on remaining with Gwen in her room during the night. The child seemed considerably better the next morning and a series of additional tests were performed to determine the cause of her hypoglycemia.

Early that evening Gwen's mother frantically ran out of the child's room screaming for help. When a nurse arrived she found the child having seizures. Emergency laboratory tests again confirmed that Gwen was markedly hypoglycemic. She had two more hypoglycemic episodes during the next week. All of her tests were negative and the cause of her disorder remained a mystery.

However, some members of the medical staff were becoming suspicious of Gwen's mother because the hypoglycemic episodes only occurred when she was present in the child's room.

One day, when Gwen's mother was in the bathroom, a nurse looked through her purse and discovered a small vial of insulin and a syringe. The mother later admitted to administering insulin to her daughter. She was barred from the hospital and Gwen did not have any further hypoglycemic episodes.

Necessary or Useful Clinical Information

- History of several previous inconclusive hospitalizations
- Repeated, unexplained physical or psychological symptoms
- Evidence that the patient is lying about some part of his or her history
- Multiple surgical scars, especially on the abdomen
- Patient has been or is a health care worker
- Patient experienced a serious illness as a child
- Patient has a fever without other evidence of active disease
- Repeated tests and evaluations yield no identifiable cause for the symptoms

Making a Diagnosis

Many patients elaborate on their illness and exaggerate their symptoms. However, this is different than an overt attempt to deceive the physician with a nonexistent illness. The core problem in making a diagnosis of Factitious Disorder is determining that the individual is consciously and intentionally faking his or her medical condition for the sole purpose of maintaining a role as a patient. This discovery usually occurs only when the patient makes a mistake, or when the clinical staff becomes suspicious of the patient's behavior or of inconsistencies in his or her illness. Unfortunately, there is no certain method of detecting patients who are feigning an illness. However, the following questions may help make the diagnosis.

1. Do the symptoms disappear when the patient is under constant observation and doesn't have access to personal belongings?

Some patients feign physical illness by taking drugs or medication, swallowing or injecting themselves with foreign material, or contaminating their urine. This may be more difficult for the patient to accomplish when he or she is under continuing observation and does not have access to personal belongings. Patients with feigned psychological illness may have a hiatus in their symptoms when they think they are being watched.

2. Is the patient excessively knowledgeable about the symptoms and suggesting appropriate tests and procedures?

Patients with a Factitious Disorder are often very knowledgeable about their disorder and frequently suggest or demand specific tests and procedures.

3. Are the patient's psychiatric symptoms unresponsive to standard treatment?

A repeated lack of response to various appropriate treatments should raise the clinician's suspicion that the patient has a Factitious Disorder.

4. Is the patient vague or lying about important elements of his or her history?

Patients who have a Factitious Disorder are often vague, secretive, or deceptive about their previous medical history. Some of their stories are obviously untrue (i.e., pseudologia fantastica). Other aspects of their history are more difficult to verify or refute. However, small inconsistencies in the patient's story may alert the medical staff to the patient's deception. The patient is usually reluctant to reveal the names of relatives, previous physicians, or facilities where he was treated. He may become angry if pressed or claim that he is unable to remember the requested information.

5. Does the patient become abusive, accuse the physician of incompetence, or abruptly leave the hospital when the medical staff becomes suspicious?

The clinical staff may become suspicious when all the medical test results are negative. The patient frequently responds to this information with angry accusations or by abruptly leaving the hospital before the staff can complete their evaluation.

Precedence of Diagnosis

Any mental disorder that better accounts for the patient's deceptive behavior takes precedence over the diagnosis of Factitious Disorder.

Discussion of Clinical Vignette

My Stomach Is Burning

Troy is a 32-year-old man who presents at the emergency room of a local hospital after an episode of vomiting blood. An extensive medical evaluation does not reveal a cause for the disorder. He accuses the physician of incompetence and abruptly leaves the hospital when she questions him in more detail about his previous medical history. Two months later she discovers that Troy was subsequently hospitalized with identical symptoms in a nearby hospital and left abruptly after he was seen drinking a small bottle of animal blood.

Troy's symptoms, behavior, and inconclusive medical evaluations meet the criteria for the diagnosis of Factitious Disorder With Predominantly Physical Signs and Symptoms. Some patients with these symptoms have a variant of the disorder called *Munchausen's syndrome,* which is characterized by pathological lying (i.e., pseudologia fantastica) and repeated visits to different hospitals, where the patient simulates a medical illness and leaves before the deception is discovered. Troy's story about being wounded in a secret mission while he was in the Marine Corps is probably an example of this type of pathological lying.

Key Diagnostic Points

The patient's only motivation for feigning illness in Factitious Disorder is to assume a sick role.

Common Questions in Making a Diagnosis

1. Keith is a 27-year-old man who was admitted to a psychiatric hospital after he complained of hearing voices telling him to hurt himself. He was treated with an antipsychotic medication but he reported that the voices continued. The dose of medication was increased without effect. One week after admission, another patient told the nurse on duty that Keith was not taking his medication and was pretending to hear voices. The physician confronted Keith but he denied faking his symptoms and stated that the voices now told him to hurt the physician. The staff made inquiries about Keith at other psychiatric facilities and discovered that he had been admitted to three hospitals in the past 2 years with the same complaint. In each case he left or was discharged with his symptoms intact. What diagnosis(es), if any, should Keith receive?

   Answer: Keith's history and behavior are consistent with Factitious Disorder. However, it is difficult to prove that he is not having auditory hallucinations unless he admits that he isn't. He may be willing to reveal that his symptoms are factitious in the context of a long-term trusting relationship with a therapist. Inconsistencies in his story may also be more evident in such a relationship.

Dissociative Disorders

Clinical Vignette

Sally and Me Make Three

Sally is an attractive 26-year-old woman who was referred to a psychiatrist for treatment of anxiety and erratic behavior. She has worked as a copywriter and editor in a large advertising agency for the past 3 years and is considered creative, intelligent, and hardworking by her employer. During that time she earned several raises and a promotion for the quality of her work. However, her friends and co-workers have recently become distressed about several unusual changes in her work and behavior. Sally also feels increasingly anxious and concerned about certain events in her life that she cannot explain. She asked her internist for help and was referred to a local psychiatrist.

In the initial session, Sally described herself as quiet, even tempered, and somewhat reserved. The psychiatrist asked her why she wanted treatment. Sally replied, "I just don't feel like myself these days. Some strange things have happened that upset me and I can't explain. I feel like I'm going crazy." Sally revealed that she had been in therapy three times before for various periods. She explained that her co-workers complain that her work is erratic and she is sometimes moody and aggressive. Sally has difficulty understanding their complaints. However, a week ago, her boss returned some of her recent work for revision with a note that said, "Sally, this work doesn't seem like you. What happened? Even your handwriting is different." When Sally looked at the copy she couldn't remember working on it. Her boss was right. The writing did not seem like her style. Its tone was far more aggressive than her normal writing.

The writing event was upsetting but far less upsetting than another event that occurred 3 weeks previously. One Saturday morning Sally woke up in bed with Arnold, a man whom she knew casually as a supervisor in another department in the agency. Sally had always found him moderately attractive but they had never dated before. She was startled to be with him and had no recollection of the previous night nor of arranging a rendezvous with him. When she questioned Arnold about the experience he seemed surprised. "You really came on strong. I never thought you could be that sexy." he said. Arnold's statement disturbed and confused her even more. As Sally dressed she did not recognize her clothes. They were far more sexually provocative than the clothes she normally wore and included a see-through blouse and a very short skirt.

Sally's therapy was uneventful for several weeks. She continued to have an erratic performance at work and experienced periods of time for which she had no memory. There were no further unusual sexual encounters and she managed to avoid Arnold at work. One day, in the middle of a therapy session, Sally suddenly became confused and complained of a headache. She looked down at her hands and remained quiet for a few moments. Then she looked up with a strange expression on her face and said, "This therapy thing is bullshit. Why don't you and I just bed down here together on the couch." The psychiatrist was startled and replied, "I don't understand what you mean, Sally." The patient replied, "Don't give me this Sally business, buster. I'm Roxy." She looked at him provocatively and licked her lips. The discussion continued for several more minutes with Roxy acting seductive and denying any knowledge of Sally.

A few minutes before the session was to end the patient again seemed briefly confused and sat back against the chair. After a minute or two she looked up and quietly said, "I'm sorry doctor. I must have fallen asleep. What were you saying?" "Sally," the psychiatrist said. "Yes," she replied. The psychiatrist continued, "Do you remember what we were talking about for the last few minutes?" Sally shook her head and the session ended.

Over the next few weeks Roxy appeared again several times. A third personality, called "Hilda the Defender," also appeared. She was angry, abrasive, and knew all about Sally and Roxy. Hilda explained that her job was to protect Sally and Roxy. She was responsible for Sally's erratic performance at work. When Hilda was the dominant personality, she pursued Sally's work with an aggressive intensity that often offended other people who didn't understand how Sally could suddenly change from a quiet, even-tempered individual to a belligerent and sometimes hostile woman. In therapy, Hilda engaged in a battle with the psychiatrist for the control of the two other personalities. Despite this struggle, the psychiatrist was able to piece together more information about Sally's past history including evidence of early physical and sexual abuse by her stepfather. Gradually, Sally became aware of the other two personalities and began the process of integrating them into her personality.

Core Concept of the Diagnostic Group

The core concept of the Dissociative Disorders is a temporary disruption in the normally integrated functions of memory, identity, or consciousness, leading to amnesia, feelings of depersonalization, or multiple distinct personalities in the same individual.

Definitions

anterograde amnesia   The inability to form new memories after the condition producing the amnesia occurs.

dissociation   The splitting off of a group of mental processes from conscious awareness.

ego-dystonic   Thoughts, affect, and behavior elements of an individual's personality that are considered unacceptable and inconsistent with the individual's total personality or self-identity.

fugue   A period of amnesia during which an individual appears to be conscious and makes rational decisions. The individual has no memory of the period on recovery.

ictus   A seizure.

interictal period   The time between seizures (the ictus).

retrograde amnesia   A loss of memory for events that occurred before the onset of the amnesia and the condition causing it.

Synopses and Diagnostic Prototypes of the Individual Disorders

The brief synopses in this section summarize the specific requirements or criteria that must be fulfilled for each of the diagnostic categories. Each of the first four specific diagnoses includes a brief vignette that provides a clinical example of the diagnosis. Each vignette is a prototype in the sense that it represents a typical patient from a specific diagnostic category. The prototypes provide a more lifelike portrayal of the diagnosis than the criteria alone. They also provide a clinical baseline that can be used in the discussion of problems associated with the diagnosis of these disorders and as a standard for comparison even if they do not exhaust all the possibilities for the clinical presentation of a specific diagnosis.

300.12   Dissociative Amnesia.   Individuals with this disorder have one or more episodes of inability to recall important personal information, usually of a trau-

matic or stressful nature, that is too extensive to be explained by ordinary forget-
fulness.

> Marcie is a 34-year-old woman who was found by the police one night wandering
> in the street. She could not remember her name, did not know where she lived, and
> did not recognize the wallet, driver's license, or other identification papers she was
> carrying. The police were initially unable to contact any family members and took
> her to a local hospital where she was examined and admitted for observation.
> Marcie had a few bruises on her head and chest but no serious injuries or physical
> symptoms of illness. Laboratory tests, including X rays of her skull, were normal.
> Her cognitive abilities were intact, with the exception of the amnesia and some
> confusion about how she had gotten to the hospital. She seemed perplexed about
> her situation and concerned that she had forgotten something.
>
> The following day the medical staff was able to contact Marcie's parents and
> brother. They rushed to the hospital. Marcie did not recognize them when they first
> arrived. Her parents told the staff that Marcie had been involved in an automobile
> accident 2 days before on her way to work with her cousin. Marcie was driving the
> car and escaped with a few bruises. Her cousin, sitting next to her in the front seat,
> was not wearing a seat belt and was severely injured when her head hit the wind-
> shield. The accident was not Marcie's fault but she seemed to blame herself. She
> became withdrawn and did not speak to anyone the remainder of the day. Later that
> evening she disappeared from her apartment. The family had been trying to locate
> her since then.
>
> Gradually, over the next few days Marcie's memory began to return. She was
> taken to see her cousin, who had regained consciousness. Marcie didn't recognize
> her at first but then began to remember details of the accident. She became de-
> pressed and began brief psychotherapy, which helped her resolve her guilt and other
> feelings about the accident.

300.13   Dissociative Fugue.   Individuals with this disorder suddenly and unex-
pectedly travel away from their home or place of work. During this period they are
unable to recall their past, have confusion about their personal identity, and may
assume a partial or complete new identity.

> Douglas is a 45-year-old man who is married with two grown children and lives in
> a small midwestern city. He owns a small furniture business that is currently doing
> poorly. Douglas and his wife have had long-term marital problems that escalated
> when their last child left home. His wife accused him of being inattentive to her
> needs and spending all his free time on his hobby, taxidermy. Douglas is proud of
> the large collection of birds that he has stuffed over the years, especially his birds
> of prey. Several of the birds decorate his home and store. When he arrives home
> after work, he immediately goes down to his taxidermy shop in the basement.
>
> Recently, after a serious argument, his wife threw out all of the stuffed birds she
> could find in the house while Douglas was at work. When he returned home he was

enraged. The next day Douglas left for work and disappeared. When he didn't return home in the evening, his wife called their children and relatives but no one had seen him. Three weeks later Douglas awoke in an inexpensive hotel room in a large city several hundred miles away from his home. He had no idea how he had gotten there and no memory of the period of time since he had left his home. He called his son, who flew to meet him. Over the next 2 days his son reconstructed the events that occurred during the 3 lost weeks.

The day after Douglas arrived in the city he went to the Museum of Natural History and volunteered to be a docent or guide in the zoology section. He seemed knowledgeable, especially about birds, and was accepted in the program. A week later he met a middle-aged woman on the museum staff who he asked out. They quickly became friends but Douglas was always vague about his past and seemed to have no visible means of support. His work at the museum and relationship with the woman continued until he awoke in his hotel room 3 weeks later with no memory of how he had gotten there.

300.14   Dissociative Identity Disorder (formerly Multiple Personality Disorder).   Individuals with this disorder have two or more distinct identities or personality states that have a relatively enduring pattern of perceiving, relating to, and thinking about the environment and self. At least two of these identities recurrently take control of the person's behavior. During these periods the individual is often unable to recall important personal information.

Sandy is a 27-year-old woman who was admitted to a local psychiatric hospital after she superficially cut one wrist in a suicide attempt following a fight with her husband. She had been hospitalized twice in the last 7 years for similar suicide gestures and attempts. Her husband reported that the couple had been married for 5 years. He described the patient as impulsive and difficult to get along with because of her need for constant reassurance and her mood swings. "One minute she acts normal and a few minutes later she's depressed and angry about something. An hour later she starts her 'baby talk' routine, calls me 'Daddy,' and wants me to take care of her," he said.

During extended interviews in the hospital, Sandy talked to the psychiatrist about feeling depressed and anxious much of the time. She agreed with her husband's report that she had a temper and often got angry at him. As the psychiatrist asked about her childhood, Sandy became quiet and looked away. "Is there something upsetting you?" she asked. Sandy looked at the psychiatrist and blinked a few times. Her eyes seemed to lose focus briefly and she said in a childlike voice, "I'm afraid of you, cause, cause, you're going to be mean to me." The psychiatrist assured Sandy that she was safe. Sandy twisted her fingers together and said, "You sure you won't be mean to me?" The psychiatrist nodded and said, "You seem different than you were a few minutes ago, Sandy. What happened?" The patient looked confused and replied, "Who's Sandy? I'm Nan. I'll be 7 next week. Can you come to my party. My mommy says if I'm good I can have a party." The psychiatrist was startled and asked, "What happens if you're not good?" Nan looked down and began to cry, "Then, then, they punish me. I don't like it when they punish me. They put me in the closet forever," she said. The interview continued for several more minutes until Nan seemed briefly distracted again for a few seconds. "What's happening, Nan," the psychiatrist asked. "My name's Sandy," the patient said.

In additional interviews over the next several days the patient switched back and forth between the two identities of Sandy and Nan several times. Neither personality seemed to be aware of the other. Each personality had private memories and internally consistent patterns of thought and behavior that were separate from the other personality.

300.6   Depersonalization Disorder.   Individuals with this disorder have persistent or recurrent experiences of feeling detached from their own thoughts or body, as if they were an outside observer. Their reality testing remains intact during these experiences.

Herman is a 33-year-old photographer who complains of frequent periods of dizziness during which he experiences several unusual and uncomfortable feelings. He describes the experience as follows. "I call them my *spells*. When they occur I feel separate from myself and my body, like I'm floating in a dream and watching myself from the outside. Sometimes other people look like robots and sometimes I feel like a robot. I begin to wonder if I'm real or if the things and people around me are real. Sometimes I think I'm losing my mind. I can't concentrate well during these spells and I can't control them."

Herman went on to report various methods he has tried to end his spells or prevent them from occurring. At various times he has held his head in a bucket of ice water, run around the block several times, and gotten drunk. None of these techniques have any effect on the spells. Herman is aware that the spells are a product of his own mind and do not actually represent reality. Therefore he does not tell people about the spells and tries to cope with them himself. Recently he has sought treatment with the hope that a psychiatrist might have some medicine that would make the spells stop.

300.15   Dissociative Disorder Not Otherwise Specified.   Individuals with this disorder have a dissociative symptom but do not meet the criteria for any specific Dissociative Disorder.

Necessary Clinical Information

- Mood swings or changes

- Unexplained changes in handwriting

- Periods of amnesia

- Episodes of unusual and uncharacteristic behavior
- Unexplained, sudden, extended trips
- Time distortions or lapses
- Erratic behavior
- The appearance of two or more distinct identities or personality states

Making a Diagnosis

Many people have experienced brief periods of dissociation when they feel separated or detached from the environment, act out of character, or forget certain events. The experiences can occur when the individual is tired, confronting a new environment, preoccupied, conflicted, or in many other situations including certain cultural and religious events. A brief sense of depersonalization or detachment is common when people walk into a busy department store or a loud, confusing celebration or gathering. In special circumstances hypnosis can produce a more extended sense of dissociation.

All of these experiences differ from the Dissociative Disorders in quality, intensity, duration, and setting. For the average person, dissociation is a transitory experience that usually can be integrated into the other parts of life. For the patient with Dissociative Disorder, the experiences are characterized by prolonged periods of amnesia, personality change, and detachment, often associated with intense affect. These episodes produce significant impairment in the patient's social, interpersonal, and occupational functioning. Often, the patient is unaware of the extent or even the nature of the problem.

Individuals with Dissociative Disorders initially seek treatment for many reasons including anxiety and depression, as well as overt dissociative symptoms such as depersonalization and amnesia. Sometimes they are motivated for treatment by the reports of other people who have detected unusual discrepancies in their behavior. Whatever the initial reason for their referral, the following questions should help provide an organized approach to identification and diagnosis of Dissociative Disorder. Specific problems in the diagnosis of these disorders will be discussed in the next section.

1. Does the individual report recurrent experiences of time distortions or lapses, unusual or ego-dystonic behavior, depersonalization, or amnesia?

Repeated time distortions or lapses, unusual or ego-dystonic behavior, depersonalization, and amnesia are all experiences typical of the Dissociative Disorders. The patient may personally observe these symptoms or be completely unaware of them. For example, individuals are usually amnestic about behavior that is distinctly different from their normal or dominant personality. In this case, the unusual behavior is observed by another individual who reports it to the patient. These characteristic symptoms may be masked by significant anxiety or depression.

2. Could the individual's symptoms be produced by drugs or a nonpsychiatric medical illness?

Many symptoms of the Dissociative Disorders can be mimicked by drugs or nonpsychiatric medical conditions. Intoxication with several drugs produce dissociative phenomenon including alcohol, hallucinogens, and sedatives. Physical disorders such as brain tumors, temporal lobe seizures, and head trauma may produce similar symptoms. Determine whether the patient has any current nonpsychiatric medical illnesses or substance-related problems. If so, deciding the relationship between these problems and the patient's psychiatric symptoms should be the first step in the diagnostic process.

Presence of nonpsychiatric medical illnesses or substance-related problems in conjunction with psychiatric symptoms does not imply the former caused the latter. The occurrence of psychiatric symptoms before the onset of a medical illness or use of a substance suggests that they have an independent etiology. Similarly, the persistence of the psychiatric symptoms after adequate treatment of the medical illness or cessation of substance use implies that the two are unrelated. Generally, symptoms that occur more than a month after an episode of drug intoxication or withdrawal are not considered to be due to the drug.

Note: Assume that an organic etiology for the patient's symptoms has been ruled out for the remaining questions in this section.

3. Does the individual report repeated experiences of feeling detached from his or her own thoughts or body?

The sense of feeling detached or separated from one's thoughts or body is typical of Depersonalization Disorder. Patients may report feeling as if they are in a dream or observing themselves from outside their body. The feeling may last for several minutes or hours. The feeling of depersonalization may also occur in many other disorders including Major Depressive Disorder, Schizophrenia, intoxication with psychotomimetic drugs, and temporal lobe seizures.

4. Has the individual experienced episodes of amnesia?

- Amnesia is a common symptom of Dissociative Amnesia, Dissociative Fugue, and Dissociative Identity Disorder (Multiple Personality Disorder) but not Depersonalization Disorder.

- If an individual has amnesia in his past history, unexpected travel away from his home or place of work, confusion about his identity or assumption of a new identity, the diagnosis is Dissociative Fugue.

- If an individual has extensive amnesia for important personal events, often including his identity, consider the diagnosis of Dissociative Amnesia.

- If an individual repeatedly displays episodes of behavior or thinking that is significantly divergent from his typical behavior and is amnestic for the episodes, consider the diagnosis of Dissociative Identity Disorder (Multiple Personality Disorder).

Common Problems in Making a Diagnosis

There are three main areas of uncertainty in the differential diagnosis of Dissociative Disorders.

1. Some patients' symptoms initially come close but don't actually fulfill the criteria for a specific diagnosis. More information or a further consideration of the diagnostic criteria may or may not resolve the problem.
2. Some patients' symptoms fulfill the diagnostic criteria for more than one, mutually exclusive, Dissociative Disorder during the course of their illness.
3. Some patients have isolated dissociative symptoms that appear with other psychiatric or general medical disorders, but do not fulfill the criteria for a specific Dissociative Disorder.

Patients Who Almost Fulfill the Diagnostic Criteria

Many people have experienced brief memory lapses, periods when they feel detached from themselves, and times when they act out of character. The diagnosis of Dissociative Disorder requires that these episodes be prolonged and intense rather than brief casual experiences. Even so, in some cases it may be difficult to determine if the patient's symptoms fulfill the criteria for a specific Dissociative Disorder. For example, a patient might complain of periods when he feels "spacey" and detached from himself. It may be difficult to determine if this symptom is of sufficient intensity and duration to fulfill the criteria for Depersonalization Disorder. The diagnosis often requires the judgment of an experienced clinician.

Example 1

Darlene is a 25-year-old woman who is in therapy with a psychiatrist. During a recent session while she was discussing her childhood, Darlene spontaneously began to talk "baby talk" and act childlike. Her speech and behavior during the episode were distinctly different than her normal mode of talking in the session. The psychiatrist asked her to describe what was happening. Darlene replied, "That's the baby part of my personality talking." After a few minutes she switched back to her normal speech and began talking more about the baby part of her personality. Darlene is able to switch back and forth between baby talk and normal speech at will. She does not have amnesia for the episodes. What diagnosis(es), if any, should Darlene receive?

Darlene has periods when she uses baby talk and acts childlike. These episodes are entirely under her conscious control and she remembers them when she reverts back to her normal speech and behavior. Darlene perceives the baby talk as a part of her personality even if it appears distinctly different from her normal speech and behavior. It does not represent a separate identity that takes control of her behavior and has its own enduring patterns of perceiving, relating to, or thinking about the environment and self.

Darlene has not had periods of amnesia and can remember the episodes of baby talk when they occur and talk about them. Because the episodes do not represent a distinct personality, she does not meet the criteria for a diagnosis of Dissociative Identity Disorder (Multiple Personality Disorder). Because she does not have periods of amnesia, depersonalization, or other dissociative symptoms, she does not meet the criteria for any Dissociative Disorder.

Patients Who Fulfill the Criteria for More Than One Dissociative Disorder

A patient may fulfill the criteria for more than one dissociative diagnosis at the same time. Usually when this occurs, the rules for the precedence of diagnosis (Table 11–1; see page 279) determine which diagnosis to use. For example, a patient who feels detached from herself and fulfills the criteria for Depersonalization Disorder cannot be given this diagnosis if her symptoms can be better explained by Dissociative Identity Disorder (Multiple Personality Disorder). An example of a situation in which the patient's feeling of detachment might be better explained by the Dissociative Identity Disorder (Multiple Personality Disorder) is if this feeling only occurred during the transition or switching between different personalities or only when one specific personality is dominant.

Example 2

Tanya is a 29-year-old woman who has been discovered several times wandering around the city, unable to remember her name or where she lives. The episodes usually occur after she has had a fight with her husband. She regains her memory soon after she is returned home by the police, but then completely forgets wandering around the city. Tanya is currently in psychiatric treatment where she has demonstrated three different personalities, each unaware of the others. Her therapist thinks that her amnestic periods correspond to the temporary emergence of one of her other personalities. What diagnosis(es), if any, should Tanya receive?

Tanya fulfills the criteria for both Dissociative Amnesia and Dissociative Identity Disorder (Multiple Personality Disorder). However, the latter diagnosis takes precedence over the former if the amnesia occurs exclusively during the course of the latter. Therefore, her diagnosis is Dissociative Identity Disorder.

Dissociative Symptoms Associated With Other Psychiatric Disorders

Dissociative symptoms are frequently found in conjunction with a number of other disturbances including substance intoxication, psychosis, depression, personality disorders, and malingering. When there is a question about the differential diagnosis of the Dissociative Disorders, the rules of diagnostic precedence (Table 11–1) will often help resolve the problem.

Example 3

A 27-year old man (John Doe) was found wandering on the street by the police. He was later identified by a woman as the man who robbed her earlier in the evening. There were no witnesses to the alleged crime. The man claims that he does not remember who he is, where he was earlier in the evening, and what he was doing. He has a moderate amount of alcohol in his blood. What diagnosis(es), if any, should the man receive?

John Doe's main clinical complaint is amnesia of indeterminate duration. There are several possible diagnoses for the individual's amnesia: Alcohol Intoxication, Alcohol Persisting Amnestic Disorder (Korsakoff's syndrome), Dissociative Amnesia, and Malingering. If the patient has Alcohol Persisting Amnestic Disorder, he should continue to have problems with his memory after he is in police custody. If the amnesia was caused by alcohol intoxication, he may not remember what occurred during the period of intoxication, but should not have continuing memory problems after he is sober.

The differential diagnosis of Dissociative Amnesia versus Malingering is difficult. In this case the patient has a potential secondary gain for the amnesia if he actually did commit the robbery. An interview using amobarbitol might help distinguish between these two diagnoses.

Example 4

Sherry is a 29-year-old woman who is considered unstable by many of her acquaintances. She has had numerous stormy relationships with men and is often moody, impulsive, angry, or suicidal. She also has a poor sense of herself and often seems to be a different person from one day to the next. What diagnosis(es), if any, should Sherry receive?

Sherry's unstable sense of her own identity is consistent with a diagnosis of Borderline Personality Disorder or Dissociative Identity Disorder (Multiple Personality Disorder). The diagnosis of the latter requires clear evidence of two or more distinct personalities that recurrently take control of the individual's behavior. A chronically unstable self-image or sense of self is not sufficient to fulfill the criteria for Dissociative Identity Disorder (Multiple Personality Disorder).

Example 5

Gilbert is a 24-year-old man who has recently begun to experience unpleasant periods during which he feels detached or separated from himself, as if he is in a dream. During these episodes he sometimes hears a woman's voice calling his name and saying things he cannot understand. Gilbert sometimes wonders if he is real during the episodes. What diagnosis(es), if any, should Gilbert receive?

Depersonalization is a symptom found in many psychiatric disorders including Schizophrenia, depression, substance intoxication, and Depersonalization Disorder. It can also be seen in patients with temporal lobe seizures or brain tumors. The diagnosis of Schizophrenia and depression can be excluded if the patient does not have the other characteristic symptoms for these disorders or if the symptoms only last for brief periods of time followed by longer periods of normalcy.

Although the voice that Gilbert hears is technically an auditory hallucination, it has little content and is not typical of the hallucinations associated with Schizophrenia or a psychotic depression. The possibility of temporal lobe seizures can be excluded by an electroencephalogram (EEG). The possibility of substance abuse should be investigated because several abused drugs may produce symptoms of depersonalization. If all of these possible etiologies are excluded, the most likely diagnosis is Depersonalization Disorder.

Precedence of Diagnosis

Several of the cases in preceding sections discuss diagnostic dilemmas that arise when patients have symptoms consistent with more than one diagnosis. The diagnoses may both be in the same diagnostic group (e.g., Dissociative Disorders) or different groups (e.g., Mood Disorders and Dissociative Disorders). When these conflicts occur, they are often resolved using the rules of diagnostic precedence that are included in the criteria for most diagnoses. These rules are

Table 11–1 Precedence of diagnosis for Dissociative Disorders	
Dissociative Disorder	**Disorders taking precedence**
Dissociative Amnesia	Does not occur exclusively during Dissociative Identity Disorder, Dissociative Fugue, Posttraumatic Stress Disorder, Acute Stress Disorder, Somatization Disorder Not due to effects of a substance or general medical condition
Dissociative Fugue	Does not occur exclusively during Dissociative Identity Disorder Not due to effects of a substance or general medical condition
Dissociative Identity Disorder (Multiple Personality Disorder)	Not due to effects of a substance or general medical condition
Depersonalization Disorder	Does not occur exclusively during another mental disorder Not due to effects of a substance or general medical condition
Dissociative Disorder NOS	Does not meet criteria for any specific Dissociative Disorder
Note. NOS = Not Otherwise Specified.	

summarized in Table 11–1. Each of the diagnoses in the right-hand column should be considered and excluded before a specific Dissociative Disorder diagnosis is made.

Discussion of Clinical Vignette

Sally and Me Make Three

Sally is a 26-year-old woman who is anxious about several unusual personal experiences that she cannot easily explain. These include promiscuous and aggressive behavior that are contrary to her normal personality. She finds her inability to remember how they occurred to be the most disturbing aspect of the episodes. The experiences are further corroborated by the reports of her co-workers and friends who have noticed discrepancies in her behavior.

These distressing events have led her to enter psychiatric treatment for the fourth time. In the therapy sessions Sally displayed sudden shifts or switches between two other, previously hidden, personalities. These personalities display the promiscuous and aggressive behavior consistent with that reported by her co-workers. Each personality has it own distinct set of memories and behaviors. Only one personality, "Hilda the Defender," is aware of the others.

The presence of three distinct personalities that each have their own enduring pattern of perceiving the world excludes the diagnosis of Borderline Personality Disorder. Sally's amnesia is consistent with several Dissociative Disorders. However, neither Dissociative Amnesia nor Dissociative Fugue include the repetitive shifts in identity that Sally displays. Her symptoms are most consistent with Dissociative Identity Disorder (Multiple Personality Disorder).

Key Diagnostic Points

- Dissociative Identity Disorder (Multiple Personality Disorder) is distinguished from Dissociative Amnesia and Dissociative Fugue because the patient has identity shifts that do not occur in the other two disorders.

- Amnesia is a symptom of Dissociative Amnesia, Dissociative Fugue, and Dissociative Identity Disorder (Multiple Personality Disorder) but not Depersonalization Disorder.

Common Questions in Making a Diagnosis

1. Iris is a 27-year-old woman who recently took an unexpected trip with a friend to a city 300 miles from her home. Four days later she was found by the police wandering around the streets. She did not remember her identity, where she was staying, or how she had gotten to the city. Iris was examined in a local hospital emergency room and released when she was not found to have trauma or a physical illness. The police identified the hotel she was staying in from her room key. They called the hotel and spoke with Iris' friend who informed them that Iris had been normal until she disappeared earlier that evening after receiving a telephone call from home informing her that her brother had been killed in an automobile accident. What diagnosis(es), if any, should Iris receive?

Answer: Iris has an episode of amnesia that does not appear to have a physical cause. Her amnesia occurred after an unexpected trip away from home. However she took the trip with her friend and had no memory problems during the initial part of the trip. The lack of amnesia during the trip excludes the diagnosis of Dissociative Fugue. Because Iris' amnesia developed after the telephone call from home informing her of her brother's death, the most likely diagnosis is Dissociative Amnesia.

2. Bruce is a 31-year-old man who complains of feeling detached or separated from his body and mind. The feeling has persisted for several months. During these times he hears a voice telling him that he is evil and should kill himself. The voice continually comments on his behavior. Bruce does not sleep much during these periods. What diagnosis(es), if any, should Bruce receive?

Answer: Bruce is experiencing periods of depersonalization accompanied by detailed auditory hallucinations that keep up a running commentary on his behavior. Depersonalization is a symptom of several psychiatric disorders including Depersonalization Disorder. However, the presence of detailed auditory hallucinations for several months in association with the symptoms of depersonalization are more consistent with a diagnosis of Schizophrenia, Paranoid Type than Depersonalization Disorder.

3. Julie is a 34-year-old woman who experiences brief dreamlike periods when she smacks her lips repeatedly, followed by a brief period of disorganized behavior. These episodes occur two or three times a month. After one recent episode, Julie disappeared and was found sitting in a park in a nearby city the next day. She had no memory of how she got there. What diagnosis(es), if any, should Julie receive?

Answer: Julie has several symptoms of Dissociative Disorder including episodes of dreamlike depersonalization, amnesia, and fugue-like states. However, the dreamlike symptoms are accompanied by automatisms (lip smacking) and followed by a brief period of disorganized behavior. These are classic symptoms of temporal lobe epilepsy that can be evaluated with an EEG. Patients with temporal lobe seizures may develop dissociative symptoms during the interictal periods of the disorder. In these cases, the diagnosis of temporal lobe seizures takes precedence.

4. Gene is a 43-year-old man who was brought to the emergency room by paramedics. They were called to treat the patient, who was found lying unconscious in the alley next to the rooming house where he lived. Gene had a bruise on his head and alcohol in his blood. When he regained consciousness he was unable to remember what had happened to him for several days previous to being found by the paramedics. Several weeks later he still did not remember that period. He had no difficulty remembering who he was and remembering the events that occurred since he awoke. What diagnosis(es), if any, should Gene receive?

Answer: Gene's main symptom is a retrograde amnesia that extends to several days before his discovery by the paramedics. However, he is able to remember who he is and remember new events that occurred after he regained consciousness. His amnesia for the lost period of time continued for several weeks after the event. Patients with Dissociative Amnesia usually have a sudden full recovery from their amnesia. The best diagnosis for Gene is Amnestic Disorder Due to a General Medical Condition.

Sexual and Gender Identity Disorders

Clinical Vignette

I Don't Think I'm a Man

Len is a 27-year-old married student who is studying for his Masters in Business Administration at a competitive local university. Recently, he made an appointment with a psychiatrist at the university health service. In the session, Len was initially very anxious and began talking vaguely about having difficulty with his identity. "I don't feel like I'm myself," he said. He looked down at the floor for a few seconds and then said, "I don't feel like a man. I want to be a woman. I want you to help me become a woman." The psychiatrist asked him to elaborate.

Len reported that he first became aware that something was wrong with him as a young child of age 8 or 9 years. His parents owned a dry cleaning store and laundry. When Len was anxious he would go into the store and look for a piece of woman's silky underwear or a smooth satiny dress. Then he would sit in the corner and rub the material against his face until he felt calm. The silky material reminded him of the blanket ("blanky") that he slept with as a young child.

As he got older he began to have fantasies of being a woman who dressed in the comforting silky material. In early adolescence he masturbated while rubbing women's silky clothes over his body. At the same time he fantasized that he was actually a woman trapped in a man's body. In high school, Len began wearing women's panties under his clothes on days when he didn't have gym or sports in school. The silky feeling of the underwear comforted him. When he felt stressed, he would dress up in a woman's bra, panties, and stockings to masturbate. While he was masturbating, he fantasized that other men found him attractive as a woman. Len felt a strong urge to dress as a woman in public but was afraid that someone he knew would see him. He also felt very guilty about his sexual feelings and tried to suppress them.

Len did not date much in high school or college but managed to have a few sexual experiences. The first was with a girl he went out with briefly in high school. One night the couple started kissing and soon were involved in mutual masturbation. Len enjoyed the experience and discovered that he was very interested in the girl's genitalia. He fantasized about having her vagina and breasts for several weeks after the episode. His second sexual experience occurred in college with Carol, the woman he later married. They engaged in sexual intercourse in his dormitory room. Len enjoyed the experience but found that he preferred to masturbate while wearing women's clothing.

He continued to date Carol and eventually they got married when he graduated from college and started working. She was warm and supportive and Len felt comfortable with her. He never told her about his sexual fantasies or cross-dressing. His need to masturbate while cross-dressing diminished in the first year or two of the marriage. Periodically, when he felt particularly stressed, he would secretly wear a pair of her panties and masturbate.

Len started business school 3 years after he was married. Neither he nor Carol anticipated the stress he would feel from his studies and the competition at school. As his anxiety increased, Len felt a strong urge to dress in women's clothes. He revealed his cross-dressing to his wife and asked if he could wear some of her underwear during sex. She was concerned about his request but finally agreed. During sexual intercourse Len fantasized that he was the woman and Carol was the man.

Len continued in school and the pressure he felt increased. His cross-dressing increased to several times a week even when he was not having sex with his wife. During his most anxious periods, Len began to fantasize about becoming a woman as a way of calming himself. He also started wearing his wife's underwear beneath his clothes during the day. Carol became increasingly distressed with this behavior and declared that she would leave him if he did not get treatment for his problems. Len became extremely anxious in response to her threat and decided that he had to immediately begin treatment to change his sex. He contacted the university health service to see a psychiatrist to begin this process.

Core Concept of the Diagnostic Group

The core concept of the Sexual and Gender Identity Disorders group is difficulty in the expression of normal sexuality. This includes confusion about gender identity, decreased sexual desire or arousal, difficulty having or timing orgasm, pain or discomfort during the sex act, the use of nonhuman objects for sexual arousal, and disturbing sexual acts and fantasies involving the production of suffering or humiliation for either sexual partner or sexual activity with children or nonconsenting adults.

Criteria Applicable to Multiple Disorders

There is one criterion that is applicable to multiple Sexual Disorders and Paraphilia diagnoses: the sexual disturbance or paraphilia causes clinically significant distress or impairment in social, occupational, or other important areas of functioning.

Definitions

cross-dressing Wearing clothes that are normally associated with individuals of the opposite sex. The term is usually applied to men who wear women's undergarments, dresses, blouses, etc.

paraphilia A condition in which an individual has persistent sexually arousing fantasies associated with 1) nonhuman objects, 2) suffering or humiliation of either partner in the sex act, or 3) sexual activity with a nonconsenting sex partner.

Synopses and Diagnostic Prototypes of the Individual Disorders

The brief synopses in this section include the specific requirements or criteria that must be fulfilled for each of the diagnostic categories. Following most of the synopses is a vignette that provides a clinical example of the diagnosis. Each vignette is a prototype in the sense that it represents a typical patient from that specific diagnostic category. The prototypes provide a more lifelike portrayal of the diagnosis than the criteria alone. They also provide a clinical baseline that can be used in the discussion of problems associated with the diagnosis of these disorders and as a standard for comparison, even if they do not exhaust all the possibilities for the clinical presentation of a specific diagnosis.

There are three large categories of Sexual and Gender Identity Disorders: 1) disorders of the physiological or physical process of sexuality including problems with sexual desire, arousal, orgasm, pain, and dysfunction due to a general medical condition or a substance (Sexual Dysfunctions); 2) disorders of the object of sexuality (Paraphilias); and 3) disorders of sexual identity (Gender Identity Disorders).

Sexual Dysfunctions

The following six subtypes apply to all Sexual Dysfunctions and should be recorded with the diagnosis. They specify the etiology, duration, and pervasiveness of the disorder.

Lifelong: The Sexual Dysfunction has been present since the onset of sexual functioning.

Acquired: The Sexual Dysfunction developed after a period of normal functioning.

Generalized: The Sexual Dysfunction is not limited to certain types of stimulation, situations, or partners.

Situational: The Sexual Dysfunction is limited to certain types of stimulation, situations, or partners.

Due to psychological factors: Psychological factors are judged to have the major role in the onset, severity, exacerbation, or maintenance of the Sexual Dysfunction. General medical factors and substances play no role in the etiology of the Sexual Dysfunction.

Due to combined factors: Psychological factors are judged to have a role in the onset, severity, exacerbation, or maintenance of the Sexual Dysfunction. A general medical condition or substance use is judged to be contributory but is not sufficient to account for the Sexual Dysfunction.

Sexual Desire Disorders

302.71   Hypoactive Sexual Desire Disorder.   Patients with this disorder have deficient or absent sexual fantasies and desire for sexual activity.

> Stanley is a 30-year-old man who got married 4 years ago after a 5-year engagement. The couple did not have sexual relations before they were married. Stanley's wife assumed that her husband avoided premarital sex because he had moral convictions similar to hers. On their wedding night she nervously awaited some sign from Stanley that he was interested in sex. Instead, he suggested that they get to sleep early so they could make their plane the next morning. She assumed he was tired and the couple went to sleep.
>
> After several days she finally confronted him about his lack of sexual interest in her. Stanley seemed surprised and said, "I'm sorry. I thought you weren't very interested in sex either." The couple had sex that night but it felt forced and was unsatisfactory. Stanley continued to show little interest in sex. His wife began to buy sexy clothes and perfume, hoping to arouse him. She arranged romantic dinners and rented pornographic videotapes. Her attempts were only marginally successful. Stanley responded halfheartedly and eventually his wife became frustrated and stopped trying to get his attention.

302.79   Sexual Aversion Disorder.   Patients with this disorder have an extreme aversion to, and avoidance of, all (or almost all) genital sexual contact with a sexual partner.

Tiffany is a 24-year-old artist who has been engaged for 2 years. She and her fiancee have dinner together several times a week and often spend the rest of the evening watching television. Tiffany enjoys the relationship except when her fiancee becomes overly passionate. She likes hugging and kissing but feels uncomfortable when they begin to pet. Tiffany tolerates petting until her fiancee tries to slip his hands under her dress and caress her thighs. Then she grabs his hand and gently, but firmly, pushes it away saying, "I told you, I don't like that." He has tried to convince her to touch his genitals several times but she resists and becomes upset.

Once, the couple drank too much wine at dinner and her fiancee got undressed and asked Tiffany to remove her clothes. When she saw him naked, Tiffany looked away and asked him to leave. Her fiancee left, but the next day he confronted her about the incident and asked why she didn't want to have sexual relations with him. Tiffany tried to avoid his questions but finally became upset and said, "It makes me uncomfortable when I see a man naked. I don't get turned on, I feel sick and slightly disgusted. I don't want anyone touching my thighs or vagina."

Sexual Arousal Disorders

302.72 Female Sexual Arousal Disorder. Women with this disorder have an inability to attain or maintain an adequate lubrication-swelling response of sexual excitement until completion of sexual activity.

Joyce is a 23-year-old, attractive actress. Recently she met a young business executive at a party. They danced and talked together most of the evening. She felt an immediate attraction to him. At one point during the party they wandered out onto a dark porch and began kissing. When the party was over he drove her home. Joyce invited him to come up to her apartment for a drink. They talked for a while and then began kissing and fondling each other. When he began unbuttoning her blouse, Joyce stiffened slightly, gently placed her hand over his and said, "Things are moving a little too fast right now. I think we should slow down." He seemed disappointed but agreed. They hugged and kissed a few more times and he left, promising to call her soon.

The next day she met her girlfriend for lunch to talk about the evening. Midway through the meal Joyce was quiet. She appeared to be struggling with her thoughts. Then she blurted out, "I don't get turned on." Her girlfriend was surprised and said, "What do you mean?" Joyce explained that when she became intimate with a man, she found herself getting tense. When they undressed, she found it difficult to become aroused and her vagina stayed dry. When she and the man began having intercourse, it was uncomfortable unless she used a lubricating jelly. Joyce admitted that she was afraid that the man would think that there was something wrong with her or that she didn't like him. This made her more tense and less likely to be aroused.

302.72 Male Erectile Disorder. Men with this disorder are unable to attain or maintain an adequate erection until completion of the sexual activity.

Jordan is a 25-year-old man who made an appointment to see a psychiatrist to talk about some "personal problems." When the meeting began he asked, "Can you help people with . . . intimate problems?" The psychiatrist asked him to describe the problems. Jordan was hesitant but continued, "You know, like sex things. I mean, I have trouble doing it sometimes." The psychiatrist asked if he could be more specific. Jordan looked embarrassed and said, "Sometimes I get soft just before I'm ready to go into the woman. Is that common? Can you fix it?"

He went on to describe his sexual experiences. Jordan explained that he was able to achieve an erection and ejaculate when he masturbated. However, he had a great deal of difficulty maintaining an erection with a woman when they were both naked. Jordan reported one successful experience with intercourse. Four years previously he broke his arm while playing football with his friends. His girlfriend drove him to the hospital and then home after his bone was set in a cast. The emergency physician gave Jordan some diazepam to help him relax that night. When the couple got home, Jordan took one of the diazepam. He soon felt very relaxed. The pain in his arm was dulled by the pain medication from the hospital. As his girlfriend kissed him, he felt aroused and began to caress her. She responded and gently helped him remove his clothes. When they were both nude, Jordan found that he still had an erection. Soon they had successful intercourse. He continued, "That was the only time I had good sex. Every other time I got soft when it was time to do it."

Orgasmic Disorders

302.73   Female Orgasmic Disorder (Inhibited Female Orgasm).   Women with this disorder have delayed or absent orgasms following a normal sexual excitement phase. The orgasm is less than would be reasonable for her age, sexual experience, and the adequacy of sexual stimulation she receives.

Catherine is a 38-year-old woman who is concerned about her relationship with her husband. The couple has been married for 10 years. In the early years of their marriage they had an active and gratifying sex life and mutual orgasms were common. Three years ago Catherine learned that her husband was having an affair with a younger woman in his office. She confronted him, he confessed, and ended the affair. The couple had no intimate relations for several months.

Her husband tried to make up for his indiscretions with thoughtful attention to Catherine's needs. She eventually softened and told him that she forgave him. Soon after the couple had sexual relations for the first time since the affair. Catherine became aroused and they had intercourse. During the intercourse Catherine felt confused. Her husband reached climax and ejaculated after a few minutes but she was unable to achieve an orgasm. Catherine was perplexed but assumed that she was rusty because of the lapse in sexual relations. However, the next few times the couple had sex, the same problem occurred. Catherine began to fake an orgasm to hide her lack of response from her husband. She felt worried that something was wrong with her. She was also aware that she was still angry with her husband and wondered if that had something to do with her problem.

302.74 Male Orgasmic Disorder (Inhibited Male Orgasm). Men with this disorder have delayed or absent orgasms following a normal sexual excitement phase that appears to be adequate in focus, intensity, and duration.

Glenn is 42-year-old man who is concerned about his sexual functioning with his wife. The couple have been married for several years. Glenn's wife has been willing but rarely eager to have sex. In the last few years she has been busy with the children and they have had sex less frequently than Glenn would like. Recently he began having an unusual problem. He describes it this way, "I get an erection and get inside her and she just lies there and doesn't move. I start to think about some of the women in my office. I keep pumping away but I can't come. Sometimes, if I keep on going, I do come, but it takes a long time." Glenn is perplexed and worried about his problem. He wonders if it means that he is getting impotent.

302.75 Premature Ejaculation. Men with this disorder ejaculate with minimal sexual stimulation before, upon, or shortly after penetration and before they wish to ejaculate. Factors such as age, duration of sexual excitement, novelty of the sexual partner or situation, and frequency of sexual activity should be taken into account in the assessment.

Conrad is a 21-year-old college student and star athlete who made an appointment to see someone at the university mental health clinic. He specifically requested to see a male therapist. When the session began Conrad broke into tears and said, "I feel so embarrassed. I know there's something wrong with me." The therapist was empathic and asked him to elaborate. Conrad looked up and continued, "Every time I have sex with a woman I get so excited that I ejaculate before I get into her. Most of the women are kind and tell me it's OK, but I feel like I want to run away and hide."

Conrad explained that the women are usually casual acquaintances and he never goes out with them again after he has failed in an attempt to have sex. He feels pressured by the talk of sex in the locker room. All of his friends discuss their sexual conquests. He spends much of his free time trying to meet new women and have sex, hoping that he can control himself better and have successful intercourse. Finally, he became convinced that there was something terribly wrong with him. He revealed his secret to the coach who suggested he seek treatment.

Sexual Pain Disorders

302.76 Dyspareunia (Not Due to a General Medical Condition). Men or women with this disorder have persistent genital pain before, during, or after sexual intercourse.

Sandy is a 36-year-old woman who is an industrial designer and who has been married for 8 years to an electrician. The couple have no children and have slowly been growing apart. Her husband has become very jealous despite or because of their growing antipathy. They have not had sex in several months. Sandy has confided her marital problems to her boss who is very sympathetic. The two often have to work late on rush projects. Sandy enjoys the projects because she is attracted to her boss and they get along well together.

A month ago Sandy and her boss had dinner together while working on the design for a new shopping mall. During dinner they had a couple of drinks. When they returned to his office, Sandy turned and found him looking directly at her. She began blushing and he kissed her gently. She liked kissing him and felt aroused. Soon they were lying on his couch with their clothes off. Sandy wanted to have sex but felt confused. She was attracted to her boss but afraid of her husband. She felt tense and ambivalent. When her boss caressed her, she felt the muscles in her pelvis and vagina tighten. She couldn't relax. They began to have intercourse but Sandy found it painful and asked him to stop. He complied and the couple slowly sat up and got dressed without looking at each other. Sandy's boss admitted that he had become very attracted to her and depended on her advice in their work. Sandy smiled, feeling flattered, and said she needed some time to think about what was happening between them.

306.51   Vaginismus (Not Due to a General Medical Condition).   Women with this disorder have recurrent or persistent involuntary spasm of the musculature of the outer third of the vagina that interferes with sexual intercourse.

Cindy is a 27-year-old single woman who owns a small dress shop. One evening as she was preparing to close, a man forced his way into the store and raped her. After he left, she called a friend and the police who took her to the hospital. She was treated and released. Cindy filed a report with the police but was unable to identify her assailant. She did not date for several months following the rape. The thought of being touched by a man made her shudder. Gradually, her negative feelings toward men subsided and she began dating.

Approximately 2 years after the rape she met Jeff. He was kind and empathic. They dated for several months, becoming more and more intimate. One night they returned to his apartment after a late movie. Jeff asked her to stay the night with him. She hesitantly agreed. When they took their clothes off and got into bed, Jeff began gently caressing her. Cindy was anxious and felt her muscles tense despite his gentleness. When they tried to have intercourse the muscles in her vagina went into spasm and he was unable to enter her. After a while they stopped trying to make love and Jeff reassured her. She began crying and told him about the rape. Over the next few weeks they tried have sex several times but each time Cindy's muscles went into spasm as they were about to have intercourse.

Sexual Dysfunction Due to a General Medical Condition

Individuals with this disorder have a clinically significant Sexual Dysfunction. There is evidence from the history, physical examination, or laboratory findings of a general medical condition judged to be etiologically related to the Sexual Dysfunction.

607.84 Male Erectile Disorder Due to . . . *[Indicate the General Medical Condition].*

608.89 Male Dyspareunia Due to . . . *[Indicate the General Medical Condition].*

Male Hypoactive Sexual Desire Disorder Due to . . . *[Indicate the General Medical Condition].*

Other Male Sexual Dysfunction Due to a General Medical Condition.

625.0 Female Dyspareunia Due to . . . *[Indicate the General Medical Condition].*

625.8 Female Hypoactive Sexual Desire Disorder Due to . . . *[Indicate the General Medical Condition].*

Other Female Sexual Dysfunction Due to . . . *[Indicate the General Medical Condition].*

> Leonard is a 55-year-old married man who recently had major surgery for prostate cancer. The cancer was caught before it spread and the doctors pronounced him cured. Before the operation they informed him of the possible adverse side effects of the surgery. The most distressing side effect was impotence caused by severing the nerves that controlled erections. Leonard felt he had no choice but to have the operation. Following the surgery he was not interested in sex for several weeks. Finally, one night 3 months later, he cautiously tried to arouse himself by masturbating. He was unable to achieve an erection. Disappointed and depressed, he telephoned his physician the next day for an appointment. The diagnosis is Male Erectile Disorder Due to Prostate Surgery (607.84)

Substance-Induced Sexual Dysfunction

Individuals with this disorder have a clinically significant Sexual Dysfunction associated with evidence from a history, physical examination, or laboratory findings that the symptoms developed within 1 month of significant substance intoxication or withdrawal, or are etiologically related to medication use or toxin exposure.

The specific codes for Substance-Induced Sexual Dysfunction are determined by the specific substance: 291.8 alcohol; 292.89 amphetamines; cocaine; opioids; sedatives, hypnotics, anxiolytics; other (or unknown) substances.

Clarence is a 27-year-old man who has been taking 500 mg of chlorpromazine a day for treatment of psychosis. Four years ago he had an acute psychotic episode that met the criteria for Brief Psychotic Disorder. The psychosis resolved in 3 weeks with medication treatment. Five months ago he had a recurrence of psychotic symptoms that responded to treatment with an increased dose of medication.

Two months after the latest psychotic episode he returned to his job as a mail sorter in the post office. Clarence sees his psychiatrist every 2 months for a medication review. At the last appointment he began complaining of sexual difficulties. He describes the problem with some emotion, "When I have sex with my girlfriend, I can't let go. You know what I mean Doc. I can't come no matter how long we go at it." The psychiatrist suspects that Clarence's problem ejaculating is due to the increased chlorpromazine, but she is reluctant to lower the dose for fear that he will have another psychotic episode. The diagnosis is Phenothiazine-Induced Sexual Dysfunction (292.89)

302.70   Sexual Dysfunction Not Otherwise Specified.   Individuals with this diagnosis have Sexual Dysfunctions that do not meet criteria for any specific Sexual Dysfunction.

Paraphilias

302.4   Exhibitionism.   Individuals with this diagnosis have a 6-month history of recurrent, intense, sexual urges and sexually arousing fantasies involving exposure of their genitals to unsuspecting strangers.

Terry is a 36-year-old married man who works as a bartender in a discotheque. Recently he was arrested on a sexual perversion charge for exposing himself. The event leading to the arrest occurred late one afternoon when Terry felt an overpowering urge to expose his genitals to an unsuspecting woman. He drove around the suburbs of a nearby city until he saw a woman walking alone down the street. Terry drove past her and parked his car around the block. He took off his pants and underwear, put on a long raincoat, got out of his car and slowly walked around the corner toward the woman. When he was 6–7 feet away from her, he yelled "Look" and opened his raincoat to reveal his genitals.

The woman stopped and appeared mildly surprised and perplexed. She looked at his genitals, shrugged, and then looked him in the face and said, "Is this some kind of political statement, or something, fella?" Terry was startled by her response. Before he could say anything or turn and run she yelled, "Henry, get this jerk out of here." A man raced off the porch of a nearby house and began chasing Terry down the street. He was caught before he could get to his car and the police arrested him. Later, Terry admitted to his lawyer that he had felt the urge to expose himself many times before and could no longer control it.

302.81   Fetishism.   Individuals with this diagnosis have a 6-month history of recurrent, intense, sexually arousing fantasies, sexual urges, or behaviors involving the use of nonliving objects.

> Barry is a 33-year-old married man who is experiencing some marital discord about his sexual needs. He has been intensely sexually aroused by women's nylon stockings for many years. As an adolescent he stole stockings from neighborhood women when they were hung out to dry on the clothesline. When he was in college, he stole stockings from the laundromat. He used the stockings to masturbate. When he got married he convinced his wife to wear nylons to bed before they had sex. Initially she complied. Eventually she began protesting saying, "You're more turned on by the stockings than by me." She refused to wear nylons several times to prove her point. Barry found it difficult to get fully aroused without the stockings.

302.89   Frotteurism.   Individuals with this diagnosis have a 6-month history of recurrent, intense, sexually arousing fantasies, sexual urges, or behaviors involving touching and rubbing against a nonconsenting person. It is the touching, not the coercive nature of the act, that is sexually exciting.

> Zack is a 24-year-old single man who is isolated and lonely. He works the evening shift as a clerk at a small bookstore. Zack's active sexual fantasy life belies his bland exterior appearance. However, he is too shy to meet and establish a relationship with a woman.
>
> Zack's only sexual outlet occurs on crowded subways and buses where he rubs his penis against the bodies of unsuspecting women. Initially they are unaware of his physical attentions. After a few seconds they seem puzzled and turn around to see Zack standing behind them reading a magazine. Most women are too embarrassed to say anything and try to move away from Zack. When this happens he switches his attentions to another woman. He is careful about making the contact seem accidental and stops when a woman seems angry. Occasionally he has been slapped or hit by one of his victims. When this occurs, he looks innocent and gets off the vehicle.

302.2   Pedophilia.   Individuals with this disorder have a 6-month history of recurrent, intense, sexually arousing fantasies, sexual urges, or behaviors involving sexual activity with a prepubescent child or children. Specify: 1) if sexually attracted to *males, females* or *both;* 2) if *limited to incest;* 3) if *exclusive* (attracted only to children, or *nonexclusive* type.

> Ian is a 26-year-old man who works as a children's clothing salesman in a large department store. He and his wife also run a short-term foster care home for young children. The court assigns children to the couple for a few months at a time, pending the child's adoption or final placement.
>
> Ian is particularly fatherly to the young boys, playing baseball with them and

taking them swimming. He often helps them get undressed for swimming, caressing their genitals as he removes their underwear. Ian is more direct with the older boys. He tells them to take off their clothes so he can examine their pubic hair for lice. If they protest, he threatens to tell the judge that they were caught stealing money and lying. "No one will ever want to adopt you if I say you steal," he tells them. The boys usually comply.

302.83   Sexual Masochism.   Individuals with this disorder have a 6-month history of recurrent, intense, sexually arousing fantasies, sexual urges, or behaviors involving the act (real, not simulated) of being humiliated, beaten, bound, or otherwise made to suffer.

> Grace is an attractive 27-year-old woman who works in an art supply store. She is friendly with Steve, one of her male co-workers, and has dated him a few times. One night, when he had driven her home after work, she invited him in for something to eat. As she was preparing the food, he massaged her neck.
>
> Suddenly she turned and kissed him on the lips. They walked into the living room, lay down on the couch, and began kissing and pressing against each other. Grace did not get aroused. She whispered to Steve, "Tie my hands together." He stopped, looked at her and said, "What do you mean tie your hands?" Grace replied, "It turns me on." She handed him a scarf and Steve began tying her hands together. Grace began to feel more aroused and pulled Steve closer. He seemed uncertain and a little confused.

302.84   Sexual Sadism.   Individuals with this disorder have a 6-month history of recurrent, intense, sexually arousing fantasies, sexual urges, or behaviors involving acts (real, not simulated) in which the psychological or physical suffering (including humiliation) of the victim is sexually exciting to the person.

> Gregory is a 32-year-old engineer who has difficulty maintaining a long-term relationship with a woman. In casual meetings he is very charming and women find him attractive. When a woman dates him Gregory is different. He begins with subtle critical comments about her clothes and makeup. Then he criticizes her ideas. Most women stop dating him at this point. A few continue to date him. The more they tolerate his critical and disparaging behavior, the more he escalates it.
>
> Some of the relationships proceed to sexual involvements. Most of the women who begin a sexual relationship with Gregory find it intolerable. He begins by making little negative comments about their appearance. When they are undressed and in bed together, he humiliates them until they are in tears. When this happens, he becomes aroused and proceeds with sexual intercourse. Few women sleep with him again after one experience.

302.82   Voyeurism.   Individuals with this disorder have a 6-month history of recurrent, intense, sexually arousing fantasies, sexual urges, or behaviors involving the act of observing an unsuspecting person who is naked, in the process of disrobing, or engaged in sexual activity.

> Dustin is a 41-year-old single man who was recently arrested for trespassing. He was discovered hiding in the bushes outside an apartment building with binoculars and a camera with a telephoto lens. When the film was developed, it contained pictures of a nude woman who lived on the fifth floor of the building. The photographs were taken through her bedroom window.
>
> Dustin's attorney asked him to see a psychiatrist before the trial. During the interview, Dustin admitted that he commonly drove through various neighborhoods looking for women who undressed in front of an open window. When possible, he masturbated while he was watching. If that was difficult, he developed the pictures at home and masturbated while looking at them.

302.3 Transvestic Fetishism. Heterosexual men with this disorder have a 6-month history of recurrent, intense, sexually arousing fantasies, sexual urges, or behaviors involving cross-dressing.

> Curtis is a 29-year-old married contractor who has a secret. When he goes to work each morning he wears a pair of women's panties. He began cross-dressing as a young boy when he would sneak into his older sister's room and put on her panties or bra. Eventually, he stole some women's underwear from the girls locker room at school. He wore the panties while he masturbated. When Curtis left home and went to college he began wearing women's panties under his clothes every day and continued to use them to masturbate.
>
> He dated infrequently in college until he met Sally. She was kind and he enjoyed being with her. Curtis had his first sexual experience with a woman when he and Sally had sex one night during his junior year. As their relationship progressed, Curtis felt he could no longer hide his secret from her. One night he told Sally that he wore women's panties under his clothes. She seemed confused about why he needed to wear the panties, but was not very upset about the fact that he wore them. Tentatively, Curtis asked her if she would be willing to let him wear the panties while they were having sex. Sally nodded and said, "I guess so, if that makes you happy." A year later they were married. During the first few years of their marriage Curtis continued to wear panties during sex. His wife periodically went shopping and brought home new panties for him as the old ones wore out.

302.9 Paraphilia Not Otherwise Specified. Individuals with this disorder have a paraphilia that does not meet the criteria for any of the specific Paraphilias.

> Stella is a 28-year-old woman who saw a psychiatrist to seek advice about her relationship with her husband. She seemed embarrassed during the interview and had difficulty beginning to talk. After several minutes she took a deep breath and started, "My husband is a good person. He loves me. But, ah . . . um, he has this

unusual sexual need that I find upsetting." Stella looked closely at the psychiatrist's face for some indication of whether to proceed. "Go on," he said.

Stella looked down and continued, "He . . . he always wants me to have a bowel movement in the bed before sex or he wants to put a finger in my butt and feel the feces. He says he can't get turned on unless he feels my shit. I know that isn't normal and it disgusts me, but I love him and don't know what to do." She looked up at the physician's face again for some reaction. "Does he know how you feel about this," the psychiatrist asked. Stella nodded, "He says he can't stop." The diagnosis is Coprophilia

302.9   Sexual Disorder Not Otherwise Specified.   Individuals with this disorder have a sexual disturbance that does not meet the criteria for any specific Sexual Disorder and is neither a dysfunction nor a paraphilia.

Gender Identity Disorders

302.6   Gender Identity Disorder in Children.   Children with this disorder have a strong and persistent cross-gender identification that is not concurrent with a physical intersexual condition and is manifested by at least four of the following:

1. Repeated stated desire to be, or insistence that he or she is, the other sex.
2. In boys, preference for cross-dressing or simulating female attire; in girls, insistence on wearing only stereotypical masculine clothing.
3. Strong and persistent preferences for cross-sex roles in make-believe play or persistent fantasies of being the other sex.
4. Intense desire to participate in the stereotypical games and pastimes of the other sex.
5. Strong preference for playmates of the other sex.

The children also have a persistent discomfort with their own sex or a sense of inappropriateness in the gender role of that sex manifested by any one of the following:

1. In boys: an assertion that his penis and testes are disgusting and will disappear or that it would be better off not to have a penis.
2. In boys: an aversion toward rough-and-tumble play and a rejection of male stereotypical toys, games, and activities.
3. In girls: rejection of urinating in a sitting position.
4. In girls: an assertion that she does not want to grow breasts or menstruate, or will grow a penis.
5. In girls: a marked aversion towards normative feminine clothing.

Cindy is a 9-year-old girl who is known as the neighborhood tomboy. Her mother reports that she has always been different than her sister. When Cindy was age 5 years she walked into the bathroom one day when her older brother was urinating. She watched him for a few seconds before he noticed she was there and chased her out. Later that day she said to her mother, "Danny stands up to pee. Why can't I stand up?" She tried to stand and urinate in front of the toilet but when the urine persistently ran down her legs, she gave up and told her mother, "It's not fair that I have to sit down."

Cindy continued to be intrigued with the activities of her brother and his friends. She refused to play with dolls and insisted that her parents buy her toy soldiers, trucks, and a football. She spent her time playing with the neighborhood boys, explaining that girls' games were "silly." Cindy would not wear girls' clothes. Instead, she wore jeans and her brother's hand-me-down shirts.

302.85   Gender Identity Disorder in Adolescents or Adults.   Adolescents or adults with this disorder have a strong and persistent cross-gender identification that is not concurrent with a physical intersexual condition and is manifested by symptoms such as a stated desire to be the other sex, frequent passing as the other sex, a desire to live or be treated as the other sex, or the conviction that one has the typical feelings and reactions of the other sex. They also have a persistent discomfort with their own sex or a sense of inappropriateness in the gender role of that sex, manifested by symptoms such as a preoccupation with getting rid of one's primary and secondary sex characteristics or a belief that they were born the wrong sex. (Specify if sexually attracted to *males, females, both,* or *neither.*)

Roy is a 28-year-old man who dresses as a woman and makes a living dancing in a bar as a drag queen. As child he remembers preferring to play with girls. In games he often played the role of a girl, the nurse helping the male doctor, or the female patient being examined by the doctor.

As he grew older, he began secretly dressing in women's clothing and imagining himself a woman. He would often push his penis and testicles out of the way between his legs and masturbate by rubbing his perineal area while fantasizing that he was a woman having sex with a man. Roy found himself sexually attracted to both men and women and had sexual relations with both, although he always fantasized he was a woman during the sexual encounter. When he had sex with women, he imagined that he was having a lesbian relationship. With men he fantasized that he was the female partner. Neither type of sexual relationship was entirely satisfactory because he could not completely think of himself as a woman during the encounters. He began to think about changing his sex so he would no longer be "living a lie." After high school, Roy got a job as a bartender in a homosexual bar. He continued his cross-dressing and preoccupations with secretly being a woman. One day the bar announced a cross-dressing contest. Roy decided to enter the contest and went shopping with a friend to buy women's clothes. He practiced walking like a woman and learned how to apply makeup. Roy won second prize in the contest.

He enjoyed the experience so much that he began to develop a persona as a cross-dressing female singer. He continued to contemplate changing his sex.

302.6   Gender Identity Disorder Not Otherwise Specified.   Individuals with this disorder have a problem in gender identity that is not classifiable as a specific Gender Identity Disorder.

Necessary Clinical Information

- History of cross-dressing
- Current preferences for sexual partner (e.g., age, sex)
- Current sexual desire
- Problems with arousal
- Problems with orgasm
- Pain associated with sex
- Current and past sexual fantasies
- Use of objects associated with the opposite sex for arousal
- Gender identity
- Unusual sexual activity (e.g., voyeurism, frotteurism)
- Coercion or humiliation in the sexual act

Making a Diagnosis

Sexuality is an important part of the life of every individual. This includes the performance of sexual acts as well as the development of sexual identity. There are three large categories of Sexual Disorders: Sexual Dysfunctions, Paraphilias, and Gender Identity Disorders. The Sexual Dysfunctions include disorders of the normal sexual cycle outlined below. The Paraphilias include disorders of the object of sexual expression. The Gender Identity Disorders are characterized by the patient's strong identification with the opposite sex and the stated preference or actual attempt to change sexual identity.

The normal sexual cycle includes four phases: appetitive, excitement, orgasm, and resolution.

1. *Appetitive:* This phase includes sexual fantasies and the desire for sexual activity.

2. *Excitement:* This phase includes feelings of sexual arousal and pleasure accompanied by specific physiological changes. Males develop an erect penis and females develop vasocongestion in the pelvis, vaginal lubrication, and swelling of the external genitalia.
3. *Orgasm:* In this phase, sexual pleasure reaches a peak, followed by a sudden release of tension, accompanied by a rhythmic contraction of the perineal muscles. In the male there is an ejaculation of semen and in females there are contractions in the wall of the vagina. Orgasm is usually accompanied by rhythmic pelvic thrusting.
4. *Resolution:* This phase includes a sense of relaxation and well-being during which the male is refractory to further erection and orgasm but the female may respond to stimulation with additional orgasms.

In Sexual Dysfunctions, problems may occur in any of the four phases of the normal sexual cycle. In Paraphilias the problem is defined by the nature of the object or situation that is the focus of desire and arousal in the first two phases of the sexual cycle. Gender Identity Disorders relate more to the individual's sexual identity and role in society than to the sexual cycle. The process of making a diagnosis of Sexual Disorder is generally straightforward and starts with the identification of the category(ies) that best describe the patient's sexual problem. The following sequence of questions provides an organized approach to the diagnosis of Sexual Disorders.

1. What is the patient's main sexual complaint?

Patients have three types of sexual complaints: 1) they have a problem functioning in a normal sexual interaction with another person, 2) they have unacceptable sexual urges that are distressing and that they may have acted on, or 3) they feel they are the wrong sex. In some cases society identifies the sexual act as unacceptable (e.g., Pedophilia, Voyeurism), but the patient is not disturbed by it and has no clinical complaint.

2. Does the patient have an Axis I disorder (other than Sexual Dysfunction) that commonly includes symptoms of sexual impairment?

Sexual problems may occur in the course of another psychiatric disorder (other than Sexual Dysfunction). For example, patients with Major Depressive Disorder, Single Episode, often have decreased sexual desire. Individuals who have Obsessive-Compulsive Disorder may have anxious, obsessive thoughts and compulsive acts associated with sexual activity that interfere with sexual functioning. Under these circumstances, the patient should not receive a diagnosis

of Sexual Dysfunction unless there is clear evidence that the sexual problems
began before the onset of the other psychiatric disorder.

3. Does the patient have a general medical condition that could produce Sexual Dysfunction?

Several general medical conditions may produce problems in sexual functioning. For example, men with chronic renal failure, diabetes mellitus, multiple
sclerosis, or other disorders may be impotent. Patients with chronic pain disorders may find it difficult to have comfortable sex because of their physical disorder, and subsequently lose the desire for sexual activity.

Women with diabetes mellitus, hypothyroidism, or other disorders may have
difficulty achieving an orgasm. These patients should receive a diagnosis of one
of the specific Sexual Dysfunctions Due to a General Medical Condition (e.g.,
Male Erectile Disorder Due to a General Medical Condition 607.84, Female
Hypoactive Sexual Disorder Due to a General Medical Condition 625.8), unless
there is clear evidence that the sexual problems began before the onset of the
general medical disorder.

4. Is the patient abusing a substance that could produce Sexual Dysfunction?

Many abused drugs produce problems with sexual functioning during intoxication (e.g., alcohol, amphetamines, cocaine, opioids, and sedatives). The problem may be a decrease in sexual desire, impotence, or difficulty achieving
orgasm. These patients should receive a diagnosis of one of the specific Substance-Induced Sexual Dysfunctions (e.g., Alcohol Sexual Dysfunction 291.8,
Cocaine Sexual Dysfunction 292.89), unless there is clear evidence that the sexual problems occur when the individual is not abusing a substance.

5. Does the patient have difficulty performing a warm, tender, and affectionate sexual act with a mutually consenting person.

Individuals with Sexual Dysfunction have difficulty participating in a warm,
tender, and affectionate sexual act with another consenting person. The problem
lies in one or more of the first three phases of the sexual cycle: appetitive, excitement, and orgasm. Individuals who are only able to perform in these three
phases of the sexual cycle when they are in pain (masochism) or when they
cause pain for another (sadism) are not included in this category of Sexual Disorders.

6. Does the patient have decreased or absent sexual desire?

- If the patient has a persistent or recurrent decrease or absence of sexual desire and fantasies, consider the diagnosis of Hypoactive Sexual Desire Disorder. Patients with this disorder have a disinterest but not a distaste for sexual contact.

- If the patient has an aversion to genital sexual contact, consider the diagnosis of Sexual Aversion Disorder. These patients have a dislike or distaste for genital sexual contact that may have been caused by previous sexual trauma, recurrent painful sexual intercourse, or a sense of shame or guilt associated with the sexual act.

7. Does the patient have difficulty becoming sexually aroused?

- If the patient is a woman who has persistent or recurrent difficulty attaining or maintaining an adequate vaginal lubrication and swelling response of sexual excitement, consider a diagnosis of Female Sexual Arousal Disorder.

- If the patient is a man who has persistent or recurrent difficulty attaining or maintaining an adequate erection until sexual activity is completed, consider the diagnosis of Male Erectile Disorder.

8. Does the patient have difficulty achieving an orgasm?

- If the patient is a woman who has a persistent delay in, or absence of, orgasm following normal sexual excitement, consider the diagnosis of Female Orgasmic Disorder.

- If the patient is a male who has a persistent or recurrent delay in, or absence of, orgasm following normal sexual excitement, consider the diagnosis of Male Orgasmic Disorder. If the patient has persistent or recurrent ejaculation with minimal sexual stimulation before, on, or shortly after penetration and before the patient wishes it, consider the diagnosis of Premature Ejaculation.

9. Does the patient experience pain during sexual intercourse?

- If the patient is a male or female who has recurrent or persistent genital pain before, during, or after sexual intercourse, consider the diagnosis of Dyspareunia.

- If a woman has recurrent or persistent genital pain before, during, or after sexual intercourse that is due to an involuntary spasm of the musculature of the outer third of the vagina, consider the diagnosis of Vaginismus.

10. Does the patient experience recurrent and intense sexual urges or fantasies involving nonhuman objects (fetishes)?

- If the patient is disturbed by or has acted on recurrent intense sexual urges and sexually arousing fantasies that involve the use of nonliving objects, consider the diagnosis of Fetishism. The most common fetish is an article of women's clothing. The patient typically holds, rubs, or smells the object while masturbating or has his partner wear the object during intercourse. Sexual arousal is dependent on the fetish object.

- If the patient is disturbed by or has acted on recurrent intense sexual urges and sexually arousing fantasies that involve wearing an item of women's clothing and masturbating while imagining that other men are attracted to him as a woman, consider the diagnosis of Transvestic Fetishism.

11. Does the patient experience recurrent, intense, and disturbing sexual urges or fantasies that involve hurting another person or violating their rights in a sexual act?

- If the patient's urges and fantasies are of exposing his or her genitals to an unsuspecting stranger, consider the diagnosis of Exhibitionism.

- If the patient's urges and fantasies are of touching and rubbing against a non-consenting person, consider the diagnosis of Frotteurism.

- If the patient's urges and fantasies involve sexual activity with a child, consider the diagnosis of Pedophilia.

- If the patient's urges and fantasies are of the psychological or physical suffering of another person that is sexually exciting, consider the diagnosis of Sexual Sadism.

- If the patient's urges and fantasies are of observing an unsuspecting person who is naked, disrobing, or engaged in sexual activity, consider the diagnosis of Voyeurism.

12. Does the patient have recurrent, intense sexual urges or fantasies that involve being made to suffer during the sexual act?

- If the patient is disturbed by or has acted on recurrent intense sexual urges and sexually arousing fantasies involving the act of being humiliated, beaten, bound, or otherwise made to suffer, consider the diagnosis of Sexual Masochism.

13. Does the patient have a strong identification with the opposite sex and persistent discomfort with his or her own sex?

- If the patient is a child who has a repeated desire to be the other sex, wear the clothes of the other sex, participate in activities as the other sex, and have playmates of the other sex, associated with a discomfort about his or her own sex, consider the diagnosis of Gender Identity Disorder in Childhood.

- If the patient is an adult or adolescent who has a repeated desire to be the other sex or to live or be treated as the other sex, associated with discomfort about his or her own sex and a conviction that he or she has the feelings and reactions of the other sex, consider the diagnosis of Gender Identity Disorder in Adolescence or Adult.

Common Problems in Making a Diagnosis

There are three main areas of uncertainty in the differential diagnosis of Sexual Disorders.

1. Some patient's symptoms initially come close but don't actually fulfill the criteria for a specific Sexual Disorder diagnosis. More information or a further consideration of the diagnostic criteria may or may not resolve the problem.
2. Some patient's symptoms fulfill the diagnostic criteria for more than one Sexual Disorder during the course of their illness.
3. Some patients have symptoms of sexual dysfunction associated with other psychiatric disorders but do not fulfill the criteria for a specific Sexual Disorder.

Patients Who Almost Fulfill the Diagnostic Criteria

Most adults have experienced a problem with sexual function at some time in their life. For example, a man may have temporary difficulty achieving an erection or a woman may not develop adequate lubrication for intercourse, or experience an orgasm. Similarly, many men have had the experience of becoming sexually aroused by seeing or feeling a women's underwear or seeing an unsuspecting woman remove her clothes. The major diagnostic question is, when are these responses and behaviors a part of the normal biological variation of sexuality, and when are they a sign of psychiatric illness.

As usual, the difficult diagnostic decisions involve patients who fall into the borderline area between normal and abnormal behavior. This uncertainty is more a problem in the diagnosis of the Sexual Dysfunctions than the Paraphilias or Gender Identity Disorders. The former leaves the determination of whether the patient experiences normal sexual desire or sexual orgasm to the judgment of the clinician. The range of normal for these sexual responses is very wide and depends on many unspecified factors, which may be judged differently by different clinicians.

Example 1

Ruth is a 33-year-old woman who has been married for 8 years. Every once in a while she experiences a 2- to 3-week interval during which she is unable to be sexually aroused and does not develop adequate vaginal lubrication to permit comfortable sexual intercourse. At other times she is sexually responsive and has enjoyable sexual intercourse with her husband, culminating in mutual orgasm. Ruth is frustrated and upset during the intervals when she cannot be aroused. What diagnosis(es), if any, should Ruth receive?

Ruth has a recurrent inability to become sexually aroused. This fulfills the letter of the criteria for Female Sexual Arousal Disorder. However, it is appropriate to ask whether these brief periods of dysfunction constitute a Sexual Disorder or merely a normal variation in human sexual response. This question is valid despite Ruth's frustration and distress because her expectations for her sexual response may be inappropriately high. The possibility that this is a normal variation in sexual response should not preclude further etiological investigations.

Example 2

Doug is a 32-year-old man who insists that his wife wear brief silk panties when they have sex. He caresses her genitals through the panties during foreplay. When they are both aroused, he takes her panties off and they have intercourse. Doug does not enjoy sex as much when his wife does not wear panties.

He has never masturbated using women's panties, but they do play an important role in his fantasies about sexual encounters with other women. Neither Doug nor his wife are particularly distressed by his demands, although his wife wishes he would be a little more flexible during lovemaking. What diagnosis(es), if any, should Doug receive?

The main diagnostic question is whether the panties are a sexual fetish. The focus of Doug's sexual interest is intercourse with his wife. The panties enhance the pleasure of the sexual experience but are not, by themselves, the object of the sexual activity. In this context they are not a typical fetish. Furthermore, neither Doug nor his wife are upset by using the panties during sex. Therefore, Doug does not fulfill the criteria for the diagnosis of Fetishism.

Example 3

Ned is a 34-year-old divorced man who has had affairs with several women. When he initially has sex with a new partner Ned becomes so sexually excited that he ejaculates a few seconds after penetration. If he continues the relationship, he is able to perform adequately, with prolonged intercourse, after two or three sexual encounters with the woman. Despite this, he is embarrassed by his brief lack of control. What diagnosis(es), if any, should Ned receive?

Ned ejaculates prematurely the first two or three times he has sex with a new woman. Subsequently, he has normal sexual intercourse. Because this is a recurrent problem, it technically fits the criteria for Premature Ejaculation. However, the use of this diagnosis should be tempered by consideration of several factors that commonly influence sexual performance. In this case the important factor is the repeated novelty of the sex partner. Because Ned has normally prolonged intercourse after the novelty wears off, it would not be appropriate to give him a diagnosis of Premature Ejaculation. The problem would not have become so apparent if Ned had not had multiple sexual partners.

Patients Who Fulfill the Diagnostic Criteria for More Than One Sexual Disorder

The individual diagnoses in the Sexual Disorders group are not mutually exclusive unless rendered obviously so by their content or target population. For example, individuals who are sadistic in their sexual activity are not usually masochistic. Certain Sexual Disorders apply to men (e.g., Premature Ejaculation) and others apply to women (e.g., Vaginismus). These exceptions aside, two or more Sexual Disorders may occur in the same patient concurrently or sequentially. For example, an individual with Pedophilia may also fulfill the criteria for Exhibitionism.

Example 4

Stewart is a 33-year-old man who works as a clerk in a supermarket. He has little interest in establishing an ongoing sexual relationship with a woman. His few mutually consenting sexual experiences have been with prostitutes. However, for several years he has used several other methods of achieving sexual release.

Stewart travels to and from work on a crowded subway. Once or twice a week he slips a condom on his penis while dressing. When he gets to the subway station he searches for a woman with large buttocks and maneuvers behind her. While they wait for the train, Stewart becomes sexually excited by fantasizing a relationship with the woman. When the train arrives and the crowd pushes toward the open door, he presses his erect penis against the woman through his clothes. Once on the subway car he continues to rub against her until he ejaculates. In the evenings, Stewart searches for women undressing in front of their windows in nearby high-rise apartments and masturbates while he watches them through a telescope from his apartment. What diagnosis(es), if any, should Stewart receive?

Stewart's symptoms fulfill the criteria for both Frotteurism and Voyeurism. Because these diagnoses are not mutually exclusive and neither takes diagnostic precedence over the other, he should receive both diagnoses.

Example 5

Patrick is age 25 years. For many years, since adolescence, he has dressed in women's clothes while masturbating. During these episodes he imagined that men were attracted to him as a woman. He had one sexual relationship with a woman who allowed him to dress in her clothing during intercourse.
   Gradually, Patrick began to fantasize about permanently dressing and living as a woman. He was convinced that he would be happier if he became a woman and investigated various hormonal and surgical methods of changing his primary and secondary sexual characteristics. What diagnosis(es), if any, should Patrick receive?

Patrick initially used cross-dressing for sexual stimulation and thereby fulfilled the criteria for Transvestic Fetishism. Later he became convinced that he should dress and live as a woman. Finally he became preoccupied with physically changing his body to acquire a woman's physical characteristics. These symptoms fulfill the criteria for the diagnosis of Adolescent or Adult Gender Identity Disorder. In this case, the Gender Identity Disorder may be concurrent with or succeed the diagnosis of Transvestic Fetishism.

Sexual Symptoms Associated With Other Psychiatric Disorders

Sexual Disorders may appear in conjunction with other nonsexual psychiatric disorders. For example, Dyspareunia and Vaginismus may be better accounted for by Somatization Disorder. The Sexual Disorder diagnosis can also be given if the sexual problem preceded Somatization Disorder. Women with a diagnosis of Histrionic Personality Disorder may appear sexually provocative but actually have Female Orgasmic Disorder (Inhibited Female Orgasm). Similarly, patients with a diagnosis of Schizoid Personality Disorder may have concomitant Hypoactive Sexual Desire Disorder. In each case, the Sexual Disorder diagnosis can be given as the Axis I diagnosis, while the Personality Disorder diagnosis is given on Axis II.

Example 6

Emily is a 35-year-old woman who has been married for 9 years and has two children. Two months ago her 8-year-old son was hit by a car while riding his bicycle.

He was hospitalized for 3 weeks with several broken bones and some internal injuries. He recuperated at home for many more days and finally went back to school approximately 2 weeks ago.

Emily felt guilty and depressed about her son's accident. She blamed herself for not watching him more closely. Shortly after the accident, Emily began to develop sexual problems with her husband. She had little desire for sexual intimacy and was unable to become aroused by his caresses. Emily had never experienced similar problems in the past and had always enjoyed sexual relations with her husband. What diagnosis(es), if any, should Emily receive?

Emily fulfills the main criterion for Hypoactive Sexual Desire Disorder because she has a persistent and recurrent absence of desire for sexual activity. However, the diagnosis of Hypoactive Sexual Desire Disorder cannot be made if the patient's sexual symptoms occur exclusively in the course of another Axis I disorder. The significant change in Emily's sexual desire occurs in the context of depression and guilt about her son's accident. This emotional reaction to the stress of her son's injury fulfills the criteria for Adjustment Disorder with Depression. Therefore, the diagnosis of Hypoactive Sexual Desire Disorder cannot be made unless there is proof it began before her son's injury or it continues after the resolution of her Adjustment Disorder.

Precedence of Diagnosis

The precedence of diagnosis in the Sexual Disorders group relates mainly to the Sexual Dysfunctions rather than the Paraphilias or Gender Identity Disorders. The precedence of diagnosis for Sexual Disorders is shown in Table 12–1.

Discussion of Clinical Vignette

I Don't Think I'm a Man

Len is a 28-year-old married man who has had fantasies about being a woman since he was a young child and has been cross-dressing using women's undergarments since he was in high school. The cross-dressing commonly occurs when he is anxious and he often masturbates during the episodes. The masturbation is frequently accompanied by fantasies that other men are attracted to him in his role as a woman.

Len is currently a student in business school. He is increasingly anxious about the pressure at school and has asked his wife to let him wear her underwear during sexual intercourse. She initially agreed but finally threatened to leave him if he did not seek help for his problems. Her ultimatum made Len increasingly anxious and he became convinced that his only solution was to change his sex and become a woman.

Table 12–1   Precedence of diagnosis for Sexual Disorders

Sexual Disorder	Disorders taking precedence
Hypoactive Sexual Desire Disorder Female Sexual Arousal Disorder Male Erectile Disorder Female Orgasmic Disorder Male Orgasmic Disorder Dyspareunia Vaginismus	Does not occur exclusively during another Axis I disorder Not due to effects of a substance or general medical condition
Sexual Aversion Disorder	Does not occur exclusively during another Axis I disorder
Substance-Induced Sexual Dysfunction	Not better accounted for by any nonsubstance-induced Sexual Dysfunction
Sexual Dysfunction NOS Paraphilia NOS Sexual Disorder NOS Gender Identity Disorder NOS	Not better accounted for by any specific Sexual Dysfunction, Paraphilia, or Gender Disorder
Transvestic Fetishism	Does not occur exclusively during Gender Identity Disorder
Premature Ejaculation Sexual Dysfunction Due to a General Medical Condition Exhibitionism Fetishism Frotteurism Pedophilia Sexual Masochism Sexual Sadism Voyeurism	No other diagnosis takes precedence
Gender Identity Disorder	Not better accounted for by physi- cal intersexual condition if present

Note.   NOS = Not Otherwise Specified.

There are two related diagnostic issues in Len's case: cross-dressing and the wish to become a woman. Len meets the criteria for the diagnosis of Transvestic Fetishism because he is heterosexual and has recurrent, intense sexual urges and sexually arousing fantasies involving cross-dressing as a woman.

It is not clear whether he meets the criteria for Gender Identity Disorder. Len has a history of fantasies about becoming a woman. However he is reasonably content to be a man except during sexual activity and when he is very anxious. His response to anxiety is to fantasize that he is a woman. Len's request for help in becoming a woman appears to have been triggered by the intense anxiety associated with the pressure at school and his wife's ultimatum. It is not clear whether he would be motivated for a sex change if he was not anxious. Therefore, it is premature to make a diagnosis of Gender Identity Disorder. His feelings about his sexuality should be explored with the psychiatrist as his anxiety resolves.

Key Diagnostic Points

- In Fetishism an object is the focus of sexual excitement. In Transvestic Fetishism the individual cross-dresses in women's clothing to achieve sexual excitement, often by fantasizing that he is a woman.

- A primary diagnosis of decreased or absent sexual desire, arousal, or orgasm cannot be made if the symptoms occur exclusively during the course of another Axis I disorder (e.g., Major Depressive Disorder, Single Episode).

- The diagnosis of Dyspareunia in a woman cannot be made if the disturbance is caused exclusively by a lack of vaginal lubrication.

- The diagnostic criteria for Paraphilias require that the individual have intense sexual urges and sexually arousing fantasies that are markedly distressing but do not require that the individual perform any specific act.

Common Questions in Making a Diagnosis

1. Kurt is a 37-year-old man who likes to go to adult "peep shows" where women undress behind a window in front of him. He goes to these establishments two or three times a week. What diagnosis(es), if any, should Kurt receive?

   Answer: The diagnosis of Voyeurism requires that the individual observe an unsuspecting person who is naked, disrobing, or engaged in sexual activity. The women who perform in the "peep show" are aware that they are being watched and usually can see the man who is observing them. If Kurt fantasizes that the women are not aware of his observation and he is markedly distressed by these fantasies, he fulfills the criteria for Voyeurism. If he does not have these fantasies or is not upset about watching the women, he does not fit the criteria for Voyeurism.

2. Martin is a 33-year-old man who is a manual laborer during the day. He comes home in the evening and drinks several beers before, during, and after dinner. Recently, his wife complained that Martin is not paying attention to

her. She rubs against him when they are in bed together but he doesn't seem interested in having sexual relations with her. When she complained he replied, "I'm too tired from work. Let me sleep." She has tried to arouse him with manual stimulation several times but he seems unable to maintain an erection. His wife is convinced that he no longer loves her or is having an affair. What diagnosis(es), if any, should Martin receive?

Answer: Martin has difficulty becoming aroused and developing an erection. He does not seem particularly distressed by his problem, but his wife is. The diagnosis of Male Erectile Disorder is excluded if the disturbance is caused by the direct effects of a substance. The most likely cause of Martin's problem is alcohol intoxication. Therefore the diagnosis is Alcohol Intoxication Sexual Dysfunction With Impaired Arousal.

3. Howard is a 33-year-old man who has intrusive thoughts of choking a woman when he becomes sexually aroused. He becomes very anxious when the thoughts occur and tries to control them by counting the number of days until the next major holiday. The thoughts make it difficult for him to have sexual relations with a woman because they make it difficult for him to maintain his arousal and he often loses his erection before or during intercourse. What diagnosis(es), if any, should Howard receive?

Answer: Howard's symptoms meet the criteria for Obsessive-Compulsive Disorder. He also has a problem maintaining an erection before and during sexual intercourse. However, the diagnosis of Male Erectile Disorder cannot be made if the problem occurs during the course of another Axis I disorder. If there is evidence that his erectile disturbance started before the Obsessive-Compulsive Disorder or continues after successful treatment for that disorder, he can receive a diagnosis of Male Erectile Disorder.

4. Tom is an 18-year-old man who is involved in an ongoing sexual relationship with a 13-year-old girl. What diagnosis(es), if any, should Tom receive?

Answer: Tom's symptoms fulfill the criteria for Pedophilia, which requires that an individual have sex with a prepubescent child (usually age 13 or younger) and that the individual be at least 16 years old and at least 5 years older than the child.

5. Diane is a 35-year-old woman who complains about pain during sexual intercourse. The pain began several months ago, soon after her husband admitted that he had previously had an affair with a co-worker. Diane finds it difficult to become aroused when she is having sex with her husband. She is very concerned about the pain and wonders if there is something wrong with her. What diagnosis(es), if any, should Diane receive?

Answer: Diane meets the criteria for the diagnosis of Dyspareunia if her pain is not caused by poor vaginal lubrication secondary to her difficulty becoming aroused. If the underlying Sexual Disorder is difficulty with arousal, she could receive the diagnosis of Female Sexual Arousal Disorder. However, both the pain and lack of arousal may be due to another underlying Axis I disorder, such as depression, related to her husband's affair. In that case, neither sexual disorder could be diagnosed unless there was evidence that it occurred before the depression.

6. Alan is a 32-year-old man who has distressing fantasies of tying a woman to a bed and raping her. He has never acted on his fantasies. What diagnosis(es), if any, should Alan receive?

Answer: The diagnosis of Sexual Sadism requires that an individual have recurrent intense sexual urges and sexually arousing fantasies in which the psychological or physical suffering of a victim is sexually arousing to the individual. The individual does not have to act on the impulses to fulfill the criteria.

7. Hank is a 31-year-old man who likes to begin sexual relations with his wife by sneaking up on her and then exposing himself. She looks at his penis and responds with mock awe saying, "Oh my God, it's so big." The couple then have sexual intercourse. What diagnosis(es), if any, should Hank receive?

Answer: The diagnosis of Exhibitionism requires that the individual expose himself to an unsuspecting stranger. Hank's wife is acting the prearranged role of an unsuspecting stranger. This activity is within the realm of normal sexual activity. It does not fulfill the criteria for Exhibitionism.

Eating Disorders

Clinical Vignette

My Roommate Is Vomiting

Sally is a 23-year-old woman who finished secretarial training and began working as an executive secretary for a large company. A few months after starting work, she and Lois, another secretary in the company, decided to share a small apartment. Shortly after they moved in together, Lois began to notice that Sally had some unusual habits. Although Sally was concerned about her weight, she commonly bought large amounts of ice cream and "junk food," such as cream-filled cakes, and stored them in the kitchen cabinets. Occasionally Lois would return home in the evening after a date and find the cabinets empty and the garbage filled with empty junk-food wrappers. When she casually mentioned this one time Sally became defensive and replied, "I pigged out tonight."

Sally was also an exercise enthusiast who spent at least an hour or two each day at the local health club using the exercise machines. In the evenings, when they were making dinner, she often would ask Lois, "Do you think I put on any weight last week?" She seemed upset if Lois didn't reassure her that she hadn't gained weight.

One weekend evening Lois returned home early from a date. When she walked into the apartment she saw a number of empty food wrappers sitting on the kitchen counter. As she walked down the hall she heard the sound of someone vomiting in the bathroom. She knocked on the door and asked Sally if she needed any help. A few minutes later Sally came out of the bathroom. Lois asked her if she was sick. Sally said no and then sat down to talk with her. She told Lois that she periodically felt a craving for sweet, rich foods. She would begin by eating a few snacks and then continue eating until her stomach felt uncomfortably full. Following this she went into the bathroom and made herself vomit. On those occasions when she didn't vomit, she soon began to feel very guilty.

Core Concept of the Diagnostic Group

The core concept of the Eating Disorders group includes: 1) obsessive concern about becoming overweight or fat, 2) distorted body image, 3) inability to appropriately control food intake to maintain a healthy body weight, and 4) fluctuation of self-evaluation dependent on perceived body shape or weight. Patients may excessively restrict food intake to the point of physical illness or they may engage in binge eating, usually followed by compensatory behavior that includes excessive exercise or purging through self-induced vomiting or the misuse of laxatives or diuretics.

Criteria Applicable to Multiple Disorders

There is one criterion common to both Anorexia Nervosa and Bulimia Nervosa: the individual's self-evaluation is unduly influenced by their body weight or shape.

Definitions

anorexia   Loss of appetite accompanied by inability to eat.

binge   Excessive eating beyond the amount necessary to satisfy normal appetite.

purge   Emptying the stomach by induced vomiting or the bowels by induced evacuation with enemas or laxatives.

Synopses and Diagnostic Prototypes
of the Individual Disorders

The two main disorders in this diagnostic group are differentiated by the presence or absence of significant weight loss and binge eating.

307.1   Anorexia Nervosa.   Individuals with this disorder have an intense fear of gaining weight and refuse to maintain body weight at or above a minimal normal weight for their age and height. They also have a disturbance in the way that they experience their body weight or shape. This may include an undue influence of body weight or shape on their self-evaluation or a denial of the seriousness of the low weight. Postmenarchal women have an absence of at least three consecutive menstrual cycles. Specify one of the following types:

Restricting Type. During the episode of Anorexia Nervosa the person does not regularly engage in binge eating or purging behavior.

Binge Eating/Purging Type. During the episode of Anorexia Nervosa the person regularly engages in binge eating or purging behavior.

Alice was a perfect child. Her mother used to tell people how Alice's room was always clean when she lived at home and her school work was always neat and turned in on time. Alice's main hobby as a child was collecting dolls. She was particularly fond of Barbie dolls and used to say, "Mommy, Barbie has a perfect figure. I wish I could look like her."

When Alice was eighteen she left for college. No one in the family was aware that she was having any problems until the day she returned for summer vacation after her freshman year in college. When she stepped off the plane, her father commented that she had lost some weight. Alice looked annoyed and said, "Dad, I need to loose weight. I'm too fat." Her father was surprised and replied, "Too fat? You look too thin!" Over the next few weeks it became apparent that Alice was continuing to diet. While the family ate dinner, she ate a piece of dry toast and drank a diet Pepsi. Her mother became concerned and made an appointment for Alice with the family doctor. He found that she had lost 20 pounds from her previous weight of 115 pounds the year before. The doctor reassured Alice that she was not overweight and that she could actually harm herself if she continued to diet. However, the discussion with the doctor had little effect.

Alice continued to diet and became obsessed with food. Her menstrual periods stopped. She began buying cookbooks and preparing gourmet meals for the family. When it came time to eat the food, she sat with the family and ate a few pieces of lettuce with lemon juice and dry toast. One day her mother walked past Alice's bedroom and saw Alice standing in front of the mirror holding a Barbie doll and examining herself. When her mother entered the room, Alice turned, pinched her cheek and said "Look how chubby my face is!" Alice's eating pattern continued through the summer. Increasingly concerned, her mother called the family physician again. He referred Alice to an adolescent psychiatrist for evaluation.

307.51 Bulimia Nervosa. Individuals with this disorder have recurrent episodes of binge eating characterized by both of the following: 1) eating a significantly larger amount of food than most people would in a discrete period of time (e.g., 2 hours), and 2) a sense of lack of control over eating during the episode. Their self-evaluation is unduly influenced by body shape or weight and they use inappropriate compensatory behavior to prevent weight gain (e.g., self-induced vomiting, laxatives, diuretics, fasting, excessive exercise). The binge eating and compensatory behavior occur twice a week for 3 months but do not occur exclusively during episodes of Anorexia Nervosa.

Purging Type. The person regularly engages in self-induced vomiting or misuse of laxatives or diuretics.

Nonpurging Type.   The person uses other inappropriate compensatory behaviors, such as fasting, but does not regularly engage in self-induced vomiting or misuse of laxatives or diuretics.

Russ is a 27-year-old single man who works in a large office and models men's clothing on the side. He is very concerned about his weight and figure. During the summer he spends most of his free time on the beach with his buddies. In the winter he goes to a tanning salon near his health club to preserve his tan. Russ constantly fasts and exercises throughout the year to maintain his weight.

However, for the last year he has had a secret problem. Two or three times a week he engages in binge eating. Usually these episodes occur in a restaurant that serves a buffet dinner. Because he is a man, no one notices his frequent trips to the buffet where he piles food on his plate. After several trips to the buffet, Russ' stomach begins to hurt and he feels bloated. He goes into the bathroom and makes himself vomit by sticking his finger down his throat. When he feels less bloated he makes several more trips to the buffet.

After the bingeing, Russ feels depressed and guilty. He tries to compensate for the bingeing by excessive exercise. During work he runs up and down several flights of stairs in the office building to burn up extra calories. Several of his coworkers have admired his slim figure and asked how he keeps his weight down. Russ usually answers, "I'm careful about what and how much I eat."

307.50   Eating Disorder Not Otherwise Specified.   Individuals with this disorder have an eating disturbance that does not meet all of the criteria for a specific Eating Disorder.

Necessary Clinical Information

The diagnosis of an Eating Disorder requires the following information:

* Current and past weight

* Current and past patterns of eating

* Current and past feelings about food

* Unusual eating rituals

* Current and past appetite

* History of dieting

* Current and past feelings about weight

* Medical illnesses

* Current medications and abused substances

- Psychiatric illnesses (Schizophrenia, Major Depression, etc.)

- Psychiatric symptoms (mania, depression, anxiety, thought disorder, etc.)

- Episodes of binge eating

- Psychological conflicts related to self-evaluation (i.e., self-esteem)

- Relationship between weight and patient's self-esteem

- Family history of Eating Disorders

Making a Diagnosis

The Eating Disorders are characterized by an ever-changing interaction between the amount of food an individual consumes, the individual's perception of their weight or shape, and the relationship of this perception to their self-esteem. The following questions will help differentiate between the two specific disorders that make up this diagnostic category.

1. Does an individual's body weight or shape have an undue influence on their self-evaluation and do they fear gaining weight?

- If an individual's body weight or shape has little influence on his or her self-evaluation and/or if they don't fear gaining weight, the diagnosis of a specific Eating Disorder is excluded.

2. Does the individual refuse to maintain body weight above a minimum (e.g., 85%) of the expected normal weight for their age and height?

- If an individual maintains body weight above 85% of the expected weight for his or her age and height, the diagnosis of Anorexia Nervosa is excluded.

- If an individual does not maintain body weight above 85% of the expected minimal weight, he or she may receive a diagnosis of Anorexia Nervosa if the following requirements are also fulfilled: 1) the individual has an intense fear of gaining weight; 2) the individual's body weight and shape has a significant influence on self-evaluation; and 3) if the individual is a postmenarchal woman, she has missed three consecutive menstrual cycles.

3. Does the individual binge eat?

• If an individual has met the criteria for Anorexia Nervosa and binges, with or without purging, the diagnosis is Anorexia Nervosa Binge Eating/Purging Type.

• If an individual has not met the criteria for Anorexia Nervosa and binges using purging as a compensatory behavior to avoid gaining weight, the diagnosis is Bulimia Nervosa Purging Type.

• If an individual has not met the criteria for Anorexia Nervosa and binges using fasting and exercise instead of purging as a compensatory behavior to avoid gaining weight, the diagnosis is Bulimia Nervosa Nonpurging Type.

4. Does an individual have an eating disturbance that doesn't meet the criteria for a specific Eating Disorder?

• If an individual has an eating disturbance such as significant weight loss, bingeing, or purging but doesn't meet the criteria for a specific Eating Disorder, the diagnosis is Eating Disorder Not Otherwise Specified.

Common Problems in Making a Diagnosis

Some patients have a clear disturbance in their eating, yet may not fulfill all of the necessary criteria for a specific eating disorder. This problem can occur for both anorexic and bingeing patients. Frequently, as described in the examples below, the problem is one of interpretation rather than total absence of criteria.

Patients Who Almost Fulfill the Diagnostic Criteria

In each of the examples below the patient presents symptoms that partially fulfill some of the necessary criteria for the diagnosis of an eating disorder. An examination of the core concepts for the diagnostic group as a whole and the required criteria for the individual disorders often helps the clinician make a decision about how to use this incomplete information to make a diagnosis.

Example 1

Samantha is a 17-year-old woman who is significantly underweight. She is not fearful about gaining weight. What diagnosis (if any) should Samantha receive?

A patient who is not fearful about gaining weight cannot be given a diagnosis of Anorexia Nervosa even if she is significantly underweight. One of the core concepts underlying the diagnosis of Anorexia Nervosa is that the patient inappropriately views herself as overweight. Furthermore, the intensity of the patient's dread of gaining weight is commonly exaggerated far beyond that of a average person who is trying to avoid gaining weight.

Example 2

Alice is a 22-year-old woman who has episodes of binge eating once every week or two. What diagnosis(es) if any should Alice receive?

The frequency of Alice's eating binges do not meet the intensity criteria for Bulimia Nervosa, which requires binge eating twice a week for 3 months. However, if all of the other criteria for Bulimia Nervosa are fulfilled, with the exception of the number of eating binges in a given time period, she could be given a diagnosis of Eating Disorder Not Otherwise Specified.

In some cases a patient might have periods of frequent binge eating alternating with periods of less frequent bingeing. For these patients, the physician must decide whether the sum total of the patient's symptoms are consistent with the other criteria necessary for the diagnosis of Bulimia Nervosa even if there is borderline compliance with the intensity and duration criteria. In other cases, the patient may not reveal the full extent of their binge-purge behavior and may actually fulfill the criteria.

Example 3

Kelly is a 19-year-old woman who has lost 20 pounds in the last 2 months by dieting and now weights 115 pounds. What diagnosis(es), if any, should Kelly receive?

The criteria for the diagnosis of Anorexia Nervosa requires that the patient refuses or is unable to maintain a body weight that is over, "a minimally normal weight for age and height." A minimal normal weight is defined as 15% below the expected weight. The definition assumes that the clinician can determine the expected weight for the patient; a potentially difficult value to accurately estimate.

It is not clear what Kelly's expected weight should be. The most obvious solution is to use a standard growth chart that provides the average weight for individuals of a specific age and height. This can be effective if the patient's physique is comparable to that of the average individuals included in the chart. However, if the patient is tall and thin, her normal expected weight would fall below the average in the charts and the reduced weight necessary for the diagnosis of Anorexia Nervosa would be greater than 15% below the chart average.

Conversely, a patient with a short and heavy physique would have a normal weight above the average for individuals of her age and height. The reduced weight necessary for the diagnosis of Anorexia Nervosa for this patient would be less than 15% below the average on the growth charts. One solution is to use the value of 15% as a general guideline for estimating the necessary weight loss to validate the diagnosis. An experienced clinician will make adjustments to this value based on the examples discussed above and other relevant factors.

Example 4

Sarah is a 15-year-old adolescent girl who has been dieting excessively. Her weight fluctuates, on a weekly basis, between 10% and 15% of her previously established normal weight. What diagnosis(es), if any, should Sarah receive?

This case differs from the previous example because Sarah's normal weight has already been established. Her current weight fluctuates between 10% and 15% below the previously established normal weight. If the criteria are followed rigidly, she would have a diagnosis of Anorexia Nervosa on alternative weeks. Clearly, this would not make clinical sense.

The resolution of this problem is similar to that of the last example. The value of 15% for the weight loss is a general guideline. For some patients an average loss of 12% to 13% over several weeks would be sufficient to make the diagnosis of Anorexia Nervosa if the other criteria are fulfilled and the patient's symptoms are consistent with the core concepts of the diagnosis. These include obsessive concern about becoming fat, a feeling of being overweight despite an abnormally low weight, the inability to appropriately control food intake, and fluctuations of self-esteem linked to issues of weight.

Example 5

Carol is a 22-year-old woman who is significantly underweight from excessive dieting. She has had 1–2 months of amenorrhea followed by periods of irregular and very light menstrual bleeding. What diagnosis(es), if any, should Carol receive?

Carol's diagnosis presents a similar problem to the previous examples. In this case, a significantly underweight patient has 1–2 months of amenorrhea followed by 1–2 months of irregular and very light menstrual bleeding. Does this qualify for the diagnosis? Again, the physician must use his judgment to decide whether the other criteria are sufficiently fulfilled to make the diagnosis despite the fact that the duration or intensity of the amenorrhea does not exactly fulfill the criterion.

Example 6

Sam is a 19-year-old boy who fasts all during the day on Mondays and Fridays and then eats a dinner that is twice as large as the dinner eaten by his friends. What diagnosis(es), if any, should Sam receive?

Sam has a peculiar habit of daytime fasting 2 days a week followed by eating a dinner that is definitely larger than his friends' dinners. Although several symptoms of Bulimia Nervosa are present (i.e., fasting and frequent binge eating), an observer could reasonably ask whether the fasting is compensatory behavior for the overeating or whether the overeating was a response to the fasting.

One way of distinguishing between the two possibilities would depend on the patient's sense of control over the eating and concern about his body shape and weight. If the patient is concerned about being overweight and is fasting in order to be able to binge, the clinician might entertain a diagnosis of Bulimia Nervosa. If the patient is unconcerned about his weight and has some intellectual or quasi-religious reason for fasting, the diagnosis of an Eating Disorder would not be appropriate. In such a situation the patient's behavior might be ascribed to an unusual personal ritual.

Example 7

Tom is a 23-year-old man who occasionally binges and has pervasive problems with poor self-esteem. What diagnosis(es), if any, should Tom receive?

The criteria for Bulimia Nervosa require that the patient's body weight or shape have a strong influence on self-evaluation or self-esteem. Some patients, especially those having a personality disorder (e.g., Borderline Personality), may have a more extensive disturbance of self-esteem that is occasionally associated with episodes of binge eating. One aspect of this general defect in self-esteem may be related to the patient's body weight or shape. It is important to recognize that some elements of the criteria for this diagnosis commonly appear in other disorders. Tom may only receive the diagnosis of Bulimia Nervosa if he meets all of the criteria for the diagnosis.

Eating Symptoms Associated With Other Psychiatric Disorders

Example 8

Yvonne is a severely underweight 23-year-old woman who is depressed, anhedonic, feels worthless, has insomnia, and has recurrent thoughts about dying. What diagnosis(es), if any, should Yvonne receive?

In this case the clinician must decide if Yvonne's weight loss is caused by the Major Depression or merely accompanies it. This distinction may be difficult to make. If the patient meets the criteria for Anorexia Nervosa and Major Depression, both diagnoses may be given to the patient. If the weight loss appears to be caused by anorexia secondary to the depression, the diagnosis of Anorexia Nervosa may not be used. In the latter case, the patient is not likely to be fearful about gaining weight. She may be indifferent or actually concerned that she has lost so much weight.

Example 9

Steven is a severely underweight 19-year-old man who is psychotic. What diagnosis(es), if any, should Steven receive?

Steven may have significant weight loss associated with a diagnosis of Schizophrenia or another psychotic disorder. This weight loss may be secondary to bizarre eating habits associated with the psychotic disorder or they may represent a coexisting eating disorder. The patient can be given the additional diagnosis of Anorexia Nervosa if all of the criteria for that diagnosis are fulfilled.

Precedence of Diagnosis

The presence of any nonpsychiatric medical disorder that can cause a significant weight loss always takes precedence over the diagnosis of Anorexia Nervosa. The diagnosis of Anorexia Nervosa always takes precedence over Bulimia Nervosa. If a patient with a diagnosis of Schizophrenia has a significant weight loss and meets the criteria for Anorexia Nervosa, both diagnoses should be given. Similarly, a patient with a diagnosis of Borderline Personality Disorder who binges and meets the criteria for Bulimia Nervosa, should be given both diagnoses.

Discussion of the Clinical Vignette

My Roommate Is Vomiting

Sally has recurrent episodes of binge eating during which she consumes large amounts of sweet, rich food followed by vomiting as a compensatory behavior to avoid gaining weight. She indicates that she eats until her stomach is uncomfortably full. However, it is not clear whether she feels a lack of control over her eating during the bingeing episode. This is important to determine because it is an important part of the criteria for the diagnosis of Anorexia Nervosa. In some cases it may be difficult to decide if a patient feels a loss of control during binge eating because the patient may not acknowledge or be overtly aware of losing control. In these cases the clinician may be able to infer the loss of control if the patient continues eating to the point of feeling distinctly uncomfortable or sick as Sally does.

Sally's frequent vigorous exercise sessions accompanied by repeated requests for reassurance about her weight suggest that this is an important issue for her. It needs to be explored further to determine how much her sense of self-worth is influenced by how she and others perceive her body shape and weight. These symptoms fulfill part of the criteria for the diagnosis of Bulimia Nervosa.

The diagnosis also requires that binge eating occur at least twice a week for 3 months. If it is difficult to determine the frequency of bingeing, as discussed in the last section, or if the frequency clearly does not meet the criteria, the diagnosis is Eating Disorder Not Otherwise Specified.

Key Diagnostic Points

- The diagnosis of Anorexia Nervosa requires that a patient have an intense fear of gaining weight even though significantly underweight.

- The diagnosis of Bulimia Nervosa cannot be made if an individual fulfills the criteria for Anorexia Nervosa.

- The diagnosis of Bulimia Nervosa requires that a patient have frequent periods of binge eating associated with loss of control over eating followed by guilt, depression, or compensatory behavior.

Common Questions in Making a Diagnosis

1. A 16-year-old girl who weighs 110 pounds is 10 pounds under the average weight for her age and height. She complains that she does not have a good appetite, eats little, and has not had a menses for several months. The patient has been thin for many years and has always felt self-conscious about her low weight, considering herself unattractive. Can the patient be given a diagnosis of Anorexia Nervosa?

Answer: This patient cannot be given a diagnosis of Anorexia Nervosa. The diagnosis of Anorexia Nervosa requires that the patient refuses to maintain body weight at a minimally normal weight for their age. It also requires that they have an intense fear of gaining weight, an undue influence of their weight and shape on self-esteem, and amenorrhea. This patient weighs 9% below her normal expected weight. However, she has been thin for several years and her current weight may be her normal weight based on her body build. The patient's weight does influence her self-esteem, but this occurs in the opposite way than that required for the diagnosis of Anorexia Nervosa. She feels unattractive because she is too thin. Furthermore, she is concerned about being too thin rather than fearful of becoming too fat. The patient does have amenorrhea. However, in light of her previous history, this may be due to a nonpsychiatric medical disorder.

2. Steve is a 16-year-old student who stays after school every day to exercise and practice with his high school wrestling team for 3 hours. When he comes home he often eats three peanut butter sandwiches, a box of cookies, two apples, and drinks 2 quarts of milk before dinner. His mother comments that he acts as if he has no control over his eating. Steve is quite concerned about his physique and frequently stands in front of the mirror in his room examining his muscles. His 8-year-old sister asks, "Why does Steve eat so much food?" Should Steve be given a diagnosis of Bulimia Nervosa?

   Answer: Steve appears to fulfill many of the stated criteria for the diagnosis of Bulimia Nervosa. He frequently eats large quantities of food in a short time and appears to display little or no control over his appetite. He exercises excessively and is very concerned about his physical shape. Nevertheless, it would not be correct to give him a diagnosis of Bulimia Nervosa. Steve eats because he exercises rather than exercising as a compensatory behavior in order to avoid gaining weight. Furthermore, it is not unusual or abnormal for adolescents, especially if involved in athletics, to eat large amounts of food and be concerned about their body shape and muscle size.

3. Judy is a 23-year-old medical student who has always been concerned about her weight. She often feels a strong, sometimes uncontrollable, urge to eat large amounts of junk food such as cookies and packaged pastries. Because she is concerned about her weight, she routinely chews and spits out the food rather then swallowing it. Should Judy receive a diagnosis of Bulimia Nervosa?

   Answer: The diagnosis of Bulimia Nervosa requires that a patient actually consume the food she eats and then engage in some compensatory behavior to avoid gaining weight such as: self-induced vomiting, excessive exercise, fasting, or misuse of laxatives or diuretics. Judy's behavior does not fulfill these criteria for Bulimia Nervosa. However, her behavior of routinely spitting out chewed food to avoid gaining weight is abnormal and does fit the diagnosis of Eating Disorder Not Otherwise Specified.

4. Kelsey is a 17-year-old girl who has always been significantly underweight. What diagnosis(es), if any, should Kelsey receive?

   Answer: If Kelsey has always been significantly underweight (e.g., less than 85% of the normal body weight for her age and height), the diagnosis of Anorexia Nervosa rests on the remaining criteria. She can experience her low weight in several ways. She can be upset that she is significantly underweight and eager to gain more weight, or she can be concerned that she is fat and fearful of gaining weight. The former is a normal response, whereas the latter fulfills criteria for Anorexia Nervosa. If the patient's weight produces problems with her self-evaluation, she might feel worthless either because of her low weight or because she perceives herself as fat. Neither of these responses are examples of healthy self-esteem. However, in the latter, the patient bases her self-esteem on a distortion of her body experience. Finally, in either case, the patient may experience amenorrhea simply as a result of her abnormally low weight. Therefore, this symptom may be necessary for the diagnosis of Anorexia Nervosa but not useful in the differential diagnosis between this disorder and another physical cause for the patient's weight problem. The diagnosis of Anorexia Nervosa can be made if she is fearful of gaining weight, continues to see herself as fat despite her low weight, and is amenorrheic.

Sleep Disorders

Clinical Vignette

I Feel Sleepy All the Time

Brendan is a 26-year-old medical intern in a large urban hospital. He currently spends every third night on call in the hospital. He arrives for work at 6:00 A.M. one day and goes home at 7:00 P.M. the following day. Brendan rarely gets a chance to sleep during the night he is on call. He is responsible for a hospital ward of 12 patients. Many of the patients are acutely ill and need continual attention. Periodically during the night he is also called down to the emergency room to admit a new patient to the ward. In the morning he attends clinical rounds to present his patients to the attending physician and medical residents. Following rounds, Brendan writes medical orders for his patients, teaches the medical students, draws blood, and performs necessary medical procedures such as lumbar punctures. During the afternoon he sees his patients in the medical outpatient clinic.

Brendan has had difficulty from the start of his internship staying awake and concentrating on his duties. He tries to stay awake by drinking coffee and sometimes takes over-the-counter caffeine pills. Recently, he fell asleep early in the morning in his office and did not hear his beeper go off or a voice page summoning him to the medical unit to see a patient. As a result, the nurse had to call the medical resident to see the patient. A few weeks later, Brendan was so sleepy that he misread an electrocardiogram (ECG) the day after he was on call. The resident called the mistake to his attention in evening rounds before he had changed the patient's medication.

The attending physician has also had to speak with him twice about being late for morning rounds. Brendan explained to the physician, "When I'm on call I never seem to catch up with my sleep before I go on call again. I need 8 hours of sleep. If I don't get it, I feel sleepy all the time. Sometimes I fall asleep while I'm sitting writing progress notes in patients' charts. Maybe there's something wrong with me." The physician nodded sympathetically and said, "I know it's difficult but that's the expectation. We all had to do it. It was worse when I was an intern. We were on call every other night. You guys have it easy."

Core Concept of the Diagnostic Group

The core concept of the Sleep Disorders group is a disturbance in the process of sleep. The disturbance may include one or more of the following: difficulty initiating or maintaining sleep, difficulty sleeping at the conventional or appropriate time, excessive daytime sleepiness, or abnormal physiological or psychological events occurring during sleep.

Criteria Applicable to Multiple Disorders

There is one criterion that is applicable to multiple Sleep Disorders: the sleep disturbance causes clinically significant distress or impairment in social, occupational, or other important areas of functioning.

Definitions

apnea   Cessation of breathing.

cataplexy   Sudden loss of muscle tone that is usually associated with intense emotion and is commonly seen in patients with Narcolepsy.

DIMS   Disorders of Initiating and Maintaining Sleep (one of the four main categories in the diagnostic classification system of the Association of Sleep Disorders Centers).

DOES   Disorders of Excessive Somnolence (one of the four main categories in the diagnostic classification system of the Association of Sleep Disorders Centers).

dyssomnia   A disturbance in the amount, quality, or timing of sleep.

hypersomnia   An excessive amount of sleep.

hypnogogic   A state of arousal occurring immediately preceding sleep during which hallucinations may occur.

hypnopompic   A state of arousal occurring immediately preceding awakening during which hallucinations may occur.

insomnia   Difficulty initiating and maintaining sleep.

parasomnia   Disorders in which the predominant disturbance is an abnormal event occurring during sleep.

pavor nocturnus   Sleep terror.

somnambulism   Sleepwalking.

Synopses and Diagnostic Prototypes of the Individual Disorders

The Sleep Disorders group in DSM-IV are divided into three main categories: Primary Sleep Disorders (Dyssomnias and Parasomnias), Sleep Disorders Related to Another Mental Disorder, and Other Sleep Disorders.

Primary Sleep Disorders

Dyssomnias

307.42   Primary Insomnia.   Individuals with this disorder have difficulty initiating or maintaining sleep, or sleep that is nonrestorative, for at least 1 month.

> Irwin is a 46-year-old middle manager in a large corporation. During the last year the company has laid off several hundred workers. For 6 months there have been rumors that management people are next on the list for layoffs. Irwin has been worried about his job for several months. During that time he has had difficulty sleeping. He falls asleep at 11:00 P.M. but then awakens at 3:00 A.M. and cannot fall asleep again. He normally gets up for work at 6:30 A.M. Irwin has tried several methods to fall asleep again. Drinking milk or taking over-the-counter sleep aids have been equally ineffective. His only relief came during three nights when he was on vacation in the mountains and he slept through the entire night.

307.44   Primary Hypersomnia.   Individuals with this disorder have excessive sleepiness for at least 1 month that cannot be accounted for by an inadequate amount of sleep.

> Delia is a 25-year-old woman who works as an aid in the home of an elderly woman with Alzheimer's disease. She has worked there for 3 months. During the last 2 months Delia has become so sleepy during the day that she has had to take naps while at work. Because she is alone in the house with her charge, she has been able to sleep when the woman is resting. She does not feel sleepy during the day on weekends. Delia thinks the problem may be related to her job.

347   Narcolepsy.   Individuals with this disorder have irresistible attacks of re-
freshing sleep daily for at least 3 months. They also have cataplexy and hypnopom-
pic/hypnogogic hallucinations or sleep paralysis at the beginning or end of sleep
episodes.

> Sidney is a 16-year-old high school student who recently developed a problem with
> excessive daytime sleepiness. Periodically during the day she suddenly falls asleep
> for several seconds to a minute. Often this occurs in the middle of a class. Some-
> times she awakes to find the teacher standing over her calling her name and some
> of the other students laughing.
>
> Several of the teachers have spoken to Sidney and her parents about sleeping
> in class. She explains that she can't control the sleeping but her teachers are reluc-
> tant to believe her. The sleep episodes have made it difficult for Sidney to keep up
> with her studies because she misses important information during class. Several of
> her friends are sympathetic and help by loaning her class notes. One friend says, "I
> can always tell when you're asleep. Your mouth drops open or your head falls on
> your chest."

780.59   Breathing-Related Sleep Disorder.   Individuals with this disorder experience a disruption of sleep leading to excessive sleepiness or insomnia. The
sleep disruption is judged to be due to a sleep-related breathing condition.

> Fred is a 35-year-old obese, businessman who has difficulty staying awake in his
> office during the day. He goes to bed at 10:00 P.M. and gets up for work at 6:30 A.M.
> Despite 8½ hours of sleep, he does not feel refreshed when he awakes.
>
> Fred's wife reports that he snores so loudly during the night that he often wakes
> her. She describes a sequence of events that is particularly irritating. Fred snores
> evenly for a period of several minutes. This is followed by a choking sound and a
> prolonged period of silence that may last 20 to 30 seconds or longer. During the
> silent period, Fred begins to move and struggle. The silence ends with a sudden loud
> blast of snoring as Fred begins to breath again. Often, he wakes up during the pro-
> cess, only to quickly fall asleep again and continue snoring.

307.45   Circadian Rhythm Sleep Disorder (Sleep-Wake Schedule Disorder).
Individuals with this disorder experience a persistent and recurrent pattern of sleep
disruption, leading to excessive sleepiness or insomnia that is due to a mismatch
between the sleep-wake schedule required by the individual's environment and his
or her circadian sleep-wake pattern. (Specify one of the following: *delayed sleep
phase type; jet lag type; shift work type; unspecified type*).

> Jackie is a 25-year-old stewardess who just began working on the New York to
> Hawaii flight twice a week. She has a 2-day layover in Hawaii and then returns to
> New York. During her first month on the job, she had periods of insomnia mixed
> with somnolence. Jackie felt like she was walking around in a daze, half awake

most of the time. She asked one of her fellow stewardesses how she coped with the schedule. "Get your sleep whenever you can and don't drink alcohol." the co-worker said. Jackie continued, "How long does it take to adjust?" The other stewardess looked at her and said, "A few weeks, I guess, but some people never do make it." The diagnosis is Circadian Rhythm Sleep Disorder, Jet Lag Type

307.47   Dyssomnia Not Otherwise Specified.   Individuals with this disorder have an insomnia, hypersomnia, or circadian rhythm disturbance that does not meet criteria for any specific Dyssomnia (e.g., nocturnal myoclonus: repeated limb jerks associated with periods of arousal).

Parasomnias

307.47   Nightmare Disorder (formerly Dream Anxiety Disorder).
Individuals with this disorder have repeated awakenings from major sleep periods or naps with detailed recall of extended and highly frightening dreams, usually involving threats to survival, security, or self-esteem. The awakenings usually occur during the second half of the sleep period. On awakening from the frightening dream, the individual rapidly becomes oriented and alert.

> Linda is a 17-year-old young woman whose parents recently separated. She currently lives with her mother. Linda was very upset about the separation, even though she could see it coming for many months.
>
> The day after the separation papers were signed and her father left the house, she awoke at 4:00 A.M. with a frightening dream. In the dream she was in her car and two men were chasing her with a truck. One of the men was shooting at her with a machine gun. The driver tried to force her off the road by pulling next to her and swerving into the side of her car. As he did so, the passenger pointed the gun directly at her head and pulled the trigger. She woke up kicking the bed covers and thrashing her arms about with her heart racing. Within a few seconds Linda realized she was in her bed and sat up. She was too upset by the nightmare to go back to sleep. In the morning she explained the details of the dream to her mother who listened sympathetically. Linda experienced several similar frightening dreams over the next few weeks.

307.46   Sleep Terror Disorder.   Individuals with this disorder have recurrent episodes of abrupt awakenings from sleep, usually occurring during the first third of the major sleep episode and beginning with a panicky scream. They experience intense anxiety, signs of autonomic arousal, and are relatively unresponsive to efforts of others to comfort them during the episode. No detailed dream is recalled and there is amnesia about the episode.

> Jeremy is a 25-year-old man who has been working long hours to finish an important project in his company. He often comes home late, feeling exhausted, eats a

small dinner with his wife, and goes to bed.

In the last few weeks he has had several strange and disturbing experiences during the night. They usually occur 1–2 hours after he goes to sleep. His wife describes the episodes as follows, "Jeremy suddenly sits bolt upright in the bed, screams, and looks panicky." The first time it happened his wife was so startled that she woke up and jumped out of bed. She continued with her description, "I looked at Jeremy. His eyes were wide open, he was sweating and breathing fast. When I sat next to him I could feel his heart racing. I tried to find out what was wrong but he wouldn't respond." A minute or two later Jeremy awoke and looked at his wife. When she asked him what was wrong he replied, "I feel terrified but I don't know why." She held him for a few minutes until he fell asleep again. In the morning Jeremy did not remember anything about the episode. The succeeding episodes were similar but his wife became accustomed to them and was less startled.

307.46 Sleepwalking Disorder.   Individuals with this disorder have repeated episodes of arising from bed during sleep and walking about, usually during the first third of the major sleep episode. While sleepwalking the individual has a blank face, is relatively uncommunicative, and can only be awakened with great difficulty. Within several minutes after awakening, there is no impairment of mental activity or behavior but the individual has amnesia about the episode.

Mark is a 13-year-old boy who is spending the night at the home of his best friend Sam while his parents are away on a trip. The boys talked and watched television until midnight and then went to sleep.

Two hours later Sam awoke when he heard a noise. He looked over at the sleeping bag on the floor where Mark was sleeping. It was empty. At first he thought that Mark had gone to the bathroom. After a few minutes, when Mark hadn't returned, Sam got up to look for his friend. He found Mark wandering around the kitchen eating a banana. His friend didn't seem to notice him so he said, "Mark, what's up." Mark didn't answer. Sam tried to talk with him again but got no response. He stood in front of Mark, grabbed his shoulder, and shook it. After a few minutes Mark's head jerked and he mumbled a few words. He seemed confused for a few more minutes and then recognized Sam. "Hi Sam, where are we?" he asked. Sam led him back to the bedroom and the two boys went back to sleep. The next morning Mark had no memory of the episode. He explained, "My parents tell me that sometimes I walk around at night, but I can never remember it."

307.47 Parasomnia Not Otherwise Specified.   Individuals with this disorder have abnormal behavioral or physiological events during sleep or sleep-wake transitions that do not meet the criteria for any specific parasomnia.

Sleep Disorders Related to Another Mental Disorder

307.42   Insomnia Related to . . . *[Indicate the Axis I or Axis II Disorder].* Individuals with this disorder have difficulty initiating or maintaining sleep, or have nonrestorative sleep, for at least 1 month, that is associated with daytime fatigue or impaired daytime functioning. The sleep disturbance is judged to be related to another Axis I or Axis II disorder and is severe enough to warrant independent clinical attention.

> Carol is a 41-year-old cosmetologist. Her specialty is designer fingernails. Recently, her boss and a few customers have noticed that Carol's work has been slipping. Her designs don't have the same flair they used to have and everything she does seems to take longer than it did in the past. Carol's boss is concerned that she is upset about something and it is interfering with her work.
>
> A few days ago he called her aside and said, "You seem to be sad these days. What's wrong?" Carol looked down and said, "I feel depressed and tired all the time. I don't enjoy my job anymore and I can't concentrate on my work. The worst problem is that I can't sleep."
>
> She went on to tell her boss that she wakes each morning at 3:00 A.M. and can't go back to sleep again. "I'm so tired during the day that I can barely keep my eyes open. Sometimes I find I'm painting a customer's nails the wrong color or smearing the nail polish." The diagnosis is Insomnia Related to Major Depressive Disorder, Single Episode

307.44   Hypersomnia Related to . . . *[Indicate the Axis I or Axis II Disorder].* Individuals with this disorder have a predominant complaint of excessive sleepiness for at least 1 month that is expressed by either prolonged sleep episodes or daytime sleep episodes occurring almost daily. The hypersomnia is judged to be related to another Axis I or Axis II disorder and is severe enough to warrant independent clinical attention.

> Claire is a 43-year-old married woman who used to be very involved in public affairs in her community. For the last several months she has been bored and lies around the house all day. Her husband has repeatedly urged her to get a job or get involved in some project with her friends. Claire replies that she has no energy or self-confidence.
>
> The couple's last child, Sarah, left home 3 years ago to attend college. The daughter was particularly close to her mother. Claire explains, "I've felt depressed since Sarah left home. I don't think things will ever get better again." Claire's main complaint is that she is always tired. "I feel like sleeping all the time. Maybe I need some stimulant or something." The diagnosis is Hypersomnia Related to Dysthymic Disorder

Other Sleep Disorders

780.xx   Sleep Disorder Due to . . . *[Indicate the General Medical Condition].*
Individuals with this disorder have a prominent disturbance in sleep that is sufficiently severe to warrant independent clinical attention. There is evidence from the
history, physical examination, or laboratory findings of a general medical condition judged to be etiologically related to the sleep disturbance. Specify one of the
following types:

> *.52 Insomnia Type:*   If the predominant disturbance is insomnia.
>
> *.54 Hypersomnia Type:*   If the predominant disturbance is hypersomnia.
>
> *.59 Parasomnia Type:*   If the predominant disturbance is a parasomnia.
>
> *.59 Mixed Type:*   If more than one sleep disturbance is present but none pre-
> dominates.

> Carl is a 64-year-old retired insurance salesman who has had two mild heart attacks.
> He currently experiences periodic angina that responds well to nitroglycerin tablets.
> Carl spends much his day working in the yard or reading. He and his wife have plans
> to go on a 2-week trip to Hawaii but Carl is concerned about the trip. He recently
> saw his cardiologist and complained about a change in his angina. For the past
> several weeks he has begun to experience attacks of angina during the night that
> wake him. He finds it more and more difficult to fall asleep because he is afraid he
> will have another angina attack. As a result, he is sleepy during the day and finds it
> difficult to concentrate on the things he is doing. The diagnosis is Sleep Disorder
> Due to Angina, Insomnia Type

29x.xx Substance-Induced Sleep Disorder.   Individuals with this disorder
have a prominent disturbance in sleep that is sufficiently severe to warrant independent clinical attention. There is evidence that the symptoms developed within
1 month of significant substance intoxication or withdrawal or are etiologically
related to medication use or toxin exposure. The specific codes for Substance-Induced Sleep Disorder are determined by the specific substance: 291.8 alcohol;
292.89 amphetamines; cocaine; opioids; sedatives, hypnotics, anxiolytics; other
(or unknown) substances. Specify if onset is during intoxication or withdrawal and
specify one of the following types:

> *Insomnia Type:* If the predominant disturbance is insomnia.
>
> *Hypersomnia Type:* If the predominant disturbance is hypersomnia.
>
> *Parasomnia Type:* If the predominant disturbance is a parasomnia.
>
> *Mixed Type:* if more than one sleep disturbance is present but none predomi-
> nates.

Peter is a 27-year-old truck driver who used to do short-haul runs with a maximum distance of 400–500 miles. He usually began driving early in the morning and arrived at his destination by late in the evening. Peter dropped off his load, stayed overnight at a motel, and picked up a new load to deliver to his home base. Recently, he started driving long cross-country runs of 2,500–3,000 miles. He drove for 18-hour stretches alternating with 6 hours of sleep.

In order to stay awake during the long periods of driving, Peter began drinking more coffee than he normally did. He stopped every 2–3 hours to exercise his legs, use the bathroom, and get some coffee. On his first long run, he had 10 cups of coffee in the first 18 hours. Peter felt energized by the coffee and tireless, but also restless and nervous. He had to stop more frequently to urinate and found it difficult to sit still in his seat.

When he finally stopped for the night, he couldn't fall asleep. He tossed and turned most of the night and got up in the morning exhausted. After a few cups of coffee he felt awake again and continued driving. This pattern continued for the entire trip. When he returned home after his first trip, his wife commented that he was irritable and wandered from thought to thought when they talked together. The diagnosis is Caffeine-Induced Sleep Disorder

Necessary Clinical Information

- Insomnia or hypersomnia

- Daytime napping

- Nightmares or bad dreams

- Substance abuse

- Sleep medication (prescribed and over-the-counter)

- Excessive daytime sleepiness

- Work schedule

- Travel schedule

- Medical problems that may interfere with sleep (e.g., pulmonary, cardiac)

- Snoring

- Unusual sleep behavior (e.g., sleepwalking, episodes of terror, muscle jerks)

Making a Diagnosis

The Association of Sleep Disorders Centers categorizes sleep disturbances into four categories: Disorders of Initiating and Maintaining Sleep (DIMS); Disorders of Excessive Somnolence (DOES); Disorders of the Sleep-Wake Schedule; and Dysfunctions Associated with Sleep, Sleep Stages, or Partial Arousals (Parasomnias). DSM-IV defines only two large categories of sleep disturbances, Dyssomnias and Parasomnias. The Dyssomnias are defined as disturbances in the amount, quality, or timing of sleep. They include the first three diagnostic categories of the Association of Sleep Disorders system. In DSM-IV Parasomnias include abnormal events occurring during sleep; they are essentially identical in the two diagnostic systems.

Some of the questions below may seem redundant because the same diagnosis can be approached from more than one direction. For example, if a patient complains about excessive daytime sleepiness, the clinician might ask about snoring or a breathing disorder. On the other hand, if a patient reports that his wife complains about his loud snoring, the clinician should ask about excessive daytime sleepiness. Similarly, the identification of Major Depressive Disorder should lead the clinician to ask about a sleep disturbance, and the presence of insomnia should lead to questions about an underlying Mood or Anxiety Disorder.

1. What is the patient's main sleep complaint(s)?

The patient's sleep complaints may or may not directly correlate with one specific Sleep Disorder. For example, daytime sleepiness is a symptom of several different Sleep Disorders, whereas repeated nightmares meet the criteria for a single disorder. Patients complain about three different problems: 1) difficulty falling asleep and staying asleep (Insomnia), 2) excessive sleeping during the day (Hypersomnia) or excessive sleepiness (Hypersomnolence), and 3) disturbed sleep.

Insomnia and hypersomnia are often experienced at the same time. Individuals are consciously aware of these two problems, but may not be aware of the third. For example, patients have no memory of Sleep Terrors or Sleepwalking. They are alerted to these problems by other people who observe their behavior. Therefore, a patient's sleep complaints may actually be complaints about the patient's behavior from people who sleep, or try to sleep, nearby.

2. Does the patient have an Axis I or Axis II disorder (other than a Sleep Disorder) that could produce the sleep disturbance?

Sleep problems may occur in the course of several psychiatric disorders (other than Sleep Disorders). For example, patients with Major Depressive Disorder, Generalized Anxiety Disorder, Dysthymic Disorder, or Schizophrenia may have a sleep disturbance. If the patient's insomnia or hypersomnia is judged to be related to another Axis I or Axis II disorder, and is sufficiently severe to warrant independent clinical attention, the patient should receive a diagnosis of either Insomnia Related to [Axis I or Axis II Disorder] or Hypersomnia Related to [Axis I or Axis II Disorder].

3. Does the patient have a General Medical Condition that could produce the sleep disturbance?

Several general medical conditions can produce sleep problems including pain; tumors; and cardiac, respiratory, endocrine, or metabolic diseases. The disturbance may be an insomnia, hypersomnia, parasomnia, or mixture of more than one disturbance. Patients who have a sleep disturbance that has developed in conjunction with physical illness should receive a diagnosis of one of the specific Sleep Disorders Due to a General Medical Condition (e.g., Sleep Disorder Due to a General Medical Condition, Insomnia Type 780.52, Sleep Disorder Due to a General Medical Condition, Parasomnia Type 780.59)

4. Is the patient abusing a substance that could produce a sleep disturbance?

Intoxication with or withdrawal from many substances interferes with sleep (e.g., alcohol, amphetamines, cocaine, opioids, and sedatives). The disturbance may be an insomnia, hypersomnia, parasomnia, or mixture of more than one disturbance. If the sleep disturbance develops within a month of significant substance intoxication or withdrawal, the patient should receive a diagnosis of a specific Substance-Induced Sleep Disorder (e.g., Alcohol Sleep Disorder, Insomnia Type With Onset During Withdrawal 292.89, Cocaine Sleep Dysfunction 292.89). If the sleep disturbance had its onset before the substance use, or lasts more than a month after substance use, the patient should receive the appropriate non-substance-induced Sleep Disorder diagnosis.

5. Is the patient's main complaint difficulty falling asleep or staying asleep?

Although patients with insomnia commonly have excessive daytime sleepiness, they tend to emphasize the difficulty falling or staying asleep over the daytime sleepiness.

- If an individual complains of insomnia that is not due to the direct effect of a substance and does not occur exclusively during the course of another specific Sleep Disorder or mental disorder, consider the diagnosis of Primary Insomnia.

- If an individual complains of insomnia that is not due to the direct effect of a substance but is judged to be related to another Axis I or Axis II disorder, consider the diagnosis of Insomnia Related to [Axis I or Axis II Disorder].

- If an individual complains of insomnia and there is evidence that it is related to a general medical condition or the direct effect of a substance, consider the diagnoses of Sleep Disorder Due to a General Medical Condition, Insomnia Type or Substance-Induced Sleep Disorder, Insomnia Type.

6. Is the patient's main complaint excessive sleeping (prolonged sleep episodes) or frequent daytime sleepiness?

- If an individual complains of excessive sleepiness that is not due to the direct effect of a substance and does not occur exclusively during the course of another specific Sleep Disorder or mental disorder, consider the diagnosis of Primary Hypersomnia.

- If an individual complains of multiple irresistible attacks of daytime sleep associated with cataplexy, hypnopompic/hypnogogic hallucinations, or sleep paralysis that is not due to the direct effect of a substance, consider the diagnosis Narcolepsy.

- If an individual complains of excessive sleepiness associated with loud snoring or periods of apnea that are not due to the direct effect of a substance and do not occur exclusively during the course of another mental disorder or general medical condition, consider the diagnosis of Breathing-Related Sleep Disorder.

- If an individual complains of excessive sleepiness that is not due to the direct effect of a substance but is judged to be related to another Axis I or Axis II disorder, consider the diagnosis of Hypersomnia Related to [Axis I or Axis II Disorder].

- If an individual complains of excessive sleepiness and there is evidence that it is related to a general medical condition or the direct effect of a substance, consider the diagnosis of Sleep Disorder Due to a General Medical Condition, Hypersomnia Type or Substance-Induced Sleep Disorder, Hypersomnia Type.

7. Is the patient's main complaint sleep disruption due to an altered sleep-wake schedule?

- If an individual complains of excessive sleepiness due to an unusual sleeping schedule that is not due to the direct effect of a substance and does not occur exclusively during the course of another specific Sleep Disorder or mental disorder, consider the diagnosis of Circadian Rhythm Sleep Disorder.

- If an individual complains of insomnia due to an unusual sleeping schedule that is not due to the direct effect of a substance and does not occur exclusively during the course of another specific Sleep Disorder or mental disorder, consider the diagnosis of Circadian Rhythm Sleep Disorder.

8. Is the patient's main complaint nightmares?

If the individual's main complaint is nightmares that cause repeated awakenings and that are not due to the direct effect of a substance, consider the diagnosis of Nightmare Disorder.

9. Is the main problem a complaint about the patient's sleep behavior from another person?

- If another person has reported to the patient that they wake in the middle of the night with a panicky scream accompanied by rapid heart rate, rapid breathing or sweating, and are unresponsive, and the symptoms are not due to a substance or general medical condition, consider the diagnosis of Sleep Terror Disorder.

- If another person has reported to the patient that they wake in the middle of the night and walk around and are unresponsive, and the symptoms are not due to a substance or general medical condition, consider the diagnosis of Sleepwalking Disorder.

- If another person has reported to the patient that they snore loudly at night and periodically stop breathing, and the symptoms are not due to a substance or general medical condition, consider the diagnosis of Breathing-Related Sleep Disorder.

Common Problems in Making a Diagnosis

There are three main areas of uncertainty in the differential diagnosis of Sleep Disorders.

1. Some patients' symptoms initially come close but don't actually fulfill the criteria for a specific diagnosis. More information or a further consideration of the diagnostic criteria may or may not resolve the problem. It may be difficult to establish a single etiology for the disturbance or the individual may have an unusual type of disturbance. For example, a patient may be abusing cocaine, have nighttime angina, and have insomnia.
2. Some patients' symptoms fulfill the diagnostic criteria for more than one Sleep Disorder during the course of their illness. For example, they may have excessive daytime sleepiness associated with a Breathing-Related Sleep Disorder and a Circadian Rhythm Sleep Disorder that overlap.

3. Many patients have sleep disturbances associated with other psychiatric disorders that do not fulfill the criteria for a specific Sleep Disorder.

Patients Who Almost Fulfill the Diagnostic Criteria

Most people experience difficulty with sleep at some period in their lives. A small portion of these individuals have a diagnosable Sleep Disorder. Sometimes it is difficult to determine when an individual has passed over the line separating normal sleep fluctuations from sleep pathology. The patient may have complaints that are consistent with a Sleep Disorder but do not completely fulfill the criteria for a specific diagnosis. Frequently, further inquiry will elicit the necessary additional clinical information. At other times it may be impossible to obtain the necessary information to determine whether the patient fulfills the criteria for Sleep Disorder.

Problems in fulfilling the criteria often relate to questions of the duration and the type of symptoms the patient has experienced. For example, a patient may have episodes of hypersomnia that individually last less than 1 month or multiple problems that all contribute to the Sleep Disorder without one problem predominating. In these situations, the clinician has to use his or her judgment to decide whether the patient should receive the diagnosis despite not having completely fulfilled the criteria.

Example 1

Arnie is a 44-year-old man who complains of repeated episodes of insomnia each lasting 2–3 weeks. He does not have an Axis I psychiatric disorder or general medical condition, and does not abuse any substances. What diagnosis(es), if any, should Arnie receive?

If Arnie's insomnia is not related to an Axis I psychiatric disorder, a general medical condition, or substance abuse, the only remaining diagnosis is Primary Insomnia. The criteria for this disorder require that the sleep disturbance last for at least 1 month. Arnie's episodes of insomnia last 2–3 weeks. If the episodes occur infrequently (e.g., once or twice a year), the diagnosis would not be appropriate. However, if the episodes occur several times a year, separated by only a few weeks, the diagnosis of Primary Insomnia is probably suitable.

Example 2

Sandy is a 25-year-old woman who has experienced sudden brief episodes of falling asleep at her desk at work for the last 2 months. The episodes have been associated with a loss of muscle tone during which she slumps in her chair. Sandy has also experienced brief vivid hallucinations when falling asleep at night during the same period of time. What diagnosis(es), if any, should Sandy receive?

Sandy fulfills all of the clinical criteria for Narcolepsy except for the duration requirement of 3 months. Technically she does not meet the criteria for the diagnosis. However, her symptoms are so characteristic of the disorder that it would be appropriate to give her a working diagnosis of Narcolepsy despite the short length of time.

Patients Who Fulfill the Diagnostic Criteria for More Than One Sleep Disorder

The diagnosis of some Sleep Disorders cannot be made if they occur exclusively during the course of another Sleep Disorder (e.g., Primary Insomnia, Primary Hypersomnia, Circadian Rhythm Sleep Disorder, Substance-Induced Sleep Disorder). However, the two diagnoses can be made if they overlap so that each disorder has a period of existence independent of the other. If the two disorders occur coincidentally, both diagnoses can still be made if they do not include criteria that exclude the diagnosis when it occurs exclusively during the course of another Sleep Disorder.

For example, the diagnosis of Circadian Rhythm Sleep Disorder cannot be made if the disorder occurs exclusively during the course of another mental disorder, such as a Major Depressive Disorder. On the other hand, the diagnosis of a Breathing-Related Sleep Disorder and a Nightmare Disorder can be made at the same time because they are not mutually exclusive.

Example 3

Carl is a 35-year-old salesman who flies back and forth across the country and to Europe for business several times a month during part of the year. He stays at home the remainder of the year. Carl complains of insomnia and excessive daytime sleepiness on his trips due to jet lag. His sleep disturbance disappears if he spends more than a week in the same city on business.

At home, when he isn't traveling, Carl complains of periods of insomnia that last several weeks after he has returned and often reoccur again after brief remissions. Carl does not have a general medical condition or psychiatric disorder and does not have a substance-abuse problem. What diagnosis(es), if any, should Carl receive?

Carl presents a complicated picture of sleep disturbances. He experiences insomnia and excessive daytime sleepiness due to sleep-wake schedule changes when he travels. These symptoms fulfill the criteria for a Circadian Rhythm Sleep Disorder. Carl also complains of insomnia when he isn't traveling. The insomnia continues for several weeks after he has returned home from his last trip and then reoccurs after brief remissions. This contrasts with his experience during trips when his insomnia resolves if he spends a week in the same city. The insomnia that occurs when he is home fulfills the criteria for a Primary Insomnia. It overlaps with the Circadian Rhythm Sleep Disorder. However, the sleep disturbance continues beyond the time when his sleep-wake schedule would be restored to normal. It also reoccurs independent his travel.

Sleep Symptoms Associated With Other Psychiatric or Medical Disorders

Sleep disturbance is a common symptom of many psychiatric illnesses including Mood Disorders, Anxiety Disorders, and Adjustment Disorders. Generally, the primary psychiatric disorder takes diagnostic precedence unless the sleep disturbance is of sufficient severity to warrant independent treatment. When a sleep disturbance occurs in conjunction with a Substance-Related Disorder or a General Medical Condition the diagnosis is either Sleep Disorder Due to a General Medical Condition or Substance-Induced Sleep Disorder, unless the patient meets the criteria for a specific Sleep Disorder. However, there are situations in which Sleep Disorder overlaps or is superimposed over another psychiatric disorder. In these cases, it may be appropriate to give the patient both diagnoses.

Example 4

Eleanor is a 36-year-old woman who routinely goes to sleep at 3:00 A.M., and would sleep until 10:00 A.M if she did not have to wake up at 7:00 A.M. for a job. She feels chronically sleep-deprived but is unable to fall asleep before 3:00 A.M. Eleanor has been late to work several times because she overslept. She catches up on her sleep on weekends.

Recently, since her mother's death 5 weeks ago, Eleanor has been depressed and has also had a loss of energy, guilt about her mother's death, difficulty concentrating, and a decreased appetite. She has had difficulty falling asleep at her normal time and awakens at 6:00 A.M. feeling exhausted. She is unable to sleep longer on weekends. What diagnosis(es), if any, should Eleanor receive?

Eleanor had an established sleep-wake schedule that was persistently delayed over the standard sleep-wake schedule in society and led to occupational problems. Her symptoms meet the criteria for Circadian Rhythm Sleep Disorder. Recently she has become depressed and has many of the accompanying symptoms of depression, including insomnia and early morning awakening when compared to her earlier sleep-wake schedule.

Her symptoms fulfill the criteria for a diagnosis of Major Depressive Disorder, Single Episode, with its accompanying sleep disturbance superimposed over her previous delayed sleep-wake schedule. Because the latter disorder existed independent of her depression, she can still receive the diagnosis of Circadian Rhythm Sleep Disorder. If her insomnia becomes severe enough to warrant independent treatment, the diagnosis of Insomnia Related to Major Depressive Disorder may also be appropriate.

Example 5

Edward is a 43-year-old man who has been worried about his job for the last 9 months, ever since some of his co-workers were fired in a company reorganization plan. He finds it difficult to control worrying about his job. During this time he has also felt irritable, on edge, and has been waking up early in the morning and obsessing about finding a new job. What diagnosis(es), if any, should Edward receive?

Edward fulfills the criteria for the diagnosis of a Generalized Anxiety Disorder. His early morning awakening occurs as a symptom of the Anxiety Disorder. He can only be given a separate Sleep Disorder diagnosis if his insomnia began before the Generalized Anxiety Disorder, or if it becomes severe enough to warrant independent clinical attention.

Precedence of Diagnosis

Several of the cases in preceding sections discuss diagnostic dilemmas that arise when patients have symptoms consistent with more than one diagnosis. The diagnoses may belong to the same diagnostic group (e.g., Sleep Disorders) or different groups (e.g., Mood Disorders and Sleep Disorders). When these conflicts occur, they are often resolved using the rules of diagnostic precedence that are included in the criteria for many diagnoses.

However, these rules require clinical judgment. For example, the diagnosis of Primary Insomnia cannot usually be made if the insomnia occurs exclusively during the course of Major Depressive Disorder. However, if the insomnia is of sufficient severity to require independent treatment beyond the treatment of the depression, the patient can be given a diagnosis of Insomnia Related to Major Depressive Disorder.

Therefore, the rules of diagnostic precedence, rather than taken as hard and firm, should be seen as guidelines. They suggest other diagnoses that should be considered before a specific diagnosis is made and they indicate the circumstances under which the diagnosis in question may be excluded if the patient fulfills the criteria for other diagnoses. Table 14–1 should be used as a reminder of those diagnoses that must be considered and excluded before a specific Mood Disorder diagnosis can be made.

Discussion of Clinical Vignette

I Feel Sleepy All the Time

Brendan is a medical intern who feels sleepy all the time. He is on call every third night and often falls asleep during his call or the next day on the medical ward. He

Table 14-1   Precedence of diagnosis for Sleep Disorders

Sleep Disorder	Disorders taking precedence
Primary Insomnia	Does not occur exclusively during Circadian Rhythm Sleep Disorder, Narcolepsy, Breathing-Related Sleep Disorder, Parasomnia, or another mental disorder Not due to effects of a substance or general medical condition
Primary Hypersomnia	Does not occur exclusively during another sleep disorder or mental disorder Not better accounted for by Insomnia or inadequate amount of sleep Not due to effects of a substance or general medical condition
Narcolepsy	Not due to effects of a substance or general medical condition
Breathing-Related Sleep Disorder	Not better accounted for by another mental disorder Not due to effects of a substance or general medical condition
Circadian Rhythm Sleep Disorder	Does not occur exclusively during another sleep disorder or mental disorder Not due to effects of a substance or general medical condition
Nightmare Disorder	Does not occur exclusively during another mental disorder Not due to effects of a substance or general medical condition
Sleep Terror Disorder Sleepwalking Disorder	Not due to effects of a substance or general medical condition
Insomnia Related to Another Mental Disorder Hypersomnia Related to Another Mental Disorder	Not better accounted for by another Sleep Disorder or inadequate amount of sleep Not due to effects of a substance or general medical condition
Sleep Disorder Due to a General Medical Condition	Does not meet criteria for Breathing-Related Sleep Disorder, Narcolepsy Does not occur exclusively during Delirium Not better accounted for by another mental disorder
Substance-Induced Sleep Disorder	Any non-substance-induced Sleep Disorder

Table 14-1 Precedence of diagnosis for Sleep Disorders *(continued)*	
Sleep Disorder	**Disorders taking precedence**
Dyssomnia NOS Parasomnia NOS	Any specific Sleep Disorder

Note. NOS = Not Otherwise Specified.

also misses rounds and makes mistakes in his work because he is sleepy. Brendan's problem is related to constant changes in his work schedule when he is on call in the hospital. He does not have time to adjust his schedule and make up for the lost sleep before he is on call again.

The appropriate diagnosis is Circadian Rhythm Sleep Disorder Shift Work Type. Some people, such as Brendan's attending physician and resident, do not have as much difficulty as he does making the adjustment to a rapidly shifting sleep-wake schedule.

Key Diagnostic Points

- Individuals with Nightmare Disorder awake from sleep with a frightening dream, rapidly become alert and oriented, and remember the dream. Individuals with Sleep Terror Disorder awake from sleep with a scream, remain unresponsive, and do not remember a dream.

- The diagnosis of Insomnia and Hypersomnia Related to [Axis I or Axis II disorder] is made when the patient has a sleep disturbance related to a psychiatric disorder but the disturbance is sufficiently severe to warrant independent treatment.

- Excessive daytime sleepiness and loud snoring are defining features of Breathing-Related Sleep Disorder (sleep apnea).

Common Questions in Making a Diagnosis

1. Thomas is a 24-year-old man who frequently wakes in the middle of the night and walks around the house. He appears somewhat dazed during these episodes but is responsive if others try to communicate with him and he remembers the event. What diagnosis(es), if any, should Thomas receive?

Answer: Patients with Sleepwalking Disorder are usually unresponsive to others who try to communicate with them, can only be awakened with difficulty, and have amnesia about the episode. Thomas can easily be aroused and remembers the sleepwalking event. Therefore he does not meet the criteria for Sleepwalking Disorder or any other specific Sleep Disorder. It is not clear whether his behavior is pathological or merely a variant of normal sleep behavior. If the behavior is judged to be abnormal, he could be given a diagnosis of Parasomnia Not Otherwise Specified.

2. Jonathan is an overweight 47-year-old man who complains of excessive daytime sleepiness and repeated nightmares. The nightmares consist of frightening dreams that someone is trying to strangle him. He awakes from the dream anxious and gasping for breath. What diagnosis(es), if any, should Jonathan receive?

   Answer: Jonathan has Nightmare Disorder. However, excessive daytime sleepiness is not usually a symptom of Nightmare Disorder. The excessive sleepiness, his weight, and his gasping during the night suggest that Jonathan may also have another disorder that disturbs his sleep. The most likely candidate is Breathing-Related Sleep Disorder. This diagnosis is supported further if he snores loudly and has periods when he stops breathing for several seconds during the night.

3. Ernest is a 38-year-old man who is moderately obese. He sleeps well and is wide awake and active during the day. His wife complains that his loud snoring during the night, disturbs her sleep, leaves her sleepy during the day. What diagnosis(es), if any, should Ernest receive?

   Answer: Ernest snores loudly but does not have insomnia or excessive daytime sleepiness. Therefore he does not fulfill the criteria for Breathing-Related Sleep Disorder. Not all patients who snore have a sleep apnea syndrome. In this case, the wife has a sleep disturbance caused by Ernest's snoring.

4. Sally is a 45-year-old woman who complains of insomnia. She also admits to feeling depressed and worthless for the last several months since she lost her job. During the day she has a poor appetite and little energy or interest in her usual activities. She has never felt this way before. What diagnosis(es), if any, should Sally receive?

   Answer: Sally fulfills the criteria for Major Depressive Disorder, Single Episode. Her insomnia is a symptom of the depression. If it becomes severe enough to warrant treatment beyond that given for the depression, she could receive a diagnosis of Insomnia Related to Major Depressive Disorder.

5. Christy is a 15-year-old girl who periodically awakens in the middle of the night screaming, with rapid breathing and tachycardia. She becomes oriented after several seconds and soon calms down and returns to sleep. In the morning she remembers the dream and often talks about it at breakfast. What diagnosis(es), if any, should Christy receive?

Answer: The differential diagnosis for Christy's symptoms is Nightmare Disorder versus Sleep Terror Disorder. The latter diagnosis includes an abrupt awakening from sleep with a panicky scream, accompanied by intense anxiety and signs of autonomic arousal. However, in Sleep Terror Disorder the individual is not easily aroused and does not remember a dream or recall the episode. Christy is easily aroused and does recall the details of the dream. Therefore, her diagnosis is Nightmare Disorder.

6. Sid is a 32-year-old man who has excessive daytime sleepiness. His wife reports that he frequently kicks her in bed at night and briefly wakes up after each episode. Sid does not snore but his repeated kicking led the couple to move to twin beds from their original double bed. He does not remember kicking in the morning. What diagnosis(es), if any, should Sid receive?

Answer: Sid's persistent kicking episodes followed by a brief arousal are characteristic of nocturnal myoclonus. The lack of snoring or periods of apnea help differentiate the disorder from sleep apnea, which is also associated with hyperactivity. The diagnosis is Dyssomnia Not Otherwise Specified.

7. Joan is a 31-year-old woman who complains of insomnia. She has chronic pain from an old back injury that required surgery. She currently uses cocaine. Joan complains that her back pain keeps her awake at night and she needs pain medication and sleep medication. What diagnosis(es), if any, should Joan receive?

Answer: Joan has two possible etiologies for her insomnia. Cocaine intoxication/withdrawal and chronic pain are both associated with a sleep disturbance. Because it is difficult to determine which of these is the primary cause for her insomnia, the diagnosis is Dyssomnia Not Otherwise Specified.

Impulse-Control Disorders Not Elsewhere Classified

Clinical Vignette

I'm Just Trying to Get Even

Craig is a 32-year-old dentist with two children who is separated and undergoing bankruptcy proceedings. In retrospect, the roots of Craig's current problems were already evident during the last semester of his senior year in high school. He had been accepted to a prestigious college and had completed all of the requirements for graduation. Craig had always been a serious student with little time for anything but studying. Suddenly he had few academic responsibilities. He began spending time with a small group of friends from wealthy families who were accustomed to gambling on horses and cards. Craig didn't have much money but he found his small bets and modest winnings at poker and the race track exhilarating in a way that he had not experienced before.

Craig did well in college and was accepted to dental school. He continued to play cards and bet on the horses with a local bookmaker. By now he was a sophisticated card player and generally came out a little ahead after an evening's game. He was less successful betting on the horses, but found the process more challenging. Poker was a science but horse racing was truly a gamble. The sense that he was submitting some small element of his life to the vagaries of fate excited him even if he did not win much money.

While in dental school he began working on a system to beat the odds in horse races. His system provided little more success than random betting. In his third year of dental school Craig met his wife Betsy. They were married when he graduated. A year after they were married their first child was born, followed by a second child 18 months later. Craig opened a practice specializing in cosmetic dentistry and, within 3–4 years, was doing very well financially.

He continued to work on his system of betting. As he earned more money, he bet more on the horses using his system. Craig never told his wife how much money he spent on horse racing. To save time, he made the bets from his office using a local bookmaker. He paid careful attention to the horses' statistics, bet judiciously, and generally came out ahead in his bets.

Gradually, Craig began to increase the amount he bet. One day, after careful analysis, he bet a large sum of money on a horse that was running with 10 to 1 odds. The horse won and Craig collected an enormous amount of money. He was elated and convinced that he now had a surefire system for beating the odds. He bought his wife a new car and they took a 3-week vacation to Europe with their children.

When Craig returned from his vacation, his optimism was boundless. He no longer became excited with the careful small bets he used to make. Now, he routinely made large bets with the sure conviction that he could not lose. The heavy stakes excited him. But now his luck began to change and he lost more often than he won. He tried to cut back or stop gambling several times, but each time he became irritable and restless and eventually resumed betting.

Rather than becoming more judicious or conservative, Craig became frantic and increased his betting. He structured his life and practice around betting on the horses. He called his bookmaker several times a day to place bets and determine how he was doing. Often he stopped in the middle of caring for a patient to call the bookmaker. As his losses continued, he bet more money, trying to get even and recoup what he had lost.

Craig began spending the money in the couple's savings accounts to fund his gambling. When his wife discovered that the money was missing, she confronted him about his gambling. Craig lied to her and stated that he had used the money to invest in a small dental supply firm. His wife was suspicious but believed him.

As Craig continued to gamble and lose he began to gamble the money he needed to pay school loans, suppliers, and the mortgage. When his wife saw the mortgage default notices she confronted him again. Craig finally admitted that he was gambling and agreed to see someone in therapy. However, the therapy was unsuccessful. Craig began borrowing money from friends and then loan sharks for gambling.

Finally, after a year of financial uncertainty, his wife took the children and left. Craig's dental practice fell apart as he desperately tried to gather more money to continue betting and reclaim his losses. Finally, he declared bankruptcy. Even then he pleaded with the bookmaker to take a few small bets with the money he had in his pocket.

Core Concept of the Diagnostic Group

The core concept of Impulse-Control Disorders is the repeated expression of impulsive acts that lead to physical or financial damage to the individual or another person, and often result in a sense of relief or release of tension.

Definition

impulse   A sudden, difficult-to-resist urge or drive to perform an act that often results in a sense of relief or release of tension.

Synopses and Diagnostic Prototypes of the Individual Disorders

The brief synopses in this section include the specific requirements or criteria that must be fulfilled for each of the diagnostic categories. Following each synopsis is a vignette that provides a clinical example of the diagnosis. The Impulse-Control Disorders group contains five specific disorders that are united solely by the deleterious nature of the individual's impulsive act.

312.34   Intermittent Explosive Disorder.   Individuals with this disorder have several discrete episodes of loss of control of aggressive impulses, resulting in serious assaultive acts or destruction of property that are grossly out of proportion to the precipitating stressors.

> Ross is a 25-year-old electrician who has had difficulty keeping a job. Although he is considered a good electrician, the other men on the job find it difficult to work with him. One of Ross' co-workers recently described the problem to his supervisor. "Ross and I was working together wiring the second floor of this house. He asked me to pass him something and I didn't hear, so I says, 'Stop mumbling Ross. Open your mouth and tell me what you want.' Suddenly he jumps up and hits me in the jaw. Then he's really sorry and apologizes. Three days later he does the same thing again. I can't work with him."
>
> Ross admits that he sometimes loses his temper and refers to the episodes as "attacks" that he can't control. Despite repeated warnings, the episodes continue. Finally, he is fired. Ross also has "attacks" while driving on the expressway. These usually occur when he thinks another driver has slighted him. He usually responds by racing after the other driver and trying to cut him off. His aggressive driving has caused at least three accidents. Ross generally feels guilty or depressed after each of the episodes.

312.32   Kleptomania.   Individuals with this disorder fail to resist impulses to steal objects they do not need. The theft is not committed to express anger or vengeance, and is not a response to a delusion or hallucination. The individual experiences an increasing sense of tension before the theft and pleasure, gratification, or relief while committing the theft.

> Betty is a 33-year-old homemaker who lives in the suburbs and spends much of her free time doing volunteer work at the hospital where her husband is the chief of surgery. When she isn't at the hospital or driving her children to various

activities, she goes out with friends.

Recently Betty was shopping in the local mall. While her friend was in another part of the store she walked over to the cosmetics section. As she examined the various cosmetics Betty became tense and felt a strong urge to steal something. She initially tried to resist the impulse. Suddenly, as she watched the saleswoman turn away to help another customer, she couldn't resist further. Betty snatched a lipstick from the counter and dropped it into her purse. She immediately felt a great sense of relief and slowly walked away to join her friend.

As the two women walked out of the department store, Betty was stopped by three security guards. They insisted that she accompany them to the store manager's office. Once there, the manager asked her if she had taken anything from the store without paying for it. Betty initially said no but finally admitted the theft when the manager played a videotape showing her taking the lipstick from the counter. He stated that the store policy was to press charges against shoplifters.

Betty pleaded with him to release her, stating that she was often unable to stop herself from taking small things. She indicated that she would pay for the lipstick. The manager finally agreed to release her but insisted that she sign a statement admitting the theft and agreeing not to enter the store again. Betty signed the statement and was released. She was too embarrassed to tell her friend what she had done. Instead, she made up a story about losing her charge cards and going to the manager's office to retrieve them.

312.33   Pyromania.   Individuals with this disorder are fascinated with fires and have deliberately and purposefully set fires on more than one occasion. The individual experiences a sense of tension or affective arousal preceding the fire-setting act and pleasure, gratification, or relief once they set or witness a fire. The fire is not set for monetary gain, to make a political statement, to conceal criminal activity, to express anger or vengeance, to improve one's living circumstances, or in response to a delusion or hallucination.

Jeff is a 25-year-old man who works as a janitor in a large apartment building. He has always been fascinated with fire. As a child he set small fires in the backyard of his house and in nearby vacant lots. His fire-setting activities came to the attention of the authorities when he was 10 years old and set a fire that destroyed a deserted house in the neighborhood. Jeff stood nearby and watched as the fire trucks came to put the fire out. He was later identified by neighbors who saw him enter the house before the fire.

Three years later Jeff's family moved to another larger city. Jeff had never been a good student and did worse in his new school. He spent much of his time when he wasn't in school visiting the local fire house. During the same period he set several small fires in nearby communities but was never caught.

When he was age 18, Jeff tried to join a nearby volunteer fire company but was not accepted. He was disappointed and angry. In response he started a fire in an apartment building in a adjacent neighborhood. Jeff contrived to casually drive by the building just before the firemen arrived. Once there, he helped the inhabitants of the apartments escape. Jeff hoped that this episode would demonstrate his bravery and make the members of the volunteer fire company reconsider and accept him as a fellow fire fighter.

312.31   Pathological Gambling.   Individuals with this disorder have persistent and recurrent maladaptive gambling behavior as indicated by at least five of the following:

1. Preoccupation with gambling (e.g., preoccupied with reliving past gambling experiences, handicapping or planning the next venture, or thinking of ways to get money with which to gamble).
2. Needs to gamble with increasing amounts of money in order to achieve the desired excitement.
3. Repeated unsuccessful efforts to control, cut back , or stop gambling.
4. Restlessness or irritability when attempting to cut down or stop gambling.
5. Gambles as a way of escaping from problems or of relieving dysphoric mood (e.g., feelings of helplessness, guilt, anxiety, depression).
6. After losing money gambling, often returns another day in order to get even ("chasing" one's losses).
7. Lies to family members, therapists, or others to conceal the extent of involvement with gambling.
8. Has committed illegal acts such as forgery, fraud, theft, or embezzlement, in order to finance gambling.
9. Has jeopardized or lost a significant relationship, job, or career opportunity because of gambling.
10. Reliance on others to provide money to relieve a desperate financial situation caused by gambling.

Hank is a 19-year-old, intelligent student in his junior year at college. He grew up in a tumultuous home with an alcoholic father who could not keep a job. Hank was mildly depressed during most of his high school years and soon found that playing cards and gambling helped relieve his feelings of depression. He did reasonably well in high school because he was able to memorize large amounts of information in a relatively short time to prepare for his examinations. His performance on a nationwide test won him a small scholarship to a nearby state university.

In college he continued to gamble, spending much of his time playing pool and poker with a small group of other students. Hank skipped most of his lectures and courses during the year. He passed his courses by borrowing lecture notes from classmates and again memorizing the necessary material a few days before the final examinations. During his first 2 years in college Hank was content to gamble with his classmates. He won a moderate amount of money.

In his junior year Hank began to feel more depressed about his lack of direction and his sense that he was missing out on life. His gambling no longer produced the same excitement it had in his first 2 years. He went to the student counseling service and tried to stop gambling several times unsuccessfully. Each time he became anxious and restless.

Eventually, he became involved with a group of men in the local town who played poker and blackjack every evening. The men bet considerably more than his fellow students. Hank discovered that the high stakes restored the original excitement he had felt when he started gambling. However, the men were experienced card players and Hank often lost money playing with them. He began borrowing money from his friends and family to cover his gambling losses. When his parents became concerned, he lied and told them he needed to buy additional books and that his living expenses had increased.

312.39   Trichotillomania.   Individuals with this disorder repeatedly pull out their hair. The individual experiences an increasing sense of tension before pulling out the hair and pleasure, gratification, or relief when pulling out the hair.

Mandy is an 26-year-old married woman who is depressed and in treatment with a psychiatrist. The depression began several months ago when her marriage began to deteriorate after she discovered her husband was having an affair with another woman.

Three months after treatment began, the therapist commented that Mandy's hair looked different. Mandy admitted, for the first time, that she had a habit of pulling her hair out. She revealed a bald spot on the top of her head that she had covered by changing her hair style. Mandy explained that she started pulling her hair out when she was 8 years old and her parents went through a rancorous divorce. Following the divorce, her mother had to return to work and had little time to spend with her. Mandy began pulling her hair when she was alone. She felt a sense of tension before and a sense of relief or pleasure during and after she pulled the hair out. Mandy felt no pain when she pulled her hair. Each time she ran the few strands of hair through her mouth before throwing it away.

Mandy's hair pulling was a chronic condition that waxed and waned. In the early years of her marriage, before the fights with her husband began, she stopped the behavior and her hair regrew in the bald spots. She started pulling it again as her marriage began to fail.

312.30   Impulse-Control Disorder Not Otherwise Specified.   Individuals with this disorder have problems with impulse control that do not meet the criteria for any specific Impulse-Control Disorder.

Necessary Clinical Information

* Repeated episodes of stealing not motivated by monetary gain or vengeance

- Unexplained hair loss in unusual areas of the body

- Repeated financial difficulties in a person who appears to make adequate money

- Repeated gambling

- Sudden episodes of violence that are not warranted by the obvious stressor

- Repeated episodes of deliberate fire setting not motivated by monetary gain or vengeance

Making a Diagnosis

Impulse-Control Disorders are a heterogeneous and idiosyncratic group of syndromes that do not fit into any larger group of illnesses such as Eating Disorders, Paraphilias, and Substance-Related Disorders, that are similarly characterized by a loss of control over impulses.

The five disorders in this group are so different that it is impossible to confuse them diagnostically. Their differential diagnosis depends on distinguishing a specific disorder from illnesses with similar symptoms in other diagnostic groups. The following questions are organized to pursue a differential diagnosis for each disorder with the assumption that the behavior characteristic of that disorder has already been identified.

1. Has the individual had several episodes of sudden, serious, violent behavior that are grossly out of proportion to any precipitating event?

Aggressive and violent behavior are common symptoms of many psychiatric illnesses. Intermittent Explosive Disorder is a diagnosis of exclusion that can only be made once all other possible causes of violence are ruled out. The most obvious disorders to consider are those that include aggressive behavior as a part of their diagnostic criteria, such Antisocial Personality Disorder, Borderline Personality Disorder, and Conduct Disorder. Patients with acute Psychotic Disorder or manic episode can also display violent behavior.

Children or adolescents with Attention-Deficit/Hyperactivity Disorder can appear aggressive when they force themselves into situations with other people without respecting normal social restraints. Violent agitation also accompanies intoxication or withdrawal from a number of substances, such as phencyclidine. Finally, certain general medical conditions, such as seizures in the amygdala, are sometimes associated with violent outbursts.

2. Has the patient repeatedly stolen objects that are not needed for personal use or for their monetary value?

The main diagnostic task is differentiating between Kleptomania and other forms of stealing. The key distinguishing characteristics of Kleptomania are that the individual attempts to resist the impulse to steal, there is pleasure or relief after the theft, and the stolen items are not needed for personal use or monetary gain. Attempts to sell the stolen items are not consistent with a diagnosis of Kleptomania.

The diagnosis of Kleptomania is excluded if the individual has Conduct Disorder, Antisocial Personality Disorder, or Borderline Personality Disorder and steals for vengeance or monetary gain. The diagnosis similarly cannot be made in psychotic patients who have command hallucinations telling them to steal and cognitively impaired patients who are unaware that they are stealing. Neither of these types of patients have a sense of pleasure or relief after the theft.

3. Has the patient deliberately and purposefully set fires on several occasions?

The main diagnostic task is distinguishing between Pyromania and fire setting for profit, vengeance, or sabotage. The key distinguishing characteristic of Pyromania is the lack of any motivation other than a fascination with the fire and its associated characteristics.

The diagnosis of Pyromania is excluded if the individual has Antisocial Personality Disorder or Conduct Disorder and sets the fires for profit or vengeance. Similarly, the diagnosis of Pyromania cannot be made if an individual has Psychotic Disorder with command hallucinations telling him to set a fire, or an organic impairment with associated cognitive impairment and is unaware of setting a fire.

4. Does the person gamble excessively despite significant deleterious effects on his or her financial, social, occupational, or interpersonal activities?

The main diagnostic task is distinguishing between normal social gambling and Pathological Gambling. The latter diagnosis is excluded if the individual does not need to gamble to maintain excitement, does not experience self-esteem as intimately linked to winning and losing at gambling, and can place limits on the amount gambled and the time and effort devoted to gambling. The diagnosis is also excluded if the gambling occurs exclusively in the context of a manic episode.

5. Does the individual persistently pull out his or her hair resulting in noticeable hair loss?

The diagnosis of Trichotillomania can be excluded if an individual does not experience pleasure or a sense of relief from pulling out his or her hair. In Obsessive-Compulsive Disorders the hair pulling is not experienced as pleasurable and has a symbolic meaning beyond the act itself.

Common Problems in Making a Diagnosis

Impulse Control Disorders are such a disparate group of diagnoses that there is rarely a difficulty with a patient's symptoms fulfilling the criteria for more than one diagnosis in the group. Typically, problems may occur when a patient does not quite fulfill the criteria for a specific impulse control diagnosis or when the disorder occurs in the context of other psychiatric symptoms or disorders. In some of the latter cases, the rules of diagnostic precedence guide the diagnosis.

Patients Who Almost Fulfill the Diagnostic Criteria

One of the main challenges in the diagnosis of Impulse-Control Disorder is determining whether the individual's behavior is driven by an impulse that is difficult to resist or whether it is motivated by other factors such as vengeance, profit, or other external circumstances. For example, an individual who pulls his hair out because he is distraught over a personal loss and feels no pleasure or relief in the act, does not fulfill the criteria for Trichotillomania.

Example 1

Ginny is a 38-year-old woman who is unable to resist stealing small items. She feels tension before and relief after the theft and subsequently uses the stolen property or sells it. What diagnosis(es), if any, should Ginny receive?

The criteria for the diagnosis of Kleptomania requires that the individual steal objects that are not needed for personal use or for their monetary value. Ginny's symptoms do not appear to fulfill this part of the criteria. However, suppose the thefts are motivated by an impulse she cannot resist and subsequently she decides to keep or sell the item. The clinician must use his or her judgment to decide if the gain from the stolen objects partially motivates subsequent thefts, even if they are primarily driven by impulses. If so, the diagnosis of Kleptomania is excluded.

Example 2

Nick is a 32-year-old man who enjoys setting fires and is fascinated by all aspects of fires. He feels tense and excited before setting the fire and gratified while watching the fire. Occasionally Nick is paid to set a fire. He feels as gratified by those fires as the ones he sets spontaneously. What diagnosis(es), if any, should Nick receive?

The criteria for the diagnosis of Pyromania requires that the fires not be set for monetary gain. Nick's symptoms meet this part of the criteria for the majority of the fires he sets. However, he sets some fires to make money. Although he may fulfill the criteria for Pyromania for the fires he sets spontaneously, he does not meet the criteria for the fires he sets for profit. The latter have no psychiatric diagnosis.

Impulse Symptoms Associated With Other Psychiatric Disorders

Impulse-Control Disorders may occur in conjunction with other psychiatric symptoms or disorders. The diagnosis will often depend on whether the patient fulfills the criteria for the other disorder.

Example 3

Harold is a 37-year-old man who has felt depressed, on and off, for several years. When he feels depressed, he gambles on horses. Recently he has become more preoccupied with gambling and finds it difficult to stop despite repeated efforts. Harold becomes irritable and more depressed when he tries to stop. The gambling has significantly interfered with his work and he has had to borrow money from his brother to cover his gambling debts. What diagnosis(es), if any, should Harold receive?

Harold's symptoms fulfill the criteria for Pathological Gambling. He should also be evaluated for a Major Depressive Episode. The diagnosis of Major Depressive Disorder, Single Episode, does not exclude the diagnosis of Pathological Gambling.

Precedence of Diagnosis

Table 15–1 lists the disorders that take precedence in the diagnosis of Impulse-Control Disorders.

Table 15–1 Precedence of diagnosis for Impulse Control Disorders	
Impulse Control Disorder	**Disorders taking precedence**
Intermittent Explosive Disorder	Not better accounted for by Antisocial Personality Disorder; Borderline Personality Disorder; Psychotic Disorder
Kleptomania	Not better accounted for by Conduct Disorder, Manic Episode, or Antisocial Personality Disorder
Pyromania	Not better accounted for by Conduct Disorder, Manic Episode, or Antisocial Personality Disorder Not due to effects of a substance or general medical condition
Pathological Gambling	Not better accounted for by Manic Episode
Trichotillomania	Not better accounted for by another mental disorder Not due to a general medical condition
Impulse Control Disorder NOS	Does not meet criteria for any specific Impulse Control Disorder

Note. NOS = Not Otherwise Specified.

Discussion of Clinical Vignette

I'm Just Trying to Get Even

Craig was a hardworking student who began gambling in high school and found it exciting. Eventually he concentrated his gambling on horse races and tried to develop a system to beat the betting odds. His initial betting was restrained and judicious and he had modest winnings. One day, after he had established a successful dental practice, Craig won a substantial amount of money.

After that his pattern of gambling changed and began to fulfill the criteria for the diagnosis of Pathological Gambling. He became convinced that he could not lose and needed to bet more and more to maintain the initial excitement he had felt while gambling. Craig became careless and started to lose money, but responded by betting more money in an attempt to get even or recoup his losses. He tried to stop several times but in each instance he became irritable and restless and finally returned to gambling.

Soon the gambling began to interfere with his practice and he began using the money he needed for the mortgage and other bills to pay his gambling debts. When his wife confronted him about the money, he lied to her. Eventually, as he became desperate, Craig borrowed from friends and loan sharks to finance his gambling addiction.

Key Diagnostic Points

• The objects stolen by individuals who have Kleptomania are not needed for personal use or monetary gain.

• In Kleptomania, Pyromania, and Trichotillomania there is a sense of tension before the act, and pleasure, gratification, or relief after the act.

Common Questions in Making a Diagnosis

1. Ann is a 42-year-old woman who was caught selling several pieces of jewelry that she stole from various department stores. At the time she was arrested, she was wearing two pieces of stolen jewelry. At her trial Ann pleaded that she was a victim of Kleptomania and had no control over her stealing. What diagnosis(es), if any, should Ann receive?

   Answer: The diagnosis of Kleptomania cannot be made if the individual steals objects for personal use or monetary gain. Ann's thefts seem to be motivated by personal gain despite what she says. It would be useful to determine whether any of her thefts were planned in advance rather than a spontaneous response to impulses she could not control.

2. Sam works for the city as a building inspector. He and his fellow workers usually take a break during the afternoon to play poker for money. They also play two nights a week. Sam is restless when he can't play cards and constantly reviews the previous game in his mind to identify any mistakes he might have made. When he loses, he can't wait for the next game to recoup his losses. Generally he comes out even or slightly ahead in his gambling. The men have been discovered gambling in the past and warned that they may lose their jobs. However, they continue to play during work hours. Sam often lies to his wife about the extent of his gambling and tells her that he must work late hours in the evenings. What diagnosis(es), if any, should Sam receive?

   Answer: Sam fulfills the criteria for Pathological Gambling because of his constant preoccupation with gambling rather than any financial hardship it produces. He is involved in a work culture that encourages the gambling. It is difficult to know whether he would have difficulty stopping his gambling if he got another job. The diagnosis of Pathological Gambling usually implies that the gambling behavior is independent of the social environment.

Adjustment Disorders

Clinical Vignette

Nuts to You, Please

Chelsey is a 31-year-old married woman who went to work for a local bank after graduating from college. She did well in her job and received several promotions, finally becoming the assistant manager of one of the bank's branch offices 3 years ago. Two years ago her bank merged with a larger regional bank. A new manager was appointed to run her branch office and Chelsey's responsibilities were increased although her authority was decreased. She did not get along well with the new manager and applied for a transfer to another branch office. The transfer was not approved and the relationship with her new boss deteriorated further.

Chelsey had always had a fantasy of opening a small business of her own despite her interest and investment in her banking career. After several months of discussions with her husband, she decided to quit her job at the bank and open her own nut and candy store in a nearby shopping mall. She borrowed the necessary money and 6 months later opened a small shop called "Everybody's Nuts." Business was slow at first. For the first 6 months she did not make enough money to cover her expenses. Gradually, sales increased. Chelsey developed several clever marketing promotions, including a nut and flower bouquet for anniversaries and birthdays. By the end of her first year in business she was making a modest profit.

Business continued to improve and she began to develop a line of custom chocolates. At the end of her second year, business was good enough that Chelsey considered opening a second store in another mall. She was in the midst of planning for the second store when a candy discount store opened a few blocks from Chelsey's mall. The new store was part of a nationwide chain of large candy shops that sold assorted nuts and gourmet chocolates at low prices. The discount store did not affect Chelsey's business immediately because she had developed a number of loyal customers. However, within 4 months her sales had dropped significantly.

Chelsey became increasingly irritable and depressed. She had periods of fearfulness and difficulty sleeping. Her appetite remained intact and she actually gained 2–3 pounds from eating some of her own nuts and candy. Her husband was supportive and tried to encourage her by making suggestions that might increase her business. Chelsey tried several marketing ploys but could not effectively compete against the new store. Finally, after 3 years in business she had to close her store.

Chelsey continued to feel depressed for 3–4 months after she closed her store. She spent her time helping her husband in his business and reestablishing some of her old friendships. The couple talked about having children. Chelsey wanted to have a child but she did not want it to be a consolation prize for an unsuccessful business career. Gradually, her depression resolved and she began making plans to start another small business and have a child.

Core Concept of the Diagnostic Group

The core concept of Adjustment Disorders is the development of emotional or behavior symptoms in response to an identifiable stressor(s).

Definitions

stressor   An event or stimulus that produces a psychological, emotional, or behavioral stress response in an individual.

Synopses and Diagnostic Prototypes
of the Individual Disorders

The various diagnoses in the Adjustment Disorders group are differentiated by the type of response to the stressor(s). The diagnostic criteria are the same for all Adjustment Disorders.

Adjustment Disorders

Individuals with this disorder develop emotional or behavioral symptoms (other than during bereavement) in response to an identifiable stressor(s). The symptoms occur within 3 months of the onset of the stressor(s), last for a maximum of 6 months after termination of the stressor, and are either in excess of what would be expected from exposure to the stressor or significantly impair the individual's functioning. The disturbance does not meet the criteria for any specific Axis I disorder or represent an exacerbation of a preexisting Axis I or Axis II disorder. Specify the duration and type of disorder.

Acute: if the symptoms have persisted for less than 6 months.

Chronic: if the symptoms have persisted for 6 months or longer.

Type of Adjustment Disorder response	DSM-IV code
With Anxiety	309.24
With Depressed Mood	309.0
With Disturbance of Conduct	309.3
With Mixed Disturbance of Emotions and Conduct	309.4
With Mixed Anxiety and Depressed Mood	309.28
Unspecified	309.9

Elliott is a 67-year-old man who recently retired as the president of a large company where he had worked for the last 25 years. The Board of Trustees held a testimonial dinner for him during his last week at work. At the dinner several speakers stood up to praise his wise leadership of the company during difficult economic times. Elliott thanked them all for their kind words and explained that he was looking forward to relaxing and doing nothing for the next several months. One Board member yelled, "Sure Elliott, you're going to sit home and knit for 6 months." The audience laughed and Elliott smiled.

Elliott spent the next couple of days cleaning out his office. He began to feel a little depressed when he noticed that his secretary and staff were already accommodating to his departure. They were polite but seemed somewhat distant and were preparing for the new president. On his last day, Elliott walked around the main office and personally said good-bye to everyone. One administrator commented, "I wish I could retire and play golf all day like you." Elliott smiled but felt a queasy sensation in the pit of his stomach accompanied by some anxiety. He went home that night feeling mildly depressed and anxious about what he would do for rest of his life.

The next morning he woke up early, had breakfast, and went to his club to play golf with three business colleagues. The group played nine holes of golf, showered, and had lunch. When they finished, Elliott suggested they take a walk. One of the men laughed and said, "You're a free man Elliott. We're still part of the daily grind. I have to go back to the office." The men left and Elliott took a short walk around the grounds of the club. He felt restless and irritable. That night he had little appetite for dinner and difficulty falling asleep. He woke up at 4:30 A.M feeling anxious, worried, and depressed about his future.

Elliott avoided the club and his business friends for several weeks. He sat home and watched television, but found it difficult to sit still for more than a few minutes. Elliott's wife observed her husband's behavior for several weeks. She suggested they take a vacation or visit their children. Elliott was not interested. Finally, one night at dinner, she said, "I think you're upset about retiring. You need to find something useful to do with your life." Elliott was irritated at first by her comments and then nodded. "This isn't what I expected retirement to be like," he said. The diagnosis is Adjustment Disorders With Mixed Anxiety and Depressed Mood

Necessary Clinical Information

- Time of onset and duration of the stressor

- Time of onset and duration of the symptoms

- Inappropriate or antisocial behavior

- Depressed mood

- Anxiety

Making a Diagnosis

The diagnosis of Adjustment Disorder depends on the identification of a stressor that is causally connected to a disturbance in the patient's mood, anxiety, or conduct. The patient may or may not be consciously aware of the causal relationship between the two. The identification of this link is the crucial component of the diagnosis. The following questions provide an organized approach to the diagnosis.

1. Does the patient have a depressed mood, excessive anxiety, or a disturbance in conduct that does not meet the criteria for a specific Axis I or II disorder?

If the patient's depressed mood, excessive anxiety, or disturbance in conduct meets the criteria for a specific Axis I or Axis II disorder, the diagnosis of Adjustment Disorder is excluded. For example, if the patient meets the criteria for Major Depressive Disorder or Antisocial Personality Disorder, these diagnoses take precedence over the diagnosis of Adjustment Disorder.

2. Are the patient's emotional or behavioral symptoms a response to an identifiable stressor(s)?

The occurrence of emotional or behavioral symptoms coincident with one or more stressors does not automatically indicate that they are causally connected. The causal relationship can be confirmed by the patient or based on the physician's clinical judgment. If the stressor(s) is not related to the patient's symptoms, the diagnosis of Adjustment Disorder is excluded.

3. Have the patient's symptoms occurred within 3 months of the onset or 6 months of the termination of the stressor(s)?

- If the patient's symptoms have not occurred within 3 months of the onset of the stressor(s), they are not considered to be etiologically related for diagnostic purposes.

- If the patient's symptoms have lasted substantially longer than 6 months after the termination of the stressor(s), the diagnosis of Adjustment Disorder is excluded.

Common Problems in Making a Diagnosis

There are two main areas of uncertainty in the differential diagnosis of Adjustment Disorders.

1. Some patient's symptoms come close but don't actually fulfill the criteria for a diagnosis of Adjustment Disorder. More information or a further consideration of the diagnostic criteria may or may not resolve the problem.
2. Some patients have isolated symptoms of stress associated with other psychiatric disorders but do not fulfill the criteria for a specific Mood Disorder.

Patients Who Almost Fulfill the Diagnostic Criteria

A patient's symptoms may almost fulfill the criteria for Adjustment Disorders in two ways. It may be difficult to determine if the stressor(s) is related to the patient's symptoms or the patient's symptoms may not meet the duration criteria for Adjustment Disorder.

Example 1

Boris is a 38-year-old man who was divorced a year ago. Boris' wife initiated the divorce against Boris' wishes. He has been depressed about the divorce for the last year. What diagnosis(es), if any, should Boris receive?

Boris' depression is a response to the divorce. However, the criteria for the diagnosis of Adjustment Disorder requires that the patient's symptoms not persist for more than 6 months after the termination of the stressor. If the divorce action itself is the stressor, Boris does not meet the criteria for the diagnosis of Adjustment Disorder With Depressed Mood. Under these circumstances, the appropriate diagnosis would be Depressive Disorder Not Otherwise Specified. However, it could be argued that Boris' stressor is the condition of being divorced. In this situation the clinician must use his judgment to decide whether the criteria are met for the diagnosis of Adjustment Disorder.

Stress and Other Psychiatric Disorders

A significant stressor(s) may occur while the patient has another psychiatric disorder. Under some circumstances, it is appropriate to make an additional diagnosis of Adjustment Disorder. In other situations the precedence of diagnosis determines which diagnosis can be given to the patient.

Example 2

Monica is a 41-year-old woman who has been mildly to moderately depressed for several years. During that time she has felt inadequate, irritable, and pessimistic. Four months ago her husband of 10 years left her for a younger woman. She became increasingly depressed and began having difficulty sleeping. What diagnosis(es), if any, should Monica receive?

Monica fulfills the criteria for the diagnosis of Dysthymic Disorder. In the midst of that disorder, she became increasingly depressed and began having difficulty sleeping in response to her husband's departure. Although these symptoms would normally fulfill the criteria for the diagnosis of Adjustment Disorder With Depressed Mood, this diagnosis cannot be made in the presence of already existing Dysthymic Disorder.

Example 3

Ross is a 34-year-old scientist who is constantly suspicious of his colleagues and feels they cannot be trusted. He has accused several of his co-workers of intentionally giving him incorrect data from their experiments. Ross feels that his scientific reputation is constantly under attack by others. He is easily slighted by their casual comments even when no offense is meant.

His behavior and accusations have disrupted the cooperative work in the laboratory where he has been employed for the last 2 years. After several complaints from the staff, the manager fired Ross 3 months ago. Since that time he has been depressed. What diagnosis(es), if any, should Ross receive?

Ross meets the criteria for the diagnosis of Paranoid Personality Disorder. His depression is a response to being fired. Because depression is not a part of the criteria set for the diagnosis of Paranoid Personality Disorder, he can also receive a diagnosis of Adjustment Disorder With Depressed Mood.

Precedence of Diagnosis

If the stress-related disturbance meets the criteria for a specific Axis I disorder or bereavement, those disorders always take diagnostic precedence over the diagnosis of a specific Adjustment Disorder.

Discussion of Clinical Vignette

Nuts to You, Please

Chelsey originally hoped to establish a career in a local bank, although she had always had a fantasy of opening a small business of her own. When her job at the bank became difficult to endure, she decided to quit and open her own business. She was hopeful during the change, even though she would have preferred to stay in a banking career. Chelsey invested a significant amount of money, time, and energy building a small nut and candy store which eventually succeeded. Unfortunately, competition from a new nationwide candy store chain eventually drove her out of business.

As her business began to fail, Chelsey became irritable, depressed, tearful and had difficulty sleeping. Although her depression continued for 3–4 months after she closed her business, it did not completely fulfill the criteria for the diagnosis of Major Depressive Disorder. However, her symptoms do fulfill the criteria for the diagnosis of Adjustment Disorder with Depressed Mood because her depression is a response to an identifiable stressor, the failure of her business, and lasted less than 6 months after the termination of the stressor.

Key Diagnostic Points

- The symptoms of Adjustment Disorders must occur within 3 months of the onset of a stressor(s) and last no more than 6 months after its termination.

- The diagnosis of Adjustment Disorder with Depressed Mood cannot be made in the presence of bereavement.

Common Questions in Making a Diagnosis

1. Melinda is a 44-year-old woman who got divorced a year ago. She has been depressed since the divorce. What diagnosis(es), if any, should Melinda receive?

Answer: The diagnosis of Adjustment Disorder with Depressed Mood cannot be made more than 6 months after the termination of the stressor. If Melinda does not meet the criteria for a specific Mood Disorder, she can receive a diagnosis of Depressive Disorder Not Otherwise Specified.

2. Judy is a 32-year-old woman who feels chronically empty and forms brief intense sexual relationships with men in response. She has always been fearful of being abandoned and reacts with rage, depression, and suicidal gestures when a man leaves her. A week ago her current lover left her after 6 months. Judy became depressed and took an overdose of five vitamin pills. What diagnosis(es), if any, should Judy receive?

Answer: Judy's symptoms fulfill the criteria for the diagnosis of Borderline Personality Disorder. Depression is a common symptom of this disorder. Therefore, she cannot receive an additional diagnosis of Adjustment Disorder with Depressed Mood when she becomes depressed again after her lover departs.

Personality Disorders

Clinical Vignette

The Perfect Boss

At age 35, Lawrence is an elegant man, particularly in his own eyes. He owns a small real estate agency that employs five agents. When he walks into a room, his bearing and appearance demand attention. His hair is perfectly styled and he is always cleanly shaven, even late in the afternoon. He wears expensive suits, custom-tailored shirts, fashionable silk ties with perfect knots, and costly cologne. Lawrence buys a new sports car every year. He is obviously pleased when his secretary or one of his employees compliments him on his clothes or car. When they don't spontaneously admire his belongings, he often fishes for compliments. The agents who have lasted the longest in the company have learned to praise him frequently. He accepts the compliments with a sense of noble entitlement that some employees find difficult to tolerate and others laugh about behind his back.

Lawrence is a hard taskmaster and does little to accommodate the personal needs of his staff. He takes advantage of their dependent positions to force them to work long hours and has little sympathy for their wish to spend time with their families. In staff meetings he frequently explains that he has a mission to make the company the largest and most successful real estate agency in the state. Most of his agents do not share his fantasies of unlimited success. Lawrence's constant pressure and demands are responsible for the high turnover rate among his employees.

Lawrence does not tolerate any disagreement with his decisions or the slightest criticism of his judgment. As a result, his employees rarely inform him when he is about to make a poor decision that may lead to the loss of an important sale. Most of his current employees remember or have heard of an incident that occurred 2 years ago. Sidney had been an agent in the office for many years. He was a successful real estate salesman who had worked for Lawrence's father when he owned the business. When Lawrence took over, Sidney agreed to stay and learned to tolerate his behavior. Sidney did his work quietly and rarely commented on company policy.

However, one day Sidney was in the process of finalizing the sale of a large piece of property that he had been trying to sell for 3 years. Lawrence walked into the office and casually commented that Sidney might get a higher price for the property if he held out longer. Sidney was surprised and immediately said, "I don't think that's a good idea. This is probably the best price we can get. It's been on the market for 3 years." Lawrence jerked his head around to look directly at Sidney. With his lips barely moving he said, "Sid, I think you can probably get a higher price." Sidney replied, "Larry, I've been working on this deal for months. Let it go." Lawrence looked at him again without speaking for a minute. His face turned pale and his lips tightened. Everyone in the office turned to watch. "Sidney," he said in a cool, indifferent voice, "Come into my office." Sidney looked uncomfortable and followed Lawrence into his office. Through the closed door the entire office heard him screaming at Sidney, "Don't ever question me again. You can sell that goddamned piece of property when I say so and not before. Do you understand. Now get out of here."

Whenever Lawrence came into the office for the next several weeks, he had a critical comment or put-down for Sidney. Two months later Sidney quit. Lawrence seemed surprised and hurt. He spoke to the other agents about the importance of loyalty.

Lawrence's success with employee relations was mirrored in his personal life. He has been married and divorced twice. Both wives were attractive women who were initially awed by his cool elegance and worshipped him. Lawrence can be extremely charming and gallant when he tries to be sensitive to others. However, sensitive behavior was very taxing for him and he could rarely maintain it for more than a few hours. Eventually his wives tired of his arrogant attitudes and excessive need for admiration. Lawrence was rarely empathic to their needs and was frequently critical of the way they dressed or behaved socially. His last wife left him after announcing that she was tired of being considered a cute showpiece or doll that he carried around to make him look good. Lawrence was depressed after she left, but seemed unable to appreciate the reason for her departure. He told his secretary, "I bought them all the clothes and cars they wanted. I only expected that they live up to standards that are consistent with my position. That's not too much to demand, is it? I don't think so. They're ungrateful for all I did for them." His pain was shortlived. Within a few weeks Lawrence was dating another attractive woman.

Core Concept of the Diagnostic Group

The core concept of the Personality Disorders group is the presence of a pervasive and enduring pattern of maladaptive spontaneous behaviors, responses, and modes of thought that begin by early adulthood, often interfere with normal interpersonal relationships, and produce functional impairment or subjective distress.

Criteria Applicable to Multiple Disorders

There is one general set of diagnostic criteria applicable to all Personality Disorders.

A. An enduring pattern of inner experience and behavior that deviates markedly from the expectations of the individual's culture. This pattern is manifested in two (or more) of the following areas:

   (1) cognition (i.e., ways of perceiving and interpreting oneself, other people, and events)
   (2) affectivity (i.e., the range, intensity, lability, and appropriateness of emotional response)
   (3) interpersonal functioning
   (4) impulse control

B. The enduring pattern is inflexible and pervasive across a broad range of personal and social situations.

C. The enduring pattern leads to clinically significant distress or impairment in social, occupational, or other important areas of functioning.

D. The pattern is stable and of long duration and its onset can be traced back at least to adolescence or early adulthood.

E. The enduring pattern is not better accounted for as a manifestation or consequence of another mental disorder.

F. The enduring pattern is not due to the direct physiological effects of a substance (e.g., a drug of abuse, a medication) or a general medical condition (e.g., head trauma).

Definitions

entitlement An unreasonable expectation, communicated to others, that one is special and deserves favored treatment.

paranoid Thinking and behavior is pervasively suspiciousness, with mistrust of other people and their motives. Paranoid individuals constantly scan the people around them in an attempt to detect behaviors or comments directed toward them that they consider to be injurious.

narcissism The excessive love or investment in oneself with the corresponding inability to love another or be empathic to their concerns.

Synopses and Diagnostic Prototypes
of the Individual Disorders

Personality Disorders are divided into three clusters of disorders. The diagnoses in Cluster A are characterized by odd, eccentric, isolative, or suspicious behavior and include: Paranoid Personality Disorder, Schizoid Personality Disorder, and Schizotypal Personality Disorder. The diagnoses in Cluster B are distinguished by dramatic, emotional, erratic, or impulsive behavior, or a reduced capacity for empathy and include: Antisocial Personality Disorder, Borderline Personality Disorder, Histrionic Personality Disorder, and Narcissistic Personality Disorder. The diagnoses in Cluster C are characterized by anxious, fearful, or perfectionistic behavior and include: Avoidant Personality Disorder, Dependent Personality Disorder, and Obsessive-Compulsive Personality Disorder.

Cluster A

301.0 Paranoid Personality Disorder.   Individuals with this disorder have a pervasive distrust and suspiciousness of others and interpret their motives as malevolent. The diagnosis requires at least four of the following:

1. Suspects, without sufficient basis, that others are exploiting or deceiving him or her.
2. Preoccupied with unjustified doubts about the loyalty or trustworthiness of friends and associates.
3. Is reluctant to confide in others because of unwarranted fear that the information will be used maliciously against him or her.
4. Reads hidden demeaning or threatening meanings into benign remarks or events.
5. Persistently bears a grudge, i.e., is unforgiving of insults, injuries, or slights.
6. Perceives attacks on his or her character or reputation that are not apparent to others and is quick to react angrily or to counterattack.
7. Recurrent suspicions, without justification, regarding fidelity of a spouse or sexual partner.

Neil is a 28-year-old man who has worked as a car mechanic in the service garage of an automobile dealership for the last 2 years. He is considered a reasonably good mechanic but is difficult to work with because he is touchy, suspicious, and easily slighted. His behavior has led to a number of confrontations with other mechanics and supervisors. The dealership is reluctant to fire him because good mechanics are difficult to find.

Recently, he was called into the foreman's office after an argument with two fellow workers. The argument started when a customer brought an old car into the shop for repair. Neil was assigned to repair it. He was unhappy with the assignment, claiming it was unfair because it would take too long to get parts for the car and repair it. Neil told one co-worker that the supervisor assigned the car to him to make him look bad. When the co-worker expressed some doubt, Neil looked at him and said, "You think I'm lying. All you people are like that. You all want to get rid of me." The co-worker initially became angry, and then walked away shaking his head.

Neil started working on the car and turned in a list of parts. Several had to be ordered. He checked every day to see if the parts had arrived. After several days of inquiry, the head of the parts department told him to wait until he was called about the parts. Neil became convinced that the man was trying to disrupt his work and told him so. The parts manager replied, "You're nuts," and began working on something else. When the order finally arrived, Neil discovered that two parts were incorrect. He accused the worker and the manager of the department of sabotaging his work. The argument ended when the foreman called Neil into his office to resolve the dispute. Although this quarrel escalated more than usual, in many respects it was typical of the arguments he has with fellow workers. Neil makes some people uncomfortable even when he is calm and businesslike. He scares the women in the billing office. One of the women commented, "Whenever he's around he watches me and notices every little thing I do. It's creepy. It makes me so nervous I make mistakes. Then he gets irritated and condescending and points out my mistakes." Another woman added, "He's a real cold fish. Polite, but watch out. He got angry with me a year ago when I didn't immediately notice he was standing at my desk. He's still mad."

301.20 Schizoid Personality Disorder. Individuals with this disorder have a pervasive pattern of detachment from social relationships and a restricted range of expression of emotions in interpersonal settings. The diagnosis requires at least four of the following:

1. Neither desires nor enjoys close relationships, including being part of a family.
2. Almost always chooses solitary activities.
3. Little, if any, interest in having sexual experiences with another person.
4. Takes pleasure in few, if any, activities.
5. Lacks close friends or confidants other than first-degree relatives.
6. Appears indifferent to the praise or criticism of others.
7. Emotional coldness, detachment, or flattened affectivity.

Brad is a 33-year-old man who always liked rats and computers. As a boy he had a small collection of snakes, spiders, and mice in his bedroom. When he was age 10, he bought his first white rat. He was so fascinated with the rat that he soon he got rid of his other animals and began breeding rats in the basement. His parents were not happy. His father complained to a friend, "What kind of kid spends all his time in the basement with rats!"

When Brad was age 13 he bought his first computer kit and spent long hours in his room programming. He rarely went out with his classmates and never had a date with a girl. In school he was considered a loner; aloof and detached but harmless. He did not participate in school activities and seemed unconcerned about what others thought of him. Brad's interactions with his peers were usually uncomfortable and his occasional attempts at humor seemed strained and off target. His major academic interest was philosophy and he spend many hours reading Camus and other Existential philosophers.

After high school Brad went to college where he majored in computer sciences. The only negative incident in college occurred when the dormitory authorities discovered his rat colony and insisted that he remove it. Brad responded by moving into his own apartment so he could keep his rats. After college he took a job in a large company as a computer programmer and systems analyst. He did well, working the night shift. He remained detached, had few friends, and spent little time with his family.

301.22   Schizotypal Personality Disorder.   Individuals with this disorder have a pervasive pattern of deficits marked by discomfort with, and reduced capacity for, close relationships, as well as cognitive or perceptual distortions and eccentricities of behavior. The diagnosis requires at least five of the following:

1. Ideas of reference (excluding delusions of reference).
2. Odd beliefs or magical thinking that influence behavior and are inconsistent with subcultural norms (e.g., superstitiousness, belief in clairvoyance, telepathy).
3. Unusual perceptual experiences, including bodily illusions.
4. Odd thinking and speech (e.g., vague, circumstantial, metaphorical).
5. Suspiciousness or paranoid ideation.
6. Inappropriate or constricted affect.
7. Behavior or appearance that is odd, eccentric, or peculiar.
8. Lacks close friends or confidants other than first-degree relatives.
9. Excessive social anxiety that does not diminish with familiarity and tends to be associated with paranoid fears rather than negative judgments about self.

Lucy is a 32-year-old woman who lives alone on welfare in a small apartment. She has few friends and little family. Her neighbors consider her peculiar and the neighborhood children often tease her about her appearance. Lucy's clothes appear slightly askew and her makeup is unusual. She wears heavy eye shadow, plucks her eyebrows, and pencils thin lines in their place. The two penciled eyebrows are drawn at a slightly different angles, adding to her bizarre appearance.

Her behavior is also unusual and she is often seen watching the neighborhood children from her window, partially hidden behind the curtains. Lucy is generally suspicious of other people and often makes strange gestures when she passes people in the street. Her social worker reports that Lucy is always anxious during their meetings and has a very limited range of emotional expression. This is accompanied by unusual beliefs and patterns of thought. Lucy explains that she has special powers, "My body is a lightening rod for the thoughts of others." She believes that she knows what other people are thinking and uses this knowledge to protect herself from their attempts to control her.

Cluster B

301.7   Antisocial Personality Disorder.   Individuals with this disorder are at least age 18 years, have evidence of Conduct Disorder occurring before age 15 years, and have a pervasive pattern of disregard for and violation of the rights of others. The diagnosis requires at least three of the following:

1. Failure to conform to social norms with respect to lawful behaviors as indicated by repeatedly performing acts that are grounds for arrest.
2. Deceitfulness, as indicated by repeated lying, use of aliases, or conning others for personal profit or pleasure.
3. Impulsivity or failure to plan ahead.
4. Irritability and aggressiveness, as indicated by repeated physical fights or assaults.
5. Reckless disregard for safety of self or others.
6. Consistent irresponsibility, as indicated by repeated failure to sustain consistent work behavior or honor financial obligations.
7. Lack of remorse, as indicated by being indifferent to or rationalizing having hurt, mistreated, or stolen from another.

Vince is an unemployed 25-year-old man who has been repeatedly arrested for running illegal card games (e.g., three card monte) on the street in the large city where he lives. His victims are usually tourists. When he is asked why he tries to swindle people, he laughs and replies, "If these people are stupid enough to play my game, they deserve to have their money taken. I run a business just like they do. They don't have to shop with me. They're greedy and want to beat me."

Vince has a long history of rebellious behavior. As a child he lied to his parents, stole money from his mother, and engaged in repeated shoplifting. He was difficult to control as an adolescent and often stayed out late at night despite his parents attempts to set a curfew. Vince was arrested once for breaking into a neighbor's house with a friend.

He started using drugs at age 13 and soon was stealing and selling stolen property to make money. He dropped out of high school before graduating and moved to an apartment that he shared with two friends. Vince has held several jobs for a few weeks at a time but was unable to comply with the job requirements. Eventually, he always returns to the streets where he continues hustling people to make a living.

301.83 Borderline Personality Disorder.   Individuals with this disorder have a pervasive pattern of instability in interpersonal relationships, self-images, affects, and control over impulses. The diagnosis requires at least five of the following:

1. Frantic efforts to avoid real or imagined abandonment.
2. A pattern of unstable and intense interpersonal relationships characterized by alternating between extremes of idealization and devaluation.
3. Identity disturbance: persistent and markedly disturbed, distorted, or unstable self-image or sense of self.
4. Impulsivity in at least two areas that are potentially self-damaging (e.g., spending, sex, substance abuse, reckless driving, binge eating).
5. Recurrent suicidal behavior, gestures, or threats, or self-mutilating behavior.
6. Affective instability due to marked reactivity of mood (e.g., intense episodic dysphoria, irritability, or anxiety usually lasting a few hours and only rarely more than a few days).
7. Chronic feelings of emptiness.
8. Inappropriate, intense anger or lack of control of anger (e.g., frequent displays of temper, constant anger, recurrent physical fights).
9. Transient, stress-related paranoid ideation or severe dissociative symptoms.

Emily is a 24-year-old woman who recently arrived in a new city to begin graduate studies at a large university. She moved into an apartment with three other women graduate students who had been living together for the past 2 years. The relationship between Emily and her roommates appeared to go well initially. She became very attached to one of the woman and idealized her to the point that she began dressing like the roommate.

The woman started to feel uncomfortable when Emily confided that she felt so much like the roommate that they could be twins. The other roommates also began feeling uneasy about her behavior. She demanded more and more of their time, frequently becoming angry if one of the roommates decided not to eat dinner in the apartment with the other women. Emily seemed to need constant attention and complained of feeling bored and empty most of the time. She had mood swings, feeling elated at one moment and depressed, angry, or empty the next.

Emily was attractive and dated several men. She described each man in glowing terms initially and usually had sex with them soon after the first date. The relationships with her boyfriends were brief and intense. They usually ended after a few weeks when the boyfriend left. One of the men confided to a roommate, "I feel like she's eating me alive. I can't walk out of the apartment without her asking me where I'm going and accusing me of not caring for her."

Emily felt depressed and empty when the relationships ended. One night, following the tumultuous end of another relationship, a roommate walked into the bathroom and found Emily cutting her thigh with a razor blade. The thigh was scarred from multiple past cuts. The roommate screamed and Emily stopped and said, "Cutting helps make me feel better when I'm upset." Two days later the room-mates met and decided that Emily had to move out of the apartment. She was en-raged but agreed to go after telling them that they were all worthless and would be sorry. She moved out the next day. Subsequently, all three roommates found that several of their dresses had been slashed with a razor blade and ruined.

301.50 Histrionic Personality Disorder. Individuals with this disorder have a pervasive pattern of excessive emotionality and attention seeking. The diagnosis requires at least five of the following:

1. Is uncomfortable in situations in which he or she is not the center of atten-tion.
2. Interaction with others is often characterized by inappropriate sexually se-ductive or provocative behavior.
3. Displays rapidly shifting and shallow expression of emotions.
4. Consistently uses physical appearance to draw attention to oneself.
5. Style of speech that is excessively impressionistic and lacking in detail.
6. Self-dramatization, theatricality, and exaggerated expression of emotion.
7. Suggestibility, i.e., easily influenced by others or circumstances.
8. Considers relationships to be more intimate than they actually are.

Carla is a 35-year-old divorced woman who is heavily involved in the local art scene. She routinely holds court in a neighborhood coffeehouse where she is known for her dramatic entrances—barefoot with swirling peasant skirts and bells on her ankles. Carla finds it impossible to sit quietly and unobtrusively at any gathering of more than one person. She has an opinion about every piece of art hanging in the coffeehouse or selling in nearby galleries. Her critiques are usually based on an immediate emotional reaction to the artwork and are singularly lacking in intellec-tual details. Carla's opinions are delivered with exaggerated phrases accompanied by overly dramatic arm gestures and tosses of the head that swing her hair into the air.

   She surrounds herself with a coterie of younger men and woman who listen intently to her artistic pronouncements and appear amused by her behavior. Carla treats each of these people as close personal friends after a brief initial meeting. She embraces them at each subsequent meeting and often suggestively rubs her body against the men in a provocative sexual manner, breaking away before they can respond. Some of the men have misunderstood her friendliness and interpreted it as an invitation for further intimacy. When this occurs, Carla's warmth is rapidly trans-formed to mild irritation and she stiffens until the men rescale their affections to the appropriate level.

301.81 Narcissistic Personality Disorder. Individuals with this disorder have a pervasive pattern of grandiosity (in fantasy or behavior), need for admira-tion, and lack of empathy. The diagnosis requires at least five of the following:

1. A grandiose sense of self-importance.
2. Preoccupation with fantasies of unlimited success, power, brilliance, beauty, or ideal love.
3. Believes that he or she is "special" and unique and can only be understood by, or should associate with, other special or high-status people.
4. Requires excessive admiration.
5. A sense of entitlement.
6. Is interpersonally exploitative.
7. Lacks empathy: unwilling to recognize or identify with the feelings and needs of others.
8. Is often envious of others or believes that others are envious of him or her.
9. Arrogant, haughty behaviors, or attitudes.

> Spencer is a 51-year-old man who is the chairman of a medical department in a small medical school. His staff know him more for his wine cellar than his empathy. Each faculty member is invited to his house for dinner when they first join the department. Spencer takes them on a tour of his cellar and grandly picks a bottle of wine for the meal. During dinner his young wife carefully doles out the wine, making sure that no one takes more than their share.
>
> The discussions at dinner cover a range of topics but inevitably settle on the chairman and his experiences, achievements, goals, and aspirations. His wife sits next to her husband smiling and nodding as he talks, periodically emphasizing the importance of his achievements. Other faculty members add their appreciative comments. The chairman smiles, accepting their admiration without embarrassment.
>
> At work Spencer is less approachable. He is reluctant to spend time talking with his faculty, preferring to associate with other chairman, the Dean, and members of the Board of Trustees at the faculty club. He tells his secretary, "The Dean and the Board are the only ones who really understand my expansion plans."
>
> In reality he is an inconsistent and ineffectual administrator. His major goal is to see that the faculty bring money into the department to support his lifestyle. Spencer routinely manipulates staff to achieve his goals with minimal concerns for their needs and discomfort. He is intolerant of any criticism or opposition to his decisions. When criticized, he becomes enraged but covers his anger with superficial pleasantries and then makes plans to punish the offender.
>
> Spencer expects complete compliance with his wishes and active recognition of his achievements. He is involved in many national activities and is frequently away from the hospital at meetings. After returning, he subtly drops the names of important people he has met and emphasizes his powerful political contacts.

Cluster C

301.82   Avoidant Personality Disorder.   Individuals with this disorder have a pervasive pattern of social inhibition, feelings of inadequacy, and hypersensitivity to negative evaluation. The diagnosis requires at least four of the following:

1. Avoids occupational activities that involve significant interpersonal contact, because of fears of criticism, disapproval, or rejection.
2. Is unwilling to get involved with people unless certain of being liked.
3. Restraint within intimate relationships due to the fear of being shamed or ridiculed.
4. Preoccupation with being criticized or rejected in social situations.
5. Inhibited in new interpersonal situations because of feelings of inadequacy.
6. Belief that one is socially inept, personally unappealing, or inferior to others.
7. Is usually reluctant to take personal risks or to engage in any new activities because they may prove embarrassing.

Dennis is a 37-year-old single man who works as a clerk in the accounting department of a large bank. He is shy, dependable, and goes about his job quietly, trying to please his superiors. Although he has been working at the bank for 5 years, he has made few friends among his fellow workers and has little social contact with them outside of work.

Sally is an exception. She is a quiet, widowed woman in her early 40s who has worked as a teller at the bank for many years. Gradually, over a period of 2–3 years, Dennis and Sally became friends. Sally initiated the contact by saying, "Hello," to Dennis every time she passed his desk and asking if she could get him anything when she went out for coffee. Dennis was initially shy and chose to ignore her friendly overtures. He later told her, "I couldn't believe you wanted to talk with me. I thought you would think I was stupid and make fun of me once we started talking." Sally's persistence was finally rewarded with a few small smiles from Dennis after he became convinced that she really did like him.

Sally tried to get Dennis to be more sociable. "You just need more self-confidence," she told him. Despite her urging he was still reluctant to go to parties or bank social activities, fearing that he would spill food on someone or make some other embarrassing blunder and be criticized for being socially inept.

Dennis' lack of confidence also extended to his work. A few months ago he turned down a promotion that would have required more responsibility and involvement with bank customers. He told Sally, "I didn't think I could do the job. My boss would be watching me. If I made any mistakes with customers, he would get angry with me and get rid of me or send me back to my old job. I couldn't face that." Sally tried to be supportive but felt frustrated by Dennis' unwillingness to take chances to improve himself.

301.6 Dependent Personality Disorder. Individuals with this disorder have a pervasive and excessive need to be taken care of, leading to submissive and clinging behavior and fears of separation. The diagnosis requires at least five of the following:

1. Is unable to make everyday decisions without an excessive amount of advice and reassurance from others.
2. Needs others to assume responsibility for most major areas of his or her life.
3. Has difficulty expressing disagreement with others because of fear of loss of support or approval (*note:* do not include realistic fears of retribution).
4. Has difficulty initiating projects or doing things on his or her own (due to a lack of self-confidence in judgment or abilities rather than to a lack of motivation or energy).
5. Goes to excessive lengths to obtain nurturance and support from others, to the point of volunteering to do things that are unpleasant.
6. Feels uncomfortable or helpless when alone, because of exaggerated fears of being unable to care for himself or herself.
7. Urgently seeks another relationship as a source of care and support when a close relationship ends.
8. Unrealistic preoccupation with fears of being left to take care of himself or herself.

Florence is a 33-year-old woman who has been married for 10 years. She and her husband met in college while Florence was living at home and got married immediately after graduation. Her husband, Stan, works for a newspaper. The couple have two children, aged 5 and 7. Florence is a quiet woman who has few opinions of her own. When someone asks for her judgment about an issue, she shrugs and replies, "I don't really think about those things. I guess I'm really stupid. Why don't you ask my husband." Her husband always has an opinion about every issue and makes all of the decisions in the house. Florence has learned to agree with him no matter what he says.

Early in their marriage, before the kids were born, Florence decided to redecorate the house. She spoke to an interior decorator and went to several stores looking at paint, wallpaper, furniture, and carpeting. She called the interior decorator two or three times a day for advice. When he finally refused to speak with her more than once a week, Florence turned to her sister for advice. Her first big task was deciding what color to paint the walls. She asked her sister, "I don't know whether they should be a light purple or more neutral, like a beige. What do you think?" Her sister suggested beige. Florence called 2 hours later and asked, "Are you sure the beige will look OK? Should the trim be the same color?" Her sister wearily answered, "Beige will look fine for the walls and the trim, Sis."

After several more days of frequent telephone calls, her sister refused to help and said, "Why don't you ask Stan what he thinks? He's going to live in the house too." Her husband had little patience for her indecisiveness. He met with the interior decorator and made all the final decisions.

Since that time her husband has assumed responsibility for all the major decisions in the home. Florence is afraid to disagree with him for fear he won't approve of her behavior. She is also fearful that he might get disgusted with her and leave because she is so inept. When her husband works late or goes on a business trip,

Florence is plagued by fears that she will be unable to care for herself or that he will find another woman.

301.4 Obsessive-Compulsive Personality Disorder. Individuals with this disorder have a pervasive pattern of preoccupation with orderliness, perfectionism, and mental and interpersonal control, at the expense of flexibility, openness, and efficiency. The diagnosis requires at least four of the following:

1. Preoccupation with details, rules, lists, order, organization, or schedules to the extent that the major point of the activity is lost.
2. Perfectionism that interferes with task completion (e.g., inability to complete a project because one's own overly strict standards are not met).
3. Excessive devotion to work and productivity to the exclusion of leisure activities and friendships (not accounted for by obvious economic necessity).
4. Overconscientiousness, scrupulousness, and inflexibility about matters of morality, ethics, or values (not accounted for by cultural or religious identification).
5. Inability to discard wornout or worthless objects even when they have no sentimental value.
6. Reluctance to delegate tasks or to work with others unless they submit to exactly his or her way of doing things.
7. Adopts a miserly spending style toward both self and others; money is viewed as something to be hoarded for future catastrophes.
8. Rigidity and stubbornness.

Raymond is a 42-year-old man who is an architect in a large firm. He is known for his attention to details. His boss has been known to comment, "Give the blueprints to Raymond. If there's a screw loose or a fixture missing he'll spot it." Unfortunately, Raymond's attention to detail makes it difficult for him to complete an entire project on his own. Furthermore, none of the junior architects will work with him because he will not allow them to express their ideas in a design. He insists that they exactly follow his directions.

Despite these handicaps, the firm values Raymond for his uncompromising devotion to his work and his extreme conscientiousness. They put up with his personal quirks like his extensive collection of broken pencils, eraser nubs, bits of broken lead, and used interdepartmental envelopes. However, his rigidity has significantly limited his advancement in the firm.

301.9 Personality Disorder Not Otherwise Specified. Individuals with this disorder have a disturbance of personality functioning that does not fit the criteria for any specific Personality Disorder.

Necessary Clinical Information

The information required for the diagnosis Personality Disorder requires evidence of several of the following types of behavior and modes of thought.

- Suspiciousness or paranoia

- Excessive, poorly controlled anger or aggression

- Isolation, lack of close friends or confidants, emotional coldness

- Chronic sense of loneliness or emptiness

- Odd or psychotic thinking or speech

- Unusual perceptual experiences

- Excessive anxiety

- Excessive dependence or suggestibility

- Persistent irresponsibility, impulsivity, or deceitfulness

- Lack of remorse after having hurt, mistreated, or stolen from another

- Intense and unstable interpersonal relationships

- Frantic attempts to avoid real or imagined abandonment

- Self-dramatization and exhibitionism

- Exaggerated expression of emotions

- Grandiose sense of entitlement or self-importance, arrogance

- Lack of empathy

- Persistent exploitation of others

- Persistent sense of inferiority or inadequacy

- Preoccupation with being criticized

- Need for constant reassurance and support from others

- Excessively rigid and stubborn

- Perfectionism

Making a Diagnosis

Personality Disorder is defined by a set of abnormal or maladaptive behaviors and modes of thought expressed by an individual. Some of the behaviors that make up the criteria for specific Personality Disorders are abnormal whenever they occur (e.g., suicidal behavior, reckless disregard for safety of self and others).

Other behaviors are maladaptive but within the range of normalcy when the intensity of their expression is moderated and the target of their expression is limited to a few specific situations (e.g., suggestibility, envy of others, excessive social anxiety, suspiciousness). The mere presence of abnormal or maladaptive behavior is not sufficient for the diagnosis of Personality Disorder. Three additional factors must be taken into account for the diagnosis: 1) the pervasiveness of the behavior(s), 2) the pattern of behavior(s), and 3) the intensity of the behavior(s).

The pervasiveness of an abnormal or maladaptive behavior is a key factor in the diagnosis of Personality Disorder. A pervasive behavior is commonly and frequently exhibited by the individual in many different settings. For example, an isolated suicide attempt that occurs when a patient has Major Depressive Disorder, Single Episode, is not part of the criteria set for any Personality Disorder. However, recurrent suicidal behavior, gestures, or threats are a criterion for the diagnosis of Borderline Personality Disorder.

Similarly, periodic suggestibility, self-dramatization, or fear of criticism, although potentially maladaptive, are not part of the criteria for any Personality Disorder. It is only when the symptoms form an enduring and pervasive part of the patient's repertoire of behaviors that they fulfill criteria for Personality Disorder.

Personality Disorder also requires a pattern or set of different behaviors that present a consistent theme. Rigidity, lack of empathy, suicidal behavior, impulsivity, or similar symptoms, no matter how intense, are not sufficient in isolation to satisfy the criteria for any personality disorder. It is only when a characteristic group of behaviors appear together, and define a syndrome, that the diagnosis can be made (e.g., irritability and aggressiveness, impulsivity, reckless disregard for the safety of self or others in the diagnosis of Antisocial Personality Disorder).

Specific Personality Disorders also come in different flavors. For example, the diagnosis of Borderline Personality Disorder can be made by any combination of five of the nine possible abnormal behaviors or modes of thought listed in the criteria set. Some Borderline Personality Disorder patients may have recurrent suicidal behavior, whereas others may not. This is possible because patients may express the same core problem in several different ways. In Borderline Personality Disorder, the core problem is a pervasive pattern of instability of interpersonal relationships, self-image, affects, and control over impulses. The expression of this problem may emphasize suicidal behavior or intense and inappropriate anger.

The final factor in the diagnosis of Personality Disorder is the intensity of the abnormal behavior or mode of thought. Many people are arrogant, fearful of criticism, afraid of abandonment, aggressive, or suspicious. These behaviors, when expressed in moderation, are not necessarily indicative of Personality Disorder. The intensity of the behavior is one factor that distinguishes Personality

Disorder from a variant of normal behavior. For example, a normal person who becomes irritated at a co-worker might make an angry comment or yell. An individual with Antisocial Personality Disorder might hit the co-worker in the face and feel no remorse for the act.

Similarly, a normal individual who is slighted becomes briefly irritated at the person who insults him. An individual with Paranoid Personality Disorder often never forgives someone who slights him. He bears a persistent grudge against the person and always remains suspicious of his subsequent behavior. Therefore, in the diagnosis of Personality Disorder, the assessment of a patient's behavioral repertoire must include an evaluation of the intensity, as well as, the type, pattern, and pervasiveness of the abnormal behaviors.

There are two major steps in making the diagnosis of Personality Disorder: 1) the identification of the patient's maladaptive or abnormal behaviors, and 2) a clinical judgment of whether the pattern of behaviors constitute a recognized syndrome that is sufficiently different from normal and sufficiently pervasive and intense to fulfill the diagnostic criteria. The questions in this section provide a step-by-step method for processing the clinical information necessary to make these decisions for a typical Personality Disorder.

1. What is the patient's predominant clinical appearance or presentation?

The diagnosis of Personality Disorder starts with the identification of one or more unusual behaviors or modes of thought that are characteristic of a patient's behavioral repertoire. The behavior is unusual due to its nature (e.g., reckless disregard for the safety of self or others) or its intensity (e.g., grandiose sense of self-worth, chronic feelings of emptiness).

Some of these behaviors are representative symptoms of a specific Personality Disorder, yet do not completely fulfill the criteria for its diagnosis. For example, suspiciousness and the unwarranted perception of being attacked are important members of the criteria set for the diagnosis of Paranoid Personality Disorder but do not completely fulfill the criteria.

Once these behaviors are observed, the clinician's task is to elicit evidence of the additional features needed to fulfill the criteria. Frequently, the patient's unusual behavior is not a prominent symptom of a single specific Personality Disorder (e.g., isolative behavior, excessive anxiety). Instead, it is a general symptom that is more representative of a group of disorders that are similar.

DSM-IV defines three clusters of Personality Disorders based on a small set of common characteristic behaviors and modes of thought. The early identification of these behaviors helps narrow the diagnostic choice to one of the three clusters. Once a single Personality Disorder cluster is identified, it is often easier to distinguish between the various disorders that are contained in the cluster.

- If the patient's most prominent and pervasive behavior is odd, eccentric, isolative, or suspicious, consider the diagnoses in Cluster A (Paranoid Personality Disorder, Schizoid Personality Disorder, and Schizotypal Personality Disorder).

- If the patient's most prominent and pervasive behavior is dramatic, emotional, erratic, or impulsive, or if the patient appears to have a reduced capacity for empathy, consider the diagnoses in Cluster B (Antisocial Personality Disorder, Borderline Personality Disorder, Histrionic Personality Disorder, and Narcissistic Personality Disorder).

- If the patient's most prominent and pervasive behavior is anxious, fearful, or perfectionistic, consider the diagnoses in Cluster C (Avoidant Personality Disorder, Dependent Personality Disorder, and Obsessive-Compulsive Personality Disorder).

2. Is the patient's most prominent and pervasive behavior odd, eccentric, isolative, or suspicious (Cluster A)?

- If the patient's most prominent symptom is strikingly odd behavior or strange modes of thought (e.g., peculiarities of dress, ideas of reference, magical thinking, paranoid ideation, belief in clairvoyance, unusual speech or mannerisms) that are inconsistent with the norms of any specific subculture, consider the diagnosis of Schizotypal Personality Disorder. Although Schizoid patients have a disturbance of thinking and communication, they are not overtly psychotic. Schizotypal patients have no close friends and appear anxious, eccentric, or bizarre in most social situations. If psychotic symptoms appear they are brief and not as severe as in Schizophrenia.

- If the patient's most prominent symptom is social withdrawal, isolation, or aloofness associated with a restricted range of emotional expression, and little or no desire to have intimate relationships with other people, consider the diagnosis of Schizoid Personality Disorder. Schizoid patients generally do not experience their isolation and lack of intimate relationships as dysphoric or depressing. They are not paranoid or suspicious, which distinguishes them from patients with Paranoid Personality Disorder. Schizoid patients may seem mildly eccentric but they do not have the severe oddities of behavior, thinking, perception, or speech that are present in most Schizotypal patients.

- If the patient's most prominent symptom is suspiciousness, lack of trust, and the continual unwarranted perception of being attacked, consider the diagnosis of Paranoid Personality Disorder. Paranoid patients generally avoid intimacy, are isolative, and try to be self-sufficient. They are often jealous, argumentative, easily slighted, hypervigilant, and question the loyalty or motivations of others with little cause. Paranoid patients are also generally cold, lacking warm tender feelings, and pride themselves on being rational, objective, and un-emotional. To other people they usually appear hostile, uncompromising, stub-born, and defensive. Schizoid patients may be seen as aloof, cold, and somewhat eccentric, but they do not have the prominent paranoid ideation of patients with Paranoid Personality Disorder.

3. Is the patient's most prominent and pervasive behavior dramatic, emotional, erratic, impulsive, or a reduced capacity for empathy (Cluster B)?

• If the patient's most prominent symptom is a pervasive disregard for and vio-lation of the rights of others often associated with a lack of remorse, consider the diagnosis of Antisocial Personality Disorder. These patients' erratic or emo-tional behavior is frequently demonstrated by deceitfulness, impulsivity, and repeated outbursts of anger, accompanied by physical fights. Antisocial pa-tients have a previous history of Conduct Disorder occurring before the of age 15 years.

• If the patient's most prominent symptoms are erratic and unstable interpersonal relationships, affect, self-image, and control over impulses, consider the diag-nosis of Borderline Personality Disorder. These patients generally have chronic feelings of emptiness and may have periods of intense anger and dysphoria that are associated with suicidal behavior, gestures, or threats. They also may have transient psychotic or dissociative episodes that usually resolve within 1–2 days. The patient's erratic behavior is further demonstrated by repeated self-damaging impulsive acts such as multiple sexual partners, excessive spending, substance abuse, and reckless driving. It may be difficult to distinguish patients with Borderline Personality Disorder from patients with Antisocial or Histri-onic Personality Disorders. Key differentiating features include the Borderline Personality Disorder patient's excessive emotional demands in close relation-ships, chronic feelings of emptiness, and manipulative suicidal or self-mutilat-ing behavior. Borderline Personality Disorder patients are differentiated from Paranoid Personality Disorder patients because they do not display the extreme suspiciousness of the latter. They can be distinguished from Schizotypal Per-sonality Disorder patients because they do not have marked odd or bizarre behavior, thoughts, thinking, and speech.

• If the patient's most prominent symptoms include an exaggerated, overly dra-matic expression of emotions that are in reality shallow and rapidly shifting, and a pervasive need to be the center of attention, consider the diagnosis of Histrionic Personality Disorder. These patients are frequently sexually seduc-tive and provocative, and they dress or act in a dramatic fashion to gather at-tention. They are further characterized by superficial thinking, superficial interpersonal relationships, and a tenuous sense of their own ideas and beliefs that make them very suggestible. Histrionic Personality Disorder patients may also fulfill the criteria for the diagnosis of Borderline Personality Disorder. They may be differentiated from Borderline Personality Disorder patients who are more likely to have repeated suicide attempts, difficulty with an unstable self-image, and transient psychotic episodes.

- If the patient's most prominent symptoms are grandiosity, a sense of entitlement, a need for excessive admiration, exploitation of others, and a lack of empathy, consider the diagnosis of Narcissistic Personality Disorder. These patients are erratic in the sense that their self-esteem is often fragile, and simple criticism may provoke rage or depression. In other circumstances, their affect may fluctuate from a grandiose sense of well-being to shame and humiliation if they fail in a task or feel ignored. The distinction between patients with Narcissistic Personality Disorder and patients with Borderline, Antisocial, or Histrionic Personality Disorders can be difficult because patients may display attributes of all four personality disorders. Patients with Narcissistic Personality Disorder generally have more stable lives, a more cohesive identity, and less impulsivity than patients with Borderline Personality Disorder. Narcissistic Personality Disorder patients are also less impulsive than patients with Antisocial Personality Disorder and their exploitation of others is more likely to focus on power and control rather than outright theft and fraud to gain material wealth. They generally display less emotional exaggeration and are less dependent on others than patients with Histrionic Personality Disorder.

4. Is the patient's most prominent and pervasive behavior anxious, fearful, or perfectionistic (Cluster C)?

- If the patient's most prominent symptoms are fear of criticism and feelings of inadequacy that are associated with social inhibition, consider the diagnosis of Avoidant Personality Disorder. These patients desire human companionship but are afraid of rejection or criticism. They require an unusually strong guarantee of uncritical acceptance before they will enter into a relationship. They differ from patients with Schizoid Personality Disorder who genuinely desire to be isolated and feel uncomfortable in a close intimate relationship. The differential diagnosis between Avoidant Personality Disorder and Dependent Personality Disorder may be difficult because Avoidant Personality Disorder patients are often dependent once they form a relationship. However, Dependent Personality Disorder patients are often seen as more fearful of being abandoned than Avoidant Personality Disorder patients.

- If the patient's most prominent symptoms are dependent and submissive behavior associated with a pervasive need to be cared for, exaggerated anxieties about separation and abandonment, and fears of not being able to care for himself or herself, consider the diagnosis of Dependent Personality Disorder.

These patients often establish a long-term relationship with one person on whom they are excessively dependent. If that relationship ends, they immediately seek another relationship. They rely on other people to make important decisions for them or require excessive reassurance and advice before making everyday decisions themselves. Dependency is common in patients with Borderline Personality Disorder and Histrionic Personality Disorder. However, these patients have more unstable interpersonal relationships than patients with a diagnosis of Dependent Personality Disorder.

• If the patient's most prominent symptoms are a rigid preoccupation with orderliness, perfectionism, money, and control of themselves and others in response to anxiety, consider the diagnosis of Obsessive-Compulsive Personality Disorder. Frequently, these patients' excessive attempts at control make it difficult for the individual to finish a task or work closely with colleagues. These individuals are often seen as rigid and stubborn in their work, ethics, and values. They differ from patients with Obsessive-Compulsive Disorder who have true obsessions and compulsions.

Common Problems in Making a Diagnosis

There are three main areas of uncertainty in the diagnosis of Personality Disorders.

1. Some patients have significant personality traits but don't quite fit the criteria for a specific Personality Disorder.
2. The symptoms of various Personality Disorders often overlap one another (e.g., Avoidant Personality Disorder and Dependent Personality Disorder).
3. Many of the behaviors and modes of thought characteristic of a specific Personality Disorder may be seen in other nonpersonality psychiatric disorders.

Patients Who Almost Fulfill the Diagnostic Criteria

Every individual develops certain characteristic patterns of behavior, thought, and speech during their life. Many of these behaviors are similar or identical to those seen in various Personality Disorders. For example, a normal individual may be suggestible, impulsive, or fearful of being left to care for himself or herself. The existence of these isolated personality traits does not necessarily mean that the individual has a Personality Disorder. Two general requirements must be satisfied. First, a patient must fulfill the criteria for a specific disorder. Second, the patient's maladaptive behavior, thoughts, and speech must be pervasive and of sufficient intensity to interfere with normal interpersonal relationships and produce functional impairment or subjective distress.

Problems in diagnosis arise when a patient does not quite fulfill the criteria for a disorder or fulfills the criteria but the symptoms are not especially intense or pervasive. Another problem may occur if the patient fulfills part of the criteria for two or more Personality Disorders but does not completely fulfill the criteria for one Personality Disorder. Unfortunately, the clinical judgments necessary for the diagnosis of Personality Disorder are often subjective and may be viewed differently by different diagnosticians.

Example 1

Greg is a 37-year-old obstetrician and gynecologist who is dedicated to his work and rarely takes time for recreational activities. He is very compulsive about his practice and keeps detailed medical records on his patients. Greg is well organized, efficient, and on time when he sees patients in his office. He is inflexible in his opposition to abortion and refuses to perform the operation unless the mother's life is unequivocally in danger. Greg's dedication to his patients leads him to closely supervise his staff. Some of his colleagues and patients feel that he is excessively rigid, but others see his rigidity as a sign of responsibility and confidence about his clinical skills. Most patients trust his clinical judgment and consider him to be observant and competent. What diagnosis(es), if any, should Greg be given?

Greg is very compulsive in his work. The main diagnostic question is whether he meets the criteria for Obsessive-Compulsive Personality Disorder. Obsessive-Compulsive patients are often so preoccupied with details, rules, and lists that they lose sight of the major point of their activity. Although Greg is conscientious about keeping detailed medical records, this activity apparently does not interfere with his ability to treat his patients effectively. He is devoted to his work, rarely relaxes with leisure activities, and closely supervises his staff. His devotion to his work could be considered normal for a responsible physician. It is not clear whether he allows his staff any flexibility in the way that they perform their work.

Greg is inflexible about at least one ethical matter, his opposition to abortion. However, it is not clear that he is overconscientious or inflexible about other ethical or moral issues. Although some people consider him rigid, others interpret the same behavior as a sign of confidence and responsibility.

In summary, Greg should not receive a diagnosis of Obsessive-Compulsive Personality Disorder because he does not fulfill all the criteria and his behavior does not interfere with his functioning as a physician. He has compulsive personality traits, but these fall within the range of normal behavior. Some people would argue that his compulsivity is essential for a good physician.

Example 2

Marilyn is a 36-year-old married woman who runs a florist shop. She is competent in her business but quite emotionally dependent on her husband. Marilyn has been preoccupied with fears of being left to care for herself since she was a child. Her mother died when she was age 7 and her father was busy and had little time for her.

Marilyn is particularly anxious and fearful when her husband goes away on a business trip. She responds by working harder in her business. When she was younger, during and after college, she was involved in a number of relationships with men. When one relationship ended, she immediately sought another. Despite her emotional dependency, she did very well in school and led several student groups in various activities. What diagnosis(es), if any, should Marilyn be given?

The most striking aspect of Marilyn's personality is her emotional dependence within a relationship that contrasts with her professional independence and competence. She is uncomfortable when alone and fearful of being left to care for herself. Marilyn also needs a continuous close relationship with a man, immediately seeking a new relationship when an old one ends. Despite this dependency, Marilyn generally has self-confidence and is able to take responsibility for many areas of her life. Furthermore, she apparently does not need excessive advice and reassurance from others to initiate and complete her projects and business activities.

Marilyn's sense of emotional dependency and fear of abandonment fit three of the criteria for the diagnosis of Dependent Personality Disorder. However, her independence and competence in other areas of her life mean that the remaining necessary criteria are not fulfilled. Marilyn does not have Personality Disorder but she does have persistent and intense anxiety about loss or separation that has probably stimulated her need to have a continuous close relationship with a man for emotional support. A further diagnostic evaluation should explore the possibility of Chronic Anxiety Disorder.

Patients Who Fulfill Diagnostic Criteria for More Than One Personality Disorder

Some patients may fulfill the criteria for more than one Personality Disorder diagnosis. There are two reasons for this. First, the Personality Disorders are not mutually exclusive clinical entities. There is no reason a patient cannot have more than one Personality Disorder as long as their respective criteria are not mutually exclusive. Second, the symptoms of various Personality Disorders often overlap, reducing the number of unique criteria that differentiate between disorders, and enhancing the likelihood that a patient will fulfill more than one criteria set.

This particularly true of Personality Disorders in the same cluster (e.g., Antisocial Personality Disorder, Borderline Personality Disorder, Histrionic Personality Disorder, and Narcissistic Personality Disorder). Symptoms that are common to several Personality Disorders include isolation, eccentric behavior, impulsiveness, suspiciousness, dependency, exploitation of others, suggestibility, etc. For example, dependency is a common symptom in patients with Borderline Personality Disorder, Histrionic Personality Disorder, and Dependent Personality Disorder. If a patient meets the criteria for more than one Personality Disorder, he or she should receive all of the appropriate diagnoses. No individual Personality Disorder takes diagnostic precedence over another.

Example 3

Dennis is a 28-year-old single man who works the evening shift in the packaging division of a large company. His fellow workers consider him to be an "odd bird" who is generally suspicious, distant, displays few emotions, and has little to do with his associates. Dennis periodically announces that he knows the other workers are talking about him and attacking his reputation as a good worker. He frequently interprets their casual comments as insults and is persistently resentful of their behavior. When the foreman asks for details about his accusations, he cannot or will not be specific, other than to say that he cannot trust his co-workers.

Dennis has few friends in the factory because of his accusations and other unusual behaviors. He is always anxious and remains suspicious and unforgiving of the other workers no matter how well he knows them. During breaks he sits alone at a table in the corner of the lunchroom with his back to the wall. Dennis is an intelligent and efficient worker and the factory management feels he is worth keeping as an employee despite his unusual behavior. What diagnosis(es), if any, should Dennis receive?

Dennis is an individual whose main personality characteristic is his suspiciousness and paranoia. He suspects his co-workers of deceiving him without justification and is preoccupied with what he perceives to be their persistent demeaning remarks about him and attacks on his character. He is convinced that they are constantly talking about him behind his back. Dennis is unwilling to forgive them for these perceived slights. His lack of friends, isolative behavior, and constant anxiety in social situations make his co-workers joke about him and consider him odd.

Dennis fulfills the criteria for both Paranoid Personality Disorder and Schizotypal Personality Disorder and should receive both diagnoses because neither diagnosis has precedence over the other. His odd behavior is consistent with paranoid fears and suspicions rather than magical thinking, bizarre fantasies, or unusual thought processes and speech. If he was less paranoid and had more unusual behavior and thinking, his diagnosis would only be Schizotypal Personality Disorder.

Example 4

Lauren is a 31-year-old self-styled actress and model who supports herself by working as a waitress in a nightclub until the right professional opportunity occurs. She likes to be the center of attention and flirts with the patrons of the club who admire her sexy figure and brief costume. Lauren loves being the center of attention. What she lacks in talent, she makes up for in provocative behavior.

Lauren has had brief, impulsive sexual relationships with many men. She becomes rapidly involved with each new man, idealizes him, and begins an intense but shallow affair. As the relationship develops, she becomes more dependent and fearful of being abandoned. She begins to lose sight of her own identity and becomes more and more suggestible. Lauren's mood rapidly shifts from periods of excitement to depression as she fears that the relationship may deteriorate.

Lauren's lovers soon become disenchanted and often alarmed by her behavior. As they begin to pull away from her or try to end the relationship, Lauren makes dramatic threats that she cannot live without her lover. These have escalated to the point that she has made suicide gestures. These usually consist of scratching her wrist or taking five or six aspirin tablets. When the relationship finally ends, Lauren becomes enraged until she meets the next man. What diagnosis(es), if any, should Lauren receive?

Lauren's personality is characterized by intense, yet shallow, shifting emotions, dependency, suggestibility, and a poor sense of her own identity. She frequently becomes involved in unstable relationships that she feels are far more intimate than they really are. She uses her sexuality and physical appearance to attract men whom she idealizes and then frightens away with her dependent needs and excessive fears of abandonment. When they leave she responds with rage and dramatic manipulative acts.

This combination of symptoms demonstrates how difficult it may be to make a specific diagnosis for patients with severe Personality Disorders. Lauren fits the criteria for both Borderline Personality Disorder and Histrionic Personality Disorder. Because neither disorder has diagnostic precedence, she should receive both diagnoses. If her symptoms had emphasized chronic feelings of emptiness, self-mutilation, and transient psychotic episodes, rather than sexually provocative behavior and self-dramatization, the diagnosis would have been Borderline Personality Disorder.

Personality Symptoms Associated With Other Psychiatric Disorders

Some of the symptoms characteristic of specific Personality Disorders are part of the criteria set of other DSM-IV Axis I psychiatric disorders. In some situations, the patient should receive both the Axis I diagnosis and the Personality Disorder diagnosis. In other cases, the Axis I diagnosis takes precedence over the Personality Disorder diagnosis. For example, even if a patient's symptoms fulfill the criteria for Schizotypal Personality Disorder, they may not receive that diagnosis if they have already met the criteria for the diagnosis of Schizophrenia. The latter diagnosis always takes precedence.

Example 5

Clark is a 28-year-old garbage man who is difficult to work with. The other workers draw straws to determine who will ride on Clark's garbage truck. He is irritable and easily insulted by casual comments. He never forgives anyone who insults him and will spend an entire day on the truck without saying a single word to the person.

The men normally examine the garbage to determine whether there is anything worth salvaging. Clark is convinced that the others try to deceive him by hiding the valuables that they discover in the garbage from him. His co-workers laugh about some of Clark's peculiar notions. He is convinced that the people in certain neighborhoods put poison in their garbage so the garbage men will not go through it. Clark refuses to touch the garbage from these houses and will often try to skip them.

Some of the owners have complained about the poor service. When Clark's supervisors discuss the problem with him, he interprets their comments as an attack on his professional integrity and becomes angry. What diagnosis(es), if any, should Clark receive?

Clark's main symptoms are his suspiciousness and his delusion that some of the garbage he collects is poisoned. He is easily insulted, does not trust his fellow workers, and frequently misinterprets comments and slights directed toward him. Clark meets the criteria for the diagnosis of Delusional Disorder and Paranoid Personality Disorder. However, the diagnosis of Delusional Disorder takes precedence over the latter diagnosis. Therefore, he can only receive the diagnosis of Delusional Disorder.

Example 6

Tom is a 23-year-old man who has been drinking alcohol since he was a teenager. As an adolescent he was known as a juvenile delinquent in his neighborhood. He routinely got into fights and often bullied or threatened other teenagers. He was frequently absent from school and was caught shoplifting twice. Tom was frequently drunk and often fought with other young people while he was drinking.

As an adult Tom continued his reckless behavior, repeatedly getting into fights and driving while intoxicated. He had little regard for the rights of others and little guilt when he hurt another person. What diagnosis(es), if any, should Tom receive?

Tom has a long history of antisocial behavior that met the criteria for Conduct Disorder when he was an adolescent. As an adult, his symptoms also meet the criteria for Antisocial Personality Disorder. He has abused alcohol since his adolescence. However, substance abuse does not preclude the diagnosis of Antisocial Personality Disorder. Therefore, he should also receive the diagnosis of Alcohol Abuse.

Precedence of Diagnosis

There is no precedence of diagnosis within the Personality Disorders group. If a patient fulfills the criteria for two personality diagnoses, they should receive both diagnoses. However, the diagnosis of four specific Personality Disorders are precluded if they occur coincident with certain DSM-IV Axis I disorders. The diagnoses that take precedence are mainly Psychotic Disorders. The precedence of diagnosis for the Personality Disorders is shown in Table 17–1.

Discussion of Clinical Vignette

The Perfect Boss

Lawrence owns a small real estate agency and has grandiose fantasies that it will grow and become the largest agency in the state. He exploits his employees and has

Table 17–1 Precedence of diagnosis for Personality Disorders	
Personality Disorder	**Disorders taking precedence**
Paranoid Personality Disorder	Does not occur exclusively during Schizophrenia, Mood Disorder with Psychotic Features, any Psychotic Disorder Not due to effects of a substance or general medical condition
Schizoid Personality Disorder Schizotypal Personality Disorder	Does not occur exclusively during Schizophrenia, Mood Disorder with Psychotic Features, any Psychotic Disorder, Pervasive Developmental Disorders Not due to effects of a substance or general medical condition
Antisocial Personality Disorder	Does not occur exclusively during Schizophrenia or Manic Episode
Borderline Personality Disorder Histrionic Personality Disorder Narcissistic Personality Disorder Avoidant Personality Disorder Dependent Personality Disorder Obsessive-Compulsive Personality Disorder Personality Disorder NOS	No other disorders take precedence

Note. NOS = Not Otherwise Specified.

little sensitivity for their personal needs. As a result, they don't stay with the company for long. Lawrence's behavior is mainly characterized by a lack of empathy for other people and a need for constant attention and admiration from those around him. When his employees or wives finally leave him, he is hurt and unable to see any relationship between his behavior and their actions.

Lawrence does not consciously intend to be mean. He simply has difficulty seeing other people as independent entities with needs that are not identical to his own. These behaviors fit the criteria for the diagnosis of Narcissistic Personality Disorder. The key factors are Lawrence's need for excessive admiration and his inability to be truly empathic to the needs of other people.

Key Diagnostic Points

- Fear of rejection is the key personality trait in patients who have Avoidant Personality Disorder.

- Patients with Schizoid Personality Disorder prefer isolation. Patients with Avoidant Personality Disorder desire close relationships but are fearful of them.

- Patients with Schizotypal Personality Disorder have peculiar or odd behavior, thinking, perception, and speech that is generally more bizarre than that of patients with Schizoid Personality Disorder.

- A sense of entitlement and a lack of empathy are the hallmarks of Narcissistic Personality Disorder.

- Dependency is common in patients with Borderline Personality Disorder, Histrionic Personality Disorder, and Dependent Personality Disorder.

- Excessive anger and brief, intense, unstable relationships are characteristic of Borderline Personality Disorder.

Common Questions in Making a Diagnosis

1. Denise is a 45-year-old woman with crippling arthritis who uses a wheelchair and is dependent on her husband for most of her needs. He assumes most of the responsibility for her life, doing the shopping and making sure she gets to her doctors' appointments. Denise feels very uncomfortable when she is alone because she is afraid that she will not be able to care for herself. She has little confidence that she can initiate or complete projects on her own. Denise will not disagree with her husband because she is afraid he won't support her. Her husband admits to feeling burdened by the responsibility of caring for his wife in addition to his job. He sometimes becomes

angry with Denise, but says that he would never leave her. What diagnosis(es), if any, should Denise receive?

Answer: Denise is very dependent on her husband because of her medical condition. She fulfills the criteria for Dependent Personality Disorder. However, the core concept of this disorder is a psychological dependence based on a lifelong pattern of behavior. It is not meant to be applied to an individual who has a physical disability that realistically renders them dependent. Therefore, the diagnosis of Dependent Personality Disorder cannot be made for this patient. If her illness was cured and she was physically fit yet still remained dependent, the diagnosis might become appropriate.

2. Adrian is a 33-year-old man who works as a short-order cook on the midnight shift in a local diner. He is a quiet man who keeps to himself and seems to have no interests outside of his job, his coin collection, and his three parrots. Adrian lives alone in a small apartment. He has no close friends and appears to have no interest in making friends. One waitress at the diner described him as aloof and detached and said, "He's a good cook, but not much of a talker. He'll avoid you whenever he can and he doesn't care what you think of his cooking." What diagnosis(es), if any, should Adrian receive?

   Answer: Patients with Avoidant Personality Disorders eagerly desire social interactions and close human contact. They find it difficult to become involved with other people because they are fearful of criticism or rejection. Adrian doesn't appear to desire close contact with other people and seems indifferent to criticism. He spends his time on solitary activities at work or at home. This behavior fits the criteria for the diagnosis of Schizoid Personality Disorder.

3. Amy is a 29-year-old woman who has had several brief relationships with men. She often complains to her friend about men, "They're all worthless. All they want is sex and then they leave you rather than commit themselves to a meaningful relationship." Most of her experiences with men have been tumultuous and follow the same pattern. She meets a man who she finds attractive, establishes an intense relationship, and immediately starts sleeping with him. Initially she idealizes her lover and becomes increasingly dependent on him. Soon he begins to complain that she is too needy. Amy becomes angry and more demanding. They argue and the man leaves her. Amy responds by feeling hurt and depressed. What diagnosis(es), if any, should Amy receive?

   Answer: Amy is sexually impulsive and forms rapid, intense, idealizing relationships with men. She becomes dependent on her lover until he finally leaves her. Although this repeated pattern of behavior is maladaptive, it does not fit the criteria for any specific Personality Disorder. If Amy had a significantly reactive mood, a marked disturbance in her own self-image, suicidal behavior, or chronic feelings of emptiness, she might meet the criteria for Borderline Personality Disorder. The current diagnosis is Personality Disorder Not Otherwise Specified.

4. Glen is a 28-year-old man who has difficulty at work because he is suspicious of his co-workers and feels that they are trying to trick him into making mistakes in his work. He broods about their casual comments and is convinced that they are hidden insults attacking his character and reputation. Glen often gets angry with the individual who makes the comment and tries to intimidate him. His constant suspiciousness makes it impossible for him to develop friendships at work. At home, he behaves in a similar fashion and became convinced a year ago that his wife is having an affair with an alien creature. His accusations have led to a deterioration in their relationship. What diagnosis(es), if any, should Glen receive?

Answer: Glen's suspicions about his co-workers, perception that he is being attacked, misinterpretation of the casual comments of other, and suspicions about his wife's fidelity, fulfill the criteria for the diagnosis of Paranoid Personality Disorder. However, Glen's concern about his wife's affair with an alien creature is a psychotic delusion. The diagnosis of Psychotic Disorder takes precedence over the diagnosis of Paranoid Personality Disorder when they occur together. Glen's bizarre delusion, associated with increasing problems in the marriage and at work, fulfill the criteria for the diagnosis of Schizophrenia, Paranoid Type.

5. Vince is a 31-year-old man who is a thespian. He wears dramatic clothes on and off the stage. His favorite costume is a hat with a long pheasant feather stuck in the brim and a long dark-blue cape. He often makes a grand entrance in the local theater coffeehouse by throwing his cape open and gracefully swirling it off his shoulders in one smooth motion. If no one notices his entrance, Vince has been known to continue with grand gestures until someone says, "Alright Vince, we know you're here. Now sit down." Vince smiles and pulls up a chair. Vince has many casual acquaintances whom he considers dear, intimate friends. They hug and kiss each time they meet on the street. Among old friends and new acquaintances he is sexually provocative to both sexes but has little actual sexual contact. What diagnosis(es), if any, should Vince receive?

Answer: Vince's behavior is characterized by a need to be the center of attention, overly dramatic behavior, sexual provocation, exhibitionism, and superficiality. These behaviors fulfill the criteria for the diagnosis of Histrionic Personality Disorder.

Index

*Page numbers printed in **boldface** type refer to tables.*